PHILOSOPHICAL AND THEORETICAL PERSPECTIVES FOR ADVANCED NURSING PRACTICE

Third Edition

The Jones and Bartlett Series in Nursing

With titles in

Research

Nursing Theory

Ethics

Women's Health

Oncology

Health Policy

Leadership and Management

Community Health

Nursing Education

www.jbpub.com

PHILOSOPHICAL AND THEORETICAL PERSPECTIVES FOR ADVANCED NURSING PRACTICE

Third Edition

Edited by

Janet W. Kenney, RN, PhD

Professor
Arizona State University
College of Nursing
Tempe, Arizona

JONES AND BARTLETT PUBLISHERS
Sudbury, Massachusetts
BOSTON   TORONTO   LONDON   SINGAPORE

World Headquarters

Jones and Bartlett Publishers
40 Tall Pine Drive
Sudbury, MA 01776
(978) 443-5000
info@jbpub.com
www.jbpub.com

Jones and Bartlett Publishers International
Barb House, Barb Mews
London W6 7PA
UK

Jones and Bartlett Publishers Canada
2406 Nikanna Road
Mississauga, ON L5C 2W6
CANADA

Library of Congress Cataloging-in-Publication Data
CIP data unavailable at time of printing

Acquisition Editor: Penny M. Glynn
Associate Editor: Thomas Prindle
Production Editor: Jon Workman
Manufacturing Buyer: Therese Bräuer
Editorial Production Service: Modern Graphics, Inc.
Typesetting: Modern Graphics, Inc., Jon Workman, Philip Regan
Cover Design: Anne Spencer
Printing and Binding: Malloy Lithographing, Inc.
Cover Printing: Malloy Lithographing, Inc.

Printed in the United States of America

03 02 01 00 99   10 9 8 7 6 5 4 3 2 1

Contents

Preface

The foundation of a discipline is its unique body of specialized knowledge. Practice disciplines, such as nursing, must continually expand their knowledge base, effectively disseminate new knowledge, and determine effective ways to use this knowledge both in practice and research. Over the decades, scholars in most disciplines develop new and different philosophical and methodological perspectives, which may change or modify formerly accepted theories of practice. In the nursing discipline, it seems as though the lines have drawn between two different nursing paradigms. The 'totality' paradigm is represented by theories that examine various parts of the person to obtain a 'total' view. The newer 'simultaneity' paradigm consists of theories that use a human science perspective of the person as constantly changing during interactions with the environment.

Since the early 1970s, many nurse theorists have proposed unique models and theories. Some theories have gained greater acceptance than other theories and published research has demonstrated their usefulness in nursing practice. In 1978, Dr. Barbara Carper, introduced the importance of using all four 'way of knowing' — empirics, ethics, esthetics, and personal knowledge – to enhance holistic nursing care. Although these areas of knowledge are used in most other disciplines, this realization changed some approaches to nursing theory, education, research, and practice.

In the past two decades, there have been no new grand theories, although some theorists have modified their work. Nurse researchers continue to test various mid-range and grand theories, however, there continues to be much debate and dissension among nurse scholars as to what are acceptable research methods for testing contemporary theories. After a few contemporary nurse theorists presented their unique theories, based on their philosophy of human science, a major paradigm shift gradually occured. These theorists view humans as rationale, free-willed, persons continuously interacting and dynamically changing with their environment through their own lived experiences. Although early nurse researchers emphasized the need to used empirical methods to test nursing theories, the newer theories based on nursing as a human science required non-traditional methods. Thus, a dialogue began in nursing journals as to the validity of these new theories and research methods, and whether the theories could be effectively applied in practice as they were subject to many interpretations. This debate continues today about contemporary nursing theories.

Most graduate nursing programs require their graduate students to take a nursing theory course to acquire a greater understanding of nursing science and effectively apply nursing theories in their practice. Without knowledge of the evolution of nursing science, and the importance of understanding different philosophies, methodologies, and theories of nursing, advanced practice nurses may revert to following in the ways of 'junior' doctors or physician assistants. They may never see the 'whole' person, nor have a nursing model or theory to guide their practice, but instead rely on only the most cost effective and expedient method to treat the patient/client's health problems, and send them on their way. While this technologically efficient practice may seem temporarily effective, numerous health problems may be missed, and the variety of factors contributing to illness may not be understood, nor ever changed.

Multiple factors affect the use of nursing theories in practice. With financial restrictions from both the government (medicare and medicaid), and the demands of health maintenance organizations for high quality, yet economically efficient nursing care, the importance and application of nursing theory seems to have surrendered to high technology, standardized nursing diagnoses and treatment protocols. Evidence-based practice seems to be the latest buzzword to demonstrate nursing accountability, rather than use of critical thinking, theory-based practice and holistic care.

The 3rd edition of this book is a composite of 26 relevant articles by nurse scholars. These articles were chosen to provide a foundation for graduate nurses to understand the historical, philosophical, and theoretical evolution of nursing science today. Nursing practice is dynamically interrelated with nursing theory and research, which continue to evolve simultaneously. Future nurse leaders need a foundation in how these areas evolved, continue to change and influence the other areas, rather than relying on guidelines for nursing practice within an institution dedicated to cost effective care.

The book is organized into six parts, each with a brief overview describing the essence of the chapters that follow. Part I, "The Nursing Discipline and Development of Knowledge," explains the criteria for a professional discipline, including the structure of nursing knowledge and relevant "ways of knowing" applicable to nursing's knowledge base. The four chapters in Part II, "History and Evolution of Nursing Science," describe factors that influenced development of the nursing discipline and methodological issues in research, along with the nature and scope of nursing science.

Parts III and IV focus on the four major concepts in nursing's metaparadigm. Contemporary nurse scholars are redefining and sometimes broadening the meanings of nursing's major concepts – client/person, health, nursing, and environment. The views of these authors may be controversial, yet they challenge nurses to rethink how they define these concepts and how their definitions affect nursing practice and research. Part III, "Nursing's Metaparadigm: Conceptualizations of Nursing and Health," begins with a chapter in which five nurse theorists discuss and defend the meaning of nursing, according to their viewpoints. Three scholars present chapters expressing their views on the concept 'nursing,' including two that address a specific pattern of nursing knowledge. These chapters are followed by two on expanded views of health, well beyond all theorists' original definitions. These two chapters may challenge graduate nurses to rethink how their definitions of health may be different from the client's view, yet guides their nursing actions, and may be ineffective in altering the client's health problem or lifestyle. Part IV, "Nursing's Metaparadigm: Conceptualizations of Client and Environment," includes one chapter that proposes a new, unifying definition of client that could be used in any nursing theory, and two chapters on environment. These later chapters describe how social, political, and economic factors greatly influence both the environment, and ultimately contribute to the health problems of those living in poverty.

There are four chapters in Part V, "Contemporary Perspectives of Nursing." In the first chapter, Dr. Jacqueline Fawcett critiques the nursing discipline's lack of success in achieving her 1980s recommendations, and expresses her disappointment. Her high standards may not have been realistic considering the health care scene today. Thereafter, the other chapters explore the trend toward 'humanistic nursing science,' – a paradigm shift. This new perspective defines nursing as caring and nurturing clients by understanding their changing life patterns, which are reflected in their dynamic human-environment lived experiences. Initially, graduate students may be confused, frustrated, or delighted with these non-traditional views of nursing and wonder whether any are congruent with the reality of today's health care system. The last set of four chapters, in Part VI, "Interrelationships among Nursing Theory, Research, and Practice" begins with an article describing how the learning cycle can be applied to nursing theory, practice, and research. Then, we shift gears to an article describing why the trend toward 'evidence-based' nursing practice is unrealistic and ineffective in meeting client's health care needs. The final two chapters explain why critical thing and application of theory-based nursing practice are relevant and essential in all areas of practice. And, the last chapter describes how to select appropriate theories or models to guide nursing practice and ways to apply theories to enhance nurses' credibility and advance nursing science.

Authors

Ellen C. Birx, RN, PhD
Patricia G. Butterfield, RN, MS
Barbara A. Carper, RN, EdD
Peggy L. Chinn, RN, PhD, FAAN
William K. Cody, RN, PhD
Dorothy M. Crowley, RN, PhD
Sue K. Donaldson, RN, PhD
Joan Engebretson, RN, DrPH
Jacqueline Fawcett, RN, PhD, FAAN
Sally Gadow, RN, PhD
Mary H. Huch, RN, PhD
Joy L. Johnson, RN, PhD
Janet W. Kenney, RN, PhD
Shake' Ketefian, RN, EdD, FAAN
Hesook S. Kim, RN, PhD

Dorothy Kleffel, RN, DNSc, PhD
Gail J. Mitchell, RN, PhD
Afaf Ibrahim Meleis, RN, PhD, FAAN
Elizabeth J. Monti, RN, MSN
Nola J. Pender, RN, PhD, FAAN
John R. Phillips, RN, PhD
Steven Pryjmachuk, RMN, MSc
Dianne Pelletier Raymond, RN, MSN
Richard W. Redman, RN, PhD
Pamela G. Reed, RN, PhD, FAAN
Rozella M. Schlotfeldt, RN, PhD, FAAN
Martha S. Tingen, RN, PhD
John Wolfer, RN, PhD
Judith Wuest, RN, MN

Part I

THE NURSING DISCIPLINE AND DEVELOPMENT OF KNOWLEDGE

In 1915, Abraham Flexner, a sociologist, identified criteria, based on medicine, that must be met for a field to be considered a professional discipline. A discipline must have reached consensus on the structure, nature, and scope of its knowledge base, the rules and acceptable methods of research within its field, purposes for conducting research and desired outcomes, and the specific content and methods for educating professionals in the discipline. For nursing to be accepted as a professional discipline, it must have a unique body of knowledge based on credible methods for developing that knowledge, appropriate methods for applying the knowledge in practice, and an established process for educating and socializing students into the profession. In addition, society must also value nursing's unique knowledge and believe in nurses' integrity to benefit the public.

Over the last four decades, in their quest to become recognized as a professional discipline, nurse scholars and researchers have devoted their time and talents into developing and expanding nursing's knowledge base. For several decades, nurse scientists relied on empirical research methods to create an acceptable knowledge base and achieve credibility as a legitimate discipline. In recent decades, nurse scholars recognized the limits of traditional research and began using various phenomenological methods. According to Hesook Kim (2000), these scholars have: a) refined the discipline's four key concepts; b) identified specific nursing problems and potential solutions; c) developed multiple theories to explain human processes associated with health and illness; and d) identified the impact of environment on health and illness. Despite these advances in nursing science, and because of different philosophical beliefs, nurse scholars have not reached consensus on how to structure nursing knowledge, define the major concepts of the discipline, or agree on acceptable research methods.

Part I of this book includes five chapters that describe both classical and recent views on how to structure nursing knowledge, the nature of the nursing discipline, and essential patterns of nursing knowledge. Also, a new article presents a review of the arguments for multiple theories and models of nursing, and the final chapter presents a way to integrate and apply various nursing paradigms within current health care systems.

In her chapter on "Structuring Nursing Knowledge," Rozella Schlotfeldt identifies and prioritizes five areas for systematic inquiry. She begins with a discussion on the criteria for a profession, and recommends that nurses reach an agreement on the knowledge base essential for nursing practitioners. Dr. Schlotfelt believes that nurses must have professional knowledge about nursing science, history, philosophy and strategies, along with factors that influence human health. She describes the focus of nursing inquiry and the need to develop knowledge in these areas to advance nursing science and ultimately the discipline.

In their classic article, "The Discipline of Nursing," Sue Donaldson and Dorothy Crowley identify three major themes to guide nursing research so as to develop a unique knowledge base. These themes are still relevant today, and include "principles and laws governing optimal functioning of humans; patterns of human and environment interaction; and those processes to effect positive changes in health status." In addition, they explain how the structure of knowledge leads to different ways that academic and professional disciplines define and develop their practice, research, and education. Lastly, the authors discuss the structure of the nursing discipline, and major concepts needed in nursing theories and research.

Based on her doctoral research, Dr. Barbara Carper identified four areas of knowledge that nurses consistently use in practice, although three areas had previously been undervalued and criticized. Her article, "Fundamental Patterns of Knowing in Nursing," describes these patterns as 1) empirics – the science of nursing; 2) esthetics — the art of nursing; 3) ethics – the moral knowledge; and, 4) personal knowledge — knowing the self in relation to others. Most disciplines base their knowledge on using and integrating some or all of these patterns of knowing to provide a complete picture of reality, but only recently has nursing acknowledged other ways of knowing beyond empirics. Each pattern of knowing requires a different method to discover and validate knowledge in that area. Dr. Carper emphasizes the importance of both developing and applying all four patterns, and reinforces the value of nurse's personal knowledge, which tends to increase with experience in the field. Her work stimulated nurse scientists to examine other areas of knowledge beyond that limited to empirics.

Since the development of nursing theories and models, known as paradigms, nursing science has experienced an ongoing debate about the value of two very different views of nursing—the empiricist and interpretative paradigms. A new article, "Multiple Paradigms of Nursing Science," by Monti and Tingen, clearly present the strengths and limitations of these major paradigms, based on Kuhn's criteria. In addition, the authors discuss the advantages and disadvantages of nursing adopting a single paradigm versus using multiple paradigms, since it is impossible to reconcile ontological and epistemological differences to form a unified one. The authors recommend continued use of empirical and interpretative theories and models for development of nursing science and to expand nursing' body of knowledge.

In the continuing debate about the value of different philosophies, paradigms, and research methods, and the contradictions of combining them, some nurse scholars have begun to express concern that theories are out of touch with the reality of nursing practice in our cost effective, high technology health care system. In his chapter on "Aspects of 'Reality' and Ways of Knowing in Nursing,"

John Wolfer explains why the need for complementary types of knowledge, theory and research, based on multiple methods of inquiry. He recommends that nurses embrace a body-mind-spirit reality and develop a new paradigm that would improve integration and application of nursing knowledge. This article challenges nurse theorists to consider the practicality of their paradigms and the value of multiple methods of inquiry. Hopefully, these chapters will assist graduate students to understand the impact of contemporary issues and problems facing nursing science today.

REFERENCES

Kim, Hesook S. (2000). An integrative framework for conceptualizing clients: "A proposal for a nursing perspective in the new century." *Nursing Science Quarterly,* 13(1):37-44, p. 37.

1

Structuring Nursing Knowledge:
A Priority for Creating Nursing's Future

ROZELLA M. SCHLOTFELDT, RN, PhD, FAAN

Nursing's future will be created only as the discipline underlying nursing practices is identified, structured, and continuously updated by systematic inquiry. The kinds of knowledge contained within the discipline are identified and an approach to its structure is proposed.

There can be little doubt that one of the highest priorities for creating an appropriate future for nursing is that of identifying, structuring, and continuously advancing the knowledge that underlies the practices of professionals in the field. That statement can be made because a consensus has not yet been attained concerning the subject matter that must be mastered by those who seek to practice general and specialized nursing. Surely by the beginning of the twenty-first century, nursing's body of knowledge will be identified, selected, verified, and agreed upon by qualified professionals in the field, effectively structured, and continuously updated to reflect newly discovered knowledge. Also, knowledge judged to be erroneous, inadequate, and outdated should be deleted. This knowledge will be derived from basic and clinical scientific nursing research, both quantitative and qualitative, from philosophic and historical inquiries, and from evaluation research designed to establish valid criterion measures, devices, and approaches to establishing the efficacy and value of nursing's caring functions as they are relevant to the health, function, comfort, well-being, productivity, self-fulfillment, and happiness of human beings.

The thesis of this chapter is that only qualified professionals in the field, including general and specialist practitioners, educators, administrators, investigators, historians, philosophers, and theorists, should be given responsibility by the profession (however that is defined) to identify, verify, structure, and continuously update the extant content or subject matter that, at the minimum, should be included in the intellectual armamentaria of all professional nurses. This responsibility of the profession is essential to four functions: (a) the creation of comparable programs of study at the first professional degree level, (b) control of the profession's goals, mission, and accomplishments, (c) a valid procedure for licensing (not registering) all who quality as professionals in the field, and (d) certification of bona fide nursing specialists.

NURSING AS A PROFESSION

Two major criteria must be fulfilled by any occupational group whose members earn and

Source: Schlotfeldt, R. (1989). Structuring nursing knowledge: A priority for creating nursing's future. *Nursing Science Quarterly, 1* (1):35-38. Reprinted by permission of and copyright © 2002 Sage Publications, Inc.

achieve the status of a profession, or more appropriately for nursing, a learned helping profession. First, a profession must have an institutionalized goal or social mission. Learned professions are valued by the societies whose members give them positive sanction for two major reasons: (a) the services learned professionals render are judged to be essential and beneficial for all members of society during particular times in their lives and (b) members of each learned profession have identified and come to a consensus about the knowledge that practitioners must master and use selectively, creatively, humanely, effectively, and ethically in providing those essential services. As a second criterion, each profession must support a cadre of investigators whose role is to continuously advance its knowledge with a view toward improving its practices.

The traditional learned professions have included the clergy, lawyers, and physicians. The clergy have been valued and supported because they are expected to be knowledgeable and skillful in providing spiritual comfort and well-being for all those who consult them. Lawyers are expected to master coded law and to apply their discipline fairly and skillfully in fulfilling the goal of preserving social harmony and justice. Physicians have been valued because knowledge of human ills and disabilities and their causes and knowledge of the means to eliminate, attenuate, or manage them and alleviate their noxious consequences are considered essential to the well-being of society. Are the caring functions and mission of nurses, namely, appraising and optimizing the health, function, comfort, independence, and potential of human beings, any less valued than spiritual comfort and well-being? Are they any less desirable than social harmony and justice? Are they any less important than finding causes for, diagnosing, and treating human ills?

Unfortunately, the caring functions typically provided by nurses were for too long con-

sidered to be mere extensions of the duties and obligations of wives and mothers, for which large amounts of professional knowledge were not considered essential (Reverby, 1987). Lay members of societies have typically not recognized, and nurses themselves have been remarkably tardy in identifying and organizing the several kinds of professional knowledge that are fundamental to executing the caring functions that nurses typically provide.

The essential and often crucial nature of nurses' caring functions in promoting the health and well-being of all human beings is finally being recognized by thinking people, including scholarly nurses. There is now general agreement (at least verbal agreement) that nursing's social mission is to appraise and assist human beings in their quest to optimize their health status, health assets, and health potential (Fawcett, 1983). Furthermore, general agreement exists that there is or should be a body of structured knowledge that professionals in the field agree represents the discipline that is fundamental to general and specialty nursing practices.

Nursing scholars have discussed, described, and characterized the discipline (Donaldson & Crowley, 1978), and in the recent past the American Association of Colleges of Nursing (1986) has reported findings from a "national effort to define the essential knowledge, practice, and values that the baccalaureate nurse should possess" (p. 1). Panel members expressed the belief that the essentials so delineated can be achieved within the traditional baccalaureate degree program in nursing and that the baccalaureate represents first-level professional preparation in nursing.

The efforts that have been made toward establishing the discipline represent significant steps toward achieving the goal of identifying, organizing, and achieving a consensus concerning the specific body of extant knowledge that underlies nursing practices. It must be noted, however, that there has not yet been a concerted effort to identify and obtain agreement about the currently available knowledge that is fundamental to nursing's growing number of declared specialties or even to obtain a consensus about the requisite knowledge and skills that define what nursing's specialties are. It must be recognized also that the subject matter that constitutes the discipline has not yet been identified and structured, and agreement has not been reached concerning appropriate and needed inclusions from qualified professionals in the field. This paper presents an approach to organizing the several kinds of knowledge contained within the discipline, a possible next step toward having qualified professionals select and structure the specific extant subject matter of the discipline about which agreement is needed.

KNOWLEDGE OF THE DISCIPLINE

Figure 1.1 shows the kinds of professional knowledge contained within the discipline, which is depicted as a large sphere having a permeable and expandable membrane (represented by the second sphere) to permit the continuous addition of newly discovered knowledge and the deletion of that found through systematic inquiry to be erroneous, inadequate, or irrelevant.

The largest segment of the sphere (*a*) represents nursing's scientific subject matter. Therein belongs all of nursing science, (ie, the verified facts, principles, and laws that have been discovered through scientific inquiry to be valid, relevant, and useful for nursing practice); included also are extant scientific theories that guide scientific investigations in nursing and those that have been proposed by scholarly nurses as promising explanations of phenomena that are of particular concern to nurses.

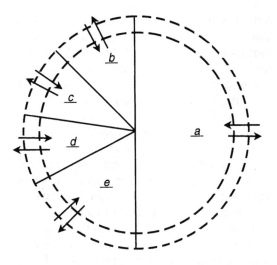

FIGURE 1.1. The nursing discipline.
a, Nursing science; *b*, nursing history; *c*, nursing philosophy; *d*, nursing strategies; *e*, factors influencing human health. Arrows denote addition and deletion of knowledge. Personal knowledge is excluded.

To date, much of nursing science has been discovered by basic scientists and subsequently found through empirical evidence and systematic study to be relevant. Nurse investigators have also been adding to nursing's scientific knowledge by testing the relevance and utility of theories generated by basic scientists in clinical nursing situations (Chinn, 1984). Few investigations have yet been reported that test scientific theories regarding human phenomena that are of particular concern to nurses but not to basic scientists (Silva, 1986). A plausible reason is that there is little agreement among nurses concerning the human phenomena that are of concern to nurses and how they should be characterized and classified and how knowledge of them should be advanced.

In general, nurses accept the notion that human beings are biopsychosocial beings (Engel, 1977). It is proposed here that the subjects nurses serve also exemplify assets of the human spirit of which relevant knowledge is inadequate. Those assets surely include human spirituality and other qualities of the human spirit, such as determination, verve, courage, beliefs, hope, and aspiration. Nurses surely hold responsibility for advancing knowledge of those health-seeking assets. In sum, human beings' health-seeking mechanisms and behaviors, beliefs, and propensities can be classified as biological, psychological (both emotional and cognitive), and sociocultural and as assets of the human spirit; all of them are directly relevant to the natural efforts by humans to seek and attain optimal health. Because so much scientific nursing knowledge remains to be discovered, it is safe to predict that nursing science will likely always represent the largest and most rapidly changing aspect of the discipline. Furthermore, nurses are increasingly recognizing the relevance of scientific knowledge from disciplines not traditionally judged to be relevant for nursing. Included, for example, are concepts, principles, and theories from economics, political science, administration and management, and computer science. The science fundamental to education has long been incorporated as an integral part of the discipline of nursing.

A second important segment of the sphere representing the nursing discipline is historical knowledge (Figure 1.1*b*). Included is knowledge of the heritage of the occupation and the developing profession of nursing, including knowledge of people, circumstances, and events that have shaped that development. Included also is the history of nursing knowledge as it has been transmitted to generations of practitioners.

The third section of the sphere (Figure 1.1*c*) represents philosophic nursing knowledge. Included are the profession's accepted values and codes of professional behavior. Included also should be the several philosophic theories that have been tested, found useful and relevant to nurses' work, and accepted as philosophic guides to practice. Illustrative are selected theories of value, justice and morality,

and ethical theories. Because nurses are encountering increasing numbers of moral and ethical dilemmas and because nurses are increasingly manifesting interest in becoming scholars in the discipline of philosophy, it is predicted that nursing knowledge henceforth will include increasing amounts of tested and relevant philosophic knowledge that will be incorporated into the discipline.

The fourth section of the sphere (Figure 1.1*d*) represents knowledge of nursing strategies, approaches, and technologies along with the scientific and artistic principles essential to their execution. Included also is knowledge of the prevailing health-care system. Relationships between the goals and caring functions of nurses and the goals and practice functions of other health professionals in the existing health-care systems represent another important segment of the discipline.

Another significant segment of nursing's body of knowledge has always been knowledge of factors that influence the health status, health assets, and health potential of human beings, both favorably and unfavorably (Figure 1.1*e*). Included is knowledge of biological, physical, and cognitive abilities with which people are naturally endowed and knowledge of environmental factors, economic and social circumstances, and changes associated with normal development, including the aging process. In the nursing perspective presented here, pathologies and medical diagnoses and treatments are factors that affect the health of human beings. Nurses must have adequate knowledge of these factors: such knowledge is an integral part of the discipline that must be mastered by nurse practitioners.

There is yet another kind of knowledge that is directly relevant to and essential for nursing practice. It is the knowledge that professionals must gain from relevant data concerning each person being served and that obtained through astute and perceptive observations. Personal knowledge of individuals and groups of persons is needed for nurses to respect the uniqueness of those for whom they provide exemplary services. For that reason, there can be no prescriptive nursing practice theories nor professional approaches to nursing care that are universally generalizable.

In summary, conceptualizing the discipline of nursing as an expandable and permeable sphere made up of segments of varying size provides an approach to classifying and organizing the several kinds of knowledge that constitute the nursing discipline. Such an approach demonstrates the vast and growing amounts of knowledge that professionals in the field must master and be able to use selectively, creatively, artistically, humanely, and skillfully to provide exemplary care.

Nursing should be recognized as a learned helping profession and a respected academic discipline. Surely nursing scholars will ensure the attainment of those goals by the beginning of the twenty-first century. Crucial to their attainment is identifying and attaining agreement about the human phenomena that are of particular concern to nurses, enhancing scholarly clinicians' involvement in generating promising relevant theories, and testing those theories as the means to discover knowledge through which to continuously improve nursing practices. Such an approach will ensure the availability of valid nursing knowledge in the twenty-first century and its currency during all centuries to come.

REFERENCES

American Association of Colleges of Nursing. (1986). *Essentials of college and university education for professional nursing.* Washington, DC: Author.

Chinn, P. (1984). From the editor. *Advances in Nursing Science, 6* (2), ix.

Donaldson, S., & Crowley, D. (1978). The discipline of nursing. *Nursing Outlook, 26,* 113-120.

Engel, G. (1977). The need for a new medical model: A challenge for biomedicine. *Science, 196,* 129-136.

Fawcett, J. (1983). Hallmarks of success in nursing theory development. In P. Chinn (Ed.), *Advances in nursing theory development* (pp. 3-17). Rockville, MD: Aspen.

Reverby, S. (1987). A caring dilemma: Womanhood and nursing in historical perspective. *Nursing Research, 36,* 5-11.

Silva, M. (1986). Research testing nursing theory: State of the art. *Advances in Nursing Science, 9* (1), 1-11.

2

The Discipline of Nursing

SUE K. DONALDSON, RN, PhD

DOROTHY M. CROWLEY, RN, PhD

All enquiry undertaken by nurses is not research that contributes to the discipline of nursing; to be nursing research, studies must be undertaken from a nursing perspective.

When one considers the gamut of research that nurses are undertaking, all of it is clearly important to the nursing profession, but the knowledge represented by the research problems and methodologies appears to be global. By definition, however, a discipline is not global; it is characterized by a unique perspective, a distinct way of viewing all phenomena, which ultimately defines the limits and nature of its inquiry.

This is the problem that plagues all of us: identification of the essence of nursing research and of the common elements and threads that give coherence to an identifiable body of knowledge. As nurse researchers, we seem to function primarily with tacit rather than explicit knowledge of the broad conceptualizations unique to nursing. We take for granted the nursing perspective as generally accepted and understood, until explanation of the particulars is required. Moreover, nursing authors tend to emphasize speculative formulations and theoretical reflections aimed at deriving the nature of nursing rather than explicating the structure of the body of

knowledge that constitutes the discipline of nursing.

Rather than expending a disproportionate amount of effort in the quest for *the* definition of the nature of nursing, it might behoove us—at least at this time—to seek relationships and commonalities in the ideas of writers whose work has influenced (and continues to influence) tacit knowledge of the scope of the field. At least since the time of Nightingale, there has been a remarkable consistency in the recurrent themes that nurse scholars use to explain what they conceive to be the essence or the core of nursing. Three general themes for enquiry emerge:

1. *Concern with principles and laws that govern the life processes, well-being, and optimum functioning of human beings—sick or well.* For example, a concern with the discovery of laws that govern health, knowledge of reparative processes, and prevention was manifest in the late nineteenth or early twentieth century in Nightingale's writings and certainly in Rogers' concern with laws and principles governing life processes in the past two decades.

2. *Concern with the patterning of human behavior in interaction with the environment in crit-*

Source: Donaldson, S. K., & Crowley, D. M. (1978). The discipline of nursing. *Nursing Outlook, 26* (2): 113-120. Used with permission from Mosby-Year Book, Inc.

ical life situations. As evidence of this theme, Rogers' writings reflect a concern with life rhythms and their relationship to environmental rhythms. Similarly, Johnson's writings in the 1960s focused attention on systems of behavior, pattern-maintenance, and pattern-disruption. The conceptual frames for most nursing curricula today include coping processes, adaptation, and supportive and non-supportive environments.

3. *Concern with the processes by which positive changes in health status are affected.* Peplau addressed herself to nursing as an interpersonal process, an educative and maturing force; whereas, Kreuter as well as Leininger and others addressed the particular type of process of support system seen as nursing's unique contribution.

These themes suggest boundaries of an area for systematic enquiry and theory development with potential for making the nature of the discipline of nursing more explicit than it is at present.

Integration of nursing research from the level of a conceptual framework for a particular study to the level of more general theories and ultimately to that of a unified body of nursing knowledge has not been pursued to any large extent. Nor have there been widespread efforts on the part of those doing research in nursing to relate individual studies to one another and, thereby, build a larger context for reference. This has contributed to fragmentation of knowledge and confusion about a perspective for nursing research.

As was the case in considering different ideas about the nature and themes of nursing, however, the goal is not to identify a single theory of nursing—rather, we would advocate pluralism. Nevertheless, it would seem desirable to be able to place such theories within the context of a discipline of nursing. More explicit identification of what we are

doing in nursing research is imperative if we are to truly function as nurse researchers, rather than as nurses conducting research in other disciplines, and if we are to have nursing theories for the professional practice of nursing. There is also a crucial need for identification of the structure of the discipline of nursing in our educational program. How can we justify doctoral programs in nursing if the discipline of nursing is not defined? Perhaps of even greater importance is the content of these doctoral programs. In fact, the very survival of the profession may be at risk unless the discipline is defined. As Armiger noted: "There exists today an unprecedented need for identification of the uniqueness of nursing science and practice, lest overriding forces in contemporary society lead to disintegration of nursing as a distinct profession."[1]

What is needed is the thinking of nurse philosophers and also some philosophizing on the part of the nurse researchers. The problem is not to devise the structure of the discipline of nursing, but to make this structure explicit. Our purpose is to make a beginning along these lines. Throughout this paper, the term *nursing* will refer to the discipline, unless otherwise clarified, and *structure* will refer to the broad conceptualizations and syntax of the discipline, rather than the theories generated within this structure.

CLASSIFICATION OF HUMAN KNOWLEDGE: DISCIPLINE

Traditionally, human knowledge and enquiry have been considered in the context of disciplines. Disciplines reflect true distinctions between bodies of knowledge per se and, as such, become the realm of learning. The *Oxford English Dictionary* defines discipline as "a branch of instruction or education, a department of learning or knowledge." Institutions of higher education are organized around these branches of knowledge into colleges, schools, and departments. Typically, disciplines have evolved as a consequence of a distinct perspective and syntax, which determine what phenomena or abstractions are of interest, in what context such phenomena are to be viewed, what questions are to be raised, what methods of study are to be used, and what canons of evidence and proof are to be required.

As a result of the complex way in which disciplines evolve, disciplines can be and have been identified and organized around a variety of characteristics and combinations of characteristics. Mathematics, for example, has been viewed as distinct from all other disciplines in that its subject matter appears to have no material existence; logic has been set apart because it is concerned with the development of canons of reasoning and evidence, which are utilized in the other disciplines. Thus, it is the unique relationship of logic to the other disciplines that sets it apart, rather than a peculiarity of its subject matter, as was the case for mathematics.

In identifying disciplines and classifying them, we are dealing with the nature and structure of the whole of human knowledge. It should be kept in mind that the number and membership of the disciplines are not agreed upon and that there is no single accepted organization of even the well-accepted disciplines. This is reflected in the diversity of organization of branches of learning in universities and colleges. The broadest classifications of disciplines depend upon a view of the inherent nature of all phenomena. A distinction on the part of the philosophers between the generality of natural phenomena and the particularity of human events leads to a distinction between such sciences as physics and sociology, which seek general laws for repeating behavior, and such disciplines as history, which

FIGURE 2.1. **Structuring of human knowledge.**

focuses on unique events, or ethics, which deals with human choices and value orientations (as shown in Figure 2.1). Among the sciences themselves, the biological sciences become distinct from physics and chemistry because they deal with the recognition of the phenomena of life and with living as opposed to nonliving things.

Nursing has both scientific aspects and aspects akin to the arts. For example, human health is considered within nursing in terms of political issues and history as well as in terms of inexorable laws of health. Therefore, nursing as a discipline is broader than nursing science and its uniqueness stems from its perspective rather than its object of enquiry or methodology.

You might well ask, Why bother with pursuing this discussion, especially since there is no agreement as to a single structure of human knowledge? There are at least two reasons: First, the discipline of nursing was not created *per se solum*, but emerged within the context of the other disciplines. Therefore, we must know its relationship to other disciplines in addition to its structure. Second, it must be remembered that the family of disciplines, be-

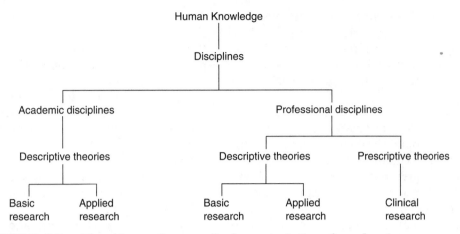

FIGURE 2.2.   Theories and research characteristics of academic and professional disciplines.

cause each of its members represents knowledge derived within a particular conceptual structure, is subject to revision in the form of fusion, extinction, and multiplication of its members as new conceptualizations emerge. Nursing as a discipline is also subject to change based upon changes in its structural conceptual base; in fact, nurse researchers and scholars have the responsibility of questioning and revising nursing's structure.

According to Shermis, the accepted academic disciplines are all characterized by an impressive body of enduring works, suitable techniques, concerns which are significant and relevant to humans, unifying and inspiring traditions, and considerable scholarly achievements. Although these are not criteria for distinguishing disciplines from nondisciplines, they do provide a basis for acceptance of a branch of learning as a discipline.

But what of emerging disciplines? In the professional field, there typically is an evolutionary process that occurs as the field moves from a vocational level, in which the art and technology are preeminent, to the rationalization of practice and the establishment of a cognitive base for professional practice. It is im-

portant to recognize that a discipline emerges as a result of creative thinking related to significant issues. Because of the vital significance of nursing's perspective, its concern with human hea-lth and well-being, and its growth through research and scholarly work, nursing will gain full acceptance in time.

For purposes of this discussion, a distinction between academic disciplines and professional disciplines will be utilized (as illustrated in Figure 2.2). The academic disciplines include sciences such as physics, physiology, and sociology, as well as liberal arts disciplines such as mathematics, history, and philosophy. The aim of academic disciplines is to know, and their theories are descriptive in nature. In contrast, professional disciplines such as law, medicine, and nursing are directed toward practical aims and thus generate prescriptive as well as descriptive theories.

For academic disciplines, the goal is to know, regardless of whether the research is basic or applied. In fact, the distinction between applied and basic research seems appropriate only in relation to descriptive theories, since applied research answers questions related to the applicability of basic theories in practical situations, rather than questions related to *how* basic theories are to be applied. Thus, applied physicists test the practical limits of theories of physics but would not derive information as to the best design for a bridge, for example.

Fields that emphasize applied research would be more correctly termed applied disciplines, or applied branches of academic disciplines, rather than professional disciplines, which have prescriptive theories in addition to descriptive ones. The prescriptive theories characteristic of professional disciplines deal with the actual implementation of knowledge in a practical sense. As Johnson has stated, ". . . professional knowledge does not consist of basic science theory which has been validated in practice."[2] In this regard, it is not correct to view professional disciplines simply as applied sciences.

Within the professional discipline there is a need "to know" and to work from descriptive theories in addition to prescriptive ones. As Gortner has pointed out, "some of the work is basic, in that it is applicable to a general understanding of human behavior or responses to illness," and other studies of nursing are applied.[3] Basic and applied research are both needed in a professional discipline because each discipline has a different practical aim which influences the perspective of that field, the way it conceptualizes the relevant world, and the questions it poses for investigation. Therefore, because of the uniqueness of each discipline's perspective and the context in which knowledge from each discipline fits, it is not possible to simply "borrow" theory or knowledge from other disciplines.

Schwab has noted that in general the statements of a given discipline are like single words of a sentence; their meanings derive more from their context than from their dictionary sense. In other words, statements of disciplines, their conclusions, are properly understood only in the context of the enquiry that produced them. They are true only in that they fit the criteria for truth in the given discipline. From this standpoint, nurse scientists may help in utilization of information from other disciplines, but this will not eliminate the need for undertaking basic research in nursing from nursing's perspective. Viewing phenomena from the perspective of healthy functioning of individuals in interaction with their environments will generate distinctive research at all levels and a defined, structured body of knowledge.

Even when useful information might be derived from the research of another discipline, the studies are not pursued, either because of lack of interest or because the conditions used invalidate the results for nursing's purpose. For example, a physiologist studying mechanisms underlying a given cellular process may work with intact cells but at a very low temperature, say 0°C, to slow the process down to allow measurement of its kinetic properties. The low temperature does not invalidate the physiologist's conclusions, but may make the data inappropriate in terms of knowing exact rates characteristic of the process at in vivo temperatures. Furthermore, animal and suborganismal, even subcellular, research is valid in its own right in physiology, whereas in nursing the information is ultimately being sought in relation to intact human beings.

Nursing cannot rely upon the academic disciplines to supply its total requirement for knowledge of laws and processes. Rather, appropriately prepared nurse researchers must generate and test descriptive theories as necessary and develop their own technology, as has been recommended for other professionals.

Another very important issue is the extent to which each discipline is dependent upon the development of the others. The Comtian view of the sciences, which is a hierarchical one, is noteworthy in this regard, since it has

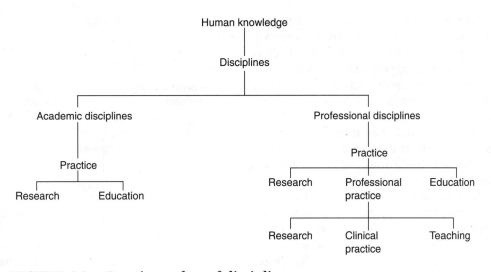

FIGURE 2.3.   Practice realms of disciplines.

influenced curricula; in turn, these curricula can lead to unwarranted views of the dependence of some disciplines on the others.

Comte held that not only human knowledge in general but also each branch of knowledge passes through states or stages of progress on its way to becoming scientific. He also conceived of the branches of knowledge as evolving in an increasingly complex organizational hierarchy ranging from the physical to the social. As a result of an arbitrary interpretation of Comte's hierarchy in curricula, physics and chemistry have been required, for example, for the mastery of biology, and so on. Although there may be increased efficiency of instruction following this plan, it should be remembered that learners influenced by such curricula may come to view all knowledge as hierarchical. Yet, the hierarchical nature of knowledge has not been demonstrated; in fact, acceptance of hierarchical structuring of knowledge can be very limiting and should be questioned.

In the first place, there is the danger that one conceive all knowledge of scientific quality as being encompassed by the academic dis-ciplines, with the professions resting on these disciplines for their cognitive base. Second, if even the potential for professional disciplines is conceded, it is difficult for proponents of the hierarchical view to envision how professional disciplines could expand their respective bodies of knowledge independently. In contrast, professional disciplines can be viewed as emerging *along with* rather than *from* academic disciplines.

This is not to imply that disciplines are totally independent of each other. Certainly, logical formulations in one discipline cannot ignore the "truths" of the others. The quality of theories and research designs and the validity of conclusions drawn within one discipline are dependent upon their congruence with all of knowledge. Therefore, knowledge in one discipline may set constraints on or enhance the process of enquiry in another. Perhaps the most obvious interrelationship of disciplines is in their associated practice realm.

Every discipline exists in part to provide knowledge which is to be utilized and thus has an associated practice realm (Figure 2.3). Accordingly, every discipline has educators and researchers who function in this realm to im-part the knowledge base to others and expand the knowledge base through research. In addi-tion, professional disciplines have practitioners who deliver a service by engaging in profes-sional practice in the form of clinical service, education, and research.

Sharing of knowledge from many disci-plines occurs in the realm of practice associated with each discipline. For example, researchers affiliated with academic disciplines may bor-row relevance or reality orientation from ob-servations of professional practitioners and use prescriptive or practice theories from profes-sional disciplines and practice. Similarly, pro-fessional disciplines derive knowledge from academic disciplines.

RELATIONSHIP OF THE DISCIPLINE TO PRACTICE

Although the discipline and the profession are inextricably linked and greatly influence each other's substance, they must be distinguished from each other. Failure to recognize the exis-tence of the discipline as a body of knowledge that is separate from the activities of practi-tioners has contributed to the fact that nursing has been viewed as a vocation rather than a profession. In turn, this has led to confusion as to whether the discipline of nursing exists.

Part of the problem in viewing a profes-sional discipline as distinct from professional practice stems from the fact that both the disci-pline and practice evolved interdependently in response to societal needs; as a result, both pos-sess a common practical aim related to these needs (Figure 2.4). Professions evolved because the service they provided was valued. Given the emphasis placed upon science and rationality in the postindustrial age, it is not surprising that there was a strong impetus for establishing a sci-entific and theoretical base for professional prac-tice. The process of upgrading professional prac-

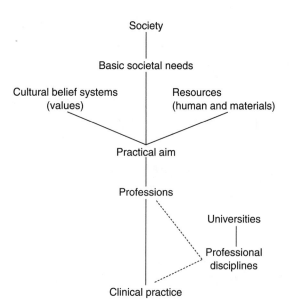

FIGURE 2.4. Interdependent evolution of discipline and practice of a profession.

tice also entailed the establishment of closer re-lations between knowledge serving as the basis of professional practice and knowledge in the academic disciplines. Since the university tradi-tionally has been the locus of development of theoretical knowledge, the professional disci-plines were eventually housed there along with the academic disciplines.

The location of professional disciplines such as nursing in institutions such as univer-sities, which are primarily concerned with human knowledge as a product rather than service, does not change the accountability of these disciplines for societal needs and the practical aim of their associated professions. As Johnson has noted, the decisions of what to study and what questions to ask necessarily have stemmed from social decisions about the profession's realm of responsibility in giving services or in clinical practice.

Florence Nightingale defined the discipline in terms of the responsibility of nursing's practitioners to promote human health based on systematic enquiry into nature's "laws of health."[4] Part of the reason for nursing's struggle in evolving stems from the slow emergence of the recognition of its social relevance. Nurses give service related to the quality of human life; this service is only recently being valued. After all, why should quality of life be considered before biological survival can be assured?

Ethical and moral values inherent in clinical practice have profoundly influenced the perspective and value orientation of the discipline. Thus, nursing has traditionally valued humanitarian service. But in addition, the self-respect and self-determination of clients are to be preserved. The goal of nursing service is to foster self-caring behavior that leads to individual health and well-being. These values and goals, which are intrinsic to professional practice, have shaped the value orientation of the discipline. As a result of this value orientation, knowledge of the basis of human choices and of methods for fostering individual independence are sought, rather than knowledge of interventions that control and directly manipulate the person per se into a societally determined state of health.

The clinical practice of nursing requires the development of prescriptive theories on the part of the discipline. Much of the early research related to the nursing profession consisted of investigations about nurses, their characteristics and behavior, but these investigations could not actually be considered nursing research. In recent years, the amount of research concerned with theories fundamental to clinical practice has increased.

A key point, however, is that the discipline of nursing should be *governing* clinical practice rather than being defined by it. Of necessity, clinical practice focuses on the individual in the here and now who has a problem requiring relevant and appropriate action. The discipline, in contrast, embodies a knowledge base relevant to all realms of professional practice and which links the past, present, and future. Its scope goes far beyond that required for current clinical practice. If the discipline were so narrowly defined, professional nursing could be limited to functioning in the realm of disaster relief rather than serving as a force in the promotion of world health. This is not meant to diminish the importance of problems encountered by nurses in current clinical practice. These problems deserve attention, but they are not the only concern of the discipline.

Part of the problem is that "clinical practice" is too often used synonymously with "professional practice," and clinical practice is narrowly defined. Professional competency goes beyond that required for delivery of health care to individuals, preparation of future practitioners, and conduct of systematic enquiry. For example, McGlothlin believes that competency includes the need on the part of professionals for social understanding of sufficient breadth to place the practice in the context of society and the need for leadership skills.

Some of the knowledge required for achieving these competencies can only come from the discipline of nursing. Prescriptive theories essential to clinical practice and the appropriate design of nursing research can only be derived from the discipline of nursing. Similarly, although knowledge from political science, history, philosophy, and other disciplines is very important for social understanding, the professional nurse cannot put nursing into a societal context without knowledge derived from the discipline of nursing. This knowledge is obtained in part from nurse philosophers and nurse historians who view nursing as it relates to other disciplines and can articulate how nursing's heritage relates to its perspective. The discipline of nursing must also provide essential components of the knowledge base for preparation of world leaders in the field of health.

The need for philosophical, historical, and similar types of enquiry within the discipline of nursing is crucial not only in terms of providing the knowledge base for professional preparation but also for the development of the discipline. It must be remembered that the discipline is defined by social relevance and value orientations rather than by empirical truths. Thus, the discipline and profession must be continually reevaluated in terms of societal needs and scientific discoveries. Similarly, the entire structure of the discipline may need to be revamped in time, and this should be done by nurse researchers.

For this reason we have been very careful not to equate the discipline of nursing with the science of nursing. As mentioned earlier, only part of nursing employs scientific method. We need doctoral preparation for nurse historians as well as nurse scientists. As Schlotfeldt has pointed out: "Nursing faculties rarely have among their members scholars who are concerned with establishing the history of nursing science and with identifying the philosophies of conceptualizations of nursing that have influenced the structure of that knowledge at various times in nursing's history."[5] Once again, the purpose in having nurse philosophers and historians is not to duplicate the efforts of other disciplines, but rather to provide these approaches from the perspective of nursing.

It should be remembered that although nursing requires researchers and scholars who utilize a variety of approaches, all research that is important to the profession of nursing is not derived from the discipline of nursing. Only information and theories stemming from nursing's perspective come from nursing per se. Nursing educators utilize information and theories from education. Even clinical practice should not be viewed as being grounded solely in the discipline of nursing.

In delivering health care, practitioners must in fact draw from many disciplines, such as business administration, medicine, education, and basic sciences. Rarely, if ever, does the skilled clinician rely only on knowledge from one discipline or even rely solely on scientific knowledge. Clinical practice is always to some extent empirical, pragmatic, intuitive, and artistic.

Once we agree that the discipline of nursing does not have to embody all, the entire whole, or knowledge utilized by the profession of nursing, then we can begin to define the discipline. Nursing is not global in its subject matter and therefore does not subsume part of any other disciplines—for example, education—just because practitioners are educated. Similarly, studies of higher education in nursing that deal with the educational process are not nursing research but educational research. In contrast, a study of the effects of educational techniques on clients' achievement of self-care is within nursing per se. Even though nursing care delivery is greatly affected by attitudes of nurses administration policies, such problems may be studied appropriately in other disciplines.

The purpose in excluding some research from nursing is not to create a ranking of importance or prestige, but rather to make the essence of nursing explicit. Nurses who conduct administrative or educational research may contribute as much to the professional practice of nursing as nurses who conduct nursing research.

In summary, the discipline and clinical practice of nursing share a common social relevance and practical aim. However, the discipline, which is a body of knowledge, must not be confused with its associated practice realm, which embodies the processes of conducting research, giving service, and educating. Furthermore, some members of the profession must engage in enquiry that is not immediately applicable to current clinical practice. As

FIGURE 2.5.   Structure of a professional discipline.

a branch of knowledge, the discipline embodies more than the science of nursing and requires researchers who employ a variety of approaches from nursing's perspective. Although the discipline provides crucial and unique content for nurse researchers, clinicians, and educators, these practitioners draw on many disciplines. Appropriately prepared nurses may elect to conduct research within other disciplines because of the critical importance of this non-nursing research to professional practice or the growth of the discipline.

STRUCTURE OF THE DISCIPLINE OF NURSING

We are now at the point of examining the structure of the discipline. According to Schwab, disciplines have both substantive and syntactical structures. The substantive structure is composed of conceptualizations which are borrowed or invented, but their inclusion is always based on their fit with the perspective of the discipline. The syntax of a discipline refers to the research methodologies and criteria used to justify the acceptance of

statements as true within the discipline (see Figure 2.5).

We have incorporated the syntax of nursing as value systems (both of science and of professional ethics) and research constraints. Such constraints include consideration of accessibility of controls, congruity with existing knowledge, manifest and latent consequences, and technological feasibility. Both values and constraints influence theory generation and actual research design. In effect, they function to ensure that enquiry will result in conclusions and statements that are appropriate, reliable, and valid for the purpose of the discipline.

Thus, the substantive structure determines primarily the scope and subject of enquiry—what is of interest; and the syntactical structure determines primarily the procedure for conducting research and criteria for acceptability of findings as truth. The findings generated by enquiry are then incorporated into the structure as concepts, theories, and facts—the statements of the discipline. In this paper, we have focused upon the structural conceptualizations, but it should be remembered that the syntax of the discipline is also important, since the syntax determines the extent to which the truth of statements of the discipline is warranted. In contrast, the substantive structure relates to the subject matter of the enquiry. The structural conceptualizations are selected for inclusion in a given discipline with its perspective as a screen.

From its perspective, nursing studies the wholeness or health of humans, recognizing that humans are in continuous interaction with their environments. Nursing's perspective evolves from the practical aim of optimizing of human environments for health. Examples of major conceptualizations in nursing deal with:

1. Distinctions between human and nonhuman beings
2. Distinctions between living and nonliving
3. Nature of environments and human-environmental interactions from cellular to societal levels
4. Illness versus health and well-being
5. Functioning of the whole human organism versus functioning of the parts
6. Levels of functioning of whole organisms
7. Human characteristics and natural processes, such as consciousness, abstraction; adaptation and healing; growth; change; self-determination; development; aging; dying; reproducing; drive satisfaction; and relating.

The structural conceptions are being utilized, but they are usually not identified or clarified, and rarely questioned. It is important, for example, to know whether health is viewed, in the context of a given theory or design, as a specific state, or as it is defined by each individual.

Depending upon the particular structural conceptualizations utilized, or combinations of them, widely different theories are proposed for testing. Such variation in theories does not lead to different bodies of knowledge, but to different aspects of a single body.

Pluralism of theories promotes productivity; in fact, without testing of a wide variety of theories, progress towards "truth" cannot be made. In physiology, for example, where knowledge of the functions and nature of vital processes of living organisms is sought, a pluralism of theories exists. Many physiologists conceive the functioning of the organism as explainable in terms of the functioning of its parts, whereas others propose an explanation utilizing a conception that the whole is more than the sum of its parts. This dual approach is very useful, regardless of the correctness of the theories, since testable theories are generated that yield empirical evidence related to knowledge of the nature of and mechanisms underlying behavior of living systems. The goal in generating theories is not just to propose an all-encompassing theory but to provide testable theories.

Research designed to test hypotheses stemming from theories is very important to the discipline and practitioners when the relationship of nursing theories to the structure of the discipline is explicit. This is the type of research that is easily identified as nursing research. Schwab calls this stable enquiry, in that there is no hesitation about what questions to ask or what structural conceptualizations to employ. For example, if the current principles of physiology are organ and function, the researcher engaged in stable enquiry discovers the function of one organ after another.

This type of stable research tends to be the most rewarded, but there is another very important realm of enquiry which must be expanded. We refer to questions relating to the structural conceptualizations and value orientations of the discipline. For example, What is the nature of health? Is health on a continuum with illness? Is health for every person a reasonable goal for society?

At least two major benefits are derived from this second type of research. First, the structural conceptualizations are clarified or altered to make them consistent with reality. They should not be accepted as givens. Second, the discipline will be continually shaped according to significant themes, those which are of vital significance to man [*sic*]. If nurse researchers are to provide the knowledge base for societal directions in relation to health, they must engage in this type of research.

For the continued growth, significance, and utility of the discipline of nursing, researchers must place their research within the context of the discipline. Theories must also be viewed in terms of the basic structural conceptualizations of the discipline. The responsibility for revising and clarifying the structural conceptions, the very framework, of the discipline of nursing rests with nurse researchers. This means lessening our preoccupation with the process of nursing and pedagogy and placing emphasis on content as substance.

REFERENCES

1. Armiger, Sister Bernadette. Scholarship in nursing. *Nurs. Outlook* 22:160-164, Mar. 1974.
2. Johnson, D. E. Development of theory: A requisite for nursing as a primary health profession. *Nurs.Res.* 23:373, Sept.-Oct. 1974.
3. Gortner, S. R. Scientific accountability in nursing. *Nurs.Outlook* 22:765, Dec. 1974.
4. Nightingale, Florence. *Notes on Nursing: What it is and What it is not.* London, Harrison, 1860.
5. Schlotfeldt, R. M. Nursing research: Reflection of values. *Nurs.Res.* 26:8, Jan.-Feb. 1977.

BIBLIOGRAPHY

Argyris, Chris, & Schon, D. A. *Theory in Practice: Increasing Professional Effectiveness.* San Francisco, Jossey-Bass, 1974.

Davies, J. T. *The Scientific Approach.* New York, Academic Press, 1965.

Gortner, S. R., & Nahm, Helen. An overview of nursing research in the United States. *Nurs.Res.* 26:10-33, Jan.-Feb. 1977.

Greenwood, E. The practice of science and the science of practice. In *The Planning of Change*, 2d edition, edited by W. G. Bennis and others. New York, Holt, Rhinehart and Winston, 1969.

Haldane, J. S. *The Sciences and Philosophy.* Garden City, N.Y., Doubleday, Doran and Co., 1929.

Henderson, Virginia. The nature of nursing. *Am. J.Nurs.* 64:62-68, Aug. 1964.

Hyde, A. The phenomenon of caring. *Nurs.Res.Rep.* 10:2-3ff, Oct. 1975.

Johnson, D. E. The significance of nursing care. *Am. J.Nurs.* 61:63-66, Nov. 1961.

Kreuter, F. R. What is good nursing care? *Nurs.Outlook* 5:302-304, May 1957.

Leininger, M. The phenomenon of caring; Part 5. Caring: the essence and central focus of nursing. *Nurs.Res.Rep.* 12:2, 14, Feb. 1977.

McGlothlin, W. J. *Patterns of Professional Education.* New York, G. P. Putnam's Sons, 1960.

Merton, R., & Lerner, D. Social scientists and research policy. In *The Planning of Change*, 2d edition, edited by W. G. Bennis and others. New York, Holt, Rhinehart and Winston, 1969.

Parsons, Talcott, & Platt, G. M. *The American University.* Cambridge, Mass., Harvard University Press, 1973.

Peplau, H. E. *Interpersonal Relations in Nursing, A Conceptual Frame of Reference for Psychodynamic Nursing.* New York, G. P. Putnam's Sons, 1952.

Rogers, M. E. *Introduction to the Theoretical Basis of Nursing.* Philadelphia, F. A. Davis Co., 1970.

Schwab, J. Structure of the disciplines: Meanings and significances. In *The Structure of Knowledge and the Curriculum*, ed. by G. W. Ford and Lawrence Pugno. Chicago, Rand McNally, 1964.

———. The structure of the natural sciences. In *The Structure of Knowledge and the Curriculum*, ed. by G. W. Ford and Lawrence Pugno. Chicago, Rand McNally, 1964.

Shermis, S. On becoming an intellectual discipline. *Phi Delta Kappan* 44:84-86, 1962.

3

Fundamental Patterns of Knowing in Nursing

BARBARA A. CARPER, RN, EdD

It is the general conception of any field of inquiry that ultimately determines the kind of knowledge the field aims to develop as well as the manner in which that knowledge is to be organized, tested, and applied. The body of knowledge that serves as the rationale for nursing practice has patterns, forms, and structure that serve as horizons of expectations and exemplify characteristic ways of thinking about phenomena. Understanding these patterns is essential for the teaching and learning of nursing. Such an understanding does not extend the range of knowledge, but rather involves critical attention to the question of what it means to know and what kinds of knowledge are held to be of most value in the discipline of nursing.

IDENTIFYING PATTERNS OF KNOWING

Four fundamental patterns of knowing have been identified from an analysis of the conceptual and syntactical structure of nursing knowledge.[1] The four patterns are distinguished according to logical type of meaning and designated as (1) empirics, the science of nursing; (2) esthetics, the art of nursing; (3) the component of a personal knowledge in

nursing; and (4) ethics, the component of moral knowledge in nursing.

Empirics: The Science of Nursing

The term *nursing science* was rarely used in the literature until the late 1950s. However, since that time there has been an increasing emphasis, one might even say a sense of urgency, regarding the development of a body of empirical knowledge specific to nursing. There seems to be general agreement that there is a critical need for knowledge about the empirical world, knowledge that is systematically organized into general laws and theories for the purpose of describing, explaining, and predicting phenomena of special concern to the discipline of nursing. Most theory development and research efforts are primarily engaged in seeking and generating explanations which are systematic and controllable by factual evidence and which can be used in the organization and classification of knowledge.

The pattern of knowing which is generally designated as "nursing science" does not presently exhibit the same degree of highly integrated abstract and systematic explanations characteristic of the more mature sciences, although nursing literature reflects this as an ideal form. Clearly there are a number of co-existing, and in a few instances competing, conceptual structures—none of which has achieved the status of what Kuhn calls a scien-

Source: Carper, B. A. (1978). Fundamental patterns of knowing in nursing. *ANS, 1* (1): 13-24. Reprinted with permission from and copyright © 1978 Aspen Publishers, Inc.

tific paradigm. That is, no single conceptual structure is as yet generally accepted as an example of actual scientific practice "which include[s] law, theory, application, and instrumentation together . . . [and] . . . provide[s] models from which spring particular coherent traditions of scientific research."[2(p10)] It could be argued that some of these conceptual structures seem to have greater potential than others for providing explanations that systematically account for observed phenomena and may ultimately permit more accurate prediction and control of them. However, this is a matter to be determined by research designed to test the validity of such explanatory concepts in the context of relevant empirical reality.

New Perspectives

What seems to be of paramount importance, at least at this stage in the development of nursing science, is that these preparadigm conceptual structures and theoretical models present new perspectives for considering the familiar phenomena of health and illness in relation to the human life process; as such they can and should be legitimately counted as discoveries in the discipline. The representation of health as more than the absence of disease is a crucial change; it permits health to be thought of as a dynamic state or process which changes over a given period of time and varies according to circumstances rather than a static either/or entity. The conceptual change in turn makes it possible to raise questions that previously would have been literally unintelligible.

The discovery that one can usefully conceptualize health as something that normally ranges along a continuum has led to attempts to observe, describe, and classify variations in health, or levels of wellness, as expressions of a human being's relationship to the internal and external environments. Related research has sought to identify behavioral responses, both physiological and psychological, that may serve as cues by which one can infer the range of normal variations of health. It has also attempted to identify and categorize significant etiological factors which serve to promote or inhibit changes in health status.

Current Stages

The science of nursing at present exhibits aspects of both the "natural history stage of inquiry" and the "stage of deductively formulated theory." The task of the natural history stage is primarily the description and classification of phenomena which are, generally speaking, ascertainable by direct observation and inspection.[3] But current nursing literature clearly reflects a shift from this descriptive and classification form to increasingly theoretical analysis which is directed toward seeking, or inventing, explanations to account for observed and classified empirical facts. This shift is reflected in the change from a largely observational vocabulary to a new, more theoretical vocabulary whose terms have a distinct meaning and definition only in the context of the corresponding explanatory theory.

Explanations in the several open-system conceptual models tend to take the form commonly labeled *functional* or *teleological*.[4] For example, the system models explain a person's level of wellness at any particular point in time as a function of current and accumulated effects of interactions with his or her internal and external environments. The concept of adaptation is central to this type of explanation. Adaptation is seen as crucial in the process of responding to environmental demands (usually classified as stressors), and enables an individual to maintain or reestablish the steady state which is designated as the goal of the system. The developmental models often exhibit a more genetic type of explanation in that certain events, the developmental tasks, are believed to be causally relevant or necessary conditions for the normal development of an individual.

Thus the first fundamental pattern of knowing in nursing is empirical, factual, descriptive, and ultimately aimed at developing abstract and theoretical explanations. It is exemplary, discursively formulated, and publicly verifiable.

Esthetics: The Art of Nursing

Few, if indeed any, familiar with the professional literature would deny that primary emphasis is placed on the development of the science of nursing. One is almost led to believe that the only valid and reliable knowledge is that which is empirical, factual, objectively descriptive, and generalizable. There seems to be a self-conscious reluctance to extend the term *knowledge* to include those aspects of knowing in nursing that are not the result of empirical investigation. There is, nonetheless, what might be described as a tacit admission that nursing is, at least in part, an art. Not much effort is made to elaborate or to make explicit this esthetic pattern of knowing in nursing—other than to vaguely associate the "art" with the general category of manual and/or technical skills involved in nursing practice.

Perhaps this reluctance to acknowledge the esthetic component as a fundamental pattern of knowing in nursing originates in the vigorous efforts made in the not-so-distant past to exorcise the image of the apprentice-type educational system. Within the apprentice system, the art of nursing was closely associated with an imitative learning style and the acquisition of knowledge by accumulation of unrationalized experiences. Another likely source of reluctance is that the definition of the term *art* has been excessively and inappropriately restricted.

Weitz suggests that art is too complex and variable to be reduced to a single definition.[5] To conceive the task of esthetic theory as definition, he says, is logically doomed to failure in that what is called art has no common properties—only recognizable similarities. This fluid and open approach to the understanding and application of the concept of art and esthetic meaning makes possible a wider consideration of conditions, situations, and experiences in nursing that may properly be called esthetic, including the creative process of discovery in the empirical pattern of knowing.

Esthetics versus Scientific Meaning

Despite this open texture of the concept of art, esthetic meanings can be distinguished from those in science in several important aspects. The recognition "that art is expressive rather than merely formal or descriptive," according to Rader, "is about as well established as any fact in the whole field of esthetics."[6(pxvi)] An esthetic experience involves the creation and/or appreciation of a singular, particular, subjective expression of imagined possibilities or equivalent realities which "resists projection into the discursive form of language."[7] Knowledge gained by empirical description is discursively formulated and publicly verifable. The knowledge gained by subjective acquaintance, the direct feeling of experience, defines discursive formulation. Although an esthetic expression required abstraction, it remains specific and unique rather than exemplary and leads us to acknowledge that "knowledge—genuine knowledge, understanding—is considerably wider than our discourse."[7(p23)]

For Wiedenbach, the art of nursing is made visible through the action taken to provide whatever the patient requires to restore or extend his [sic] ability to cope with the demands of his [sic] situation.[8] But the action taken, to have an esthetic quality, requires the active transformation of the immediate object—the patient's behavior—into a direct, nonmediated perception of what is significant in it—that is, what need is actually being expressed by the behavior. This perception of the need expressed is not only responsible for the action taken by the nurse but reflected in it.

The esthetic process described by Wiedenbach resembles what Dewey refers to as the difference between recognition and perception.[9] According to Dewey, recognition serves the purpose of identification and is satisfied when a name tag or label is attached according to some stereotype or previously formed scheme of classification. Perception, however, goes beyond recognition in that it includes an active gathering together of details and scattered particulars into an experienced whole for the purpose of seeing what is there. It is perception rather than mere recognition that results in a unity of ends and means which gives the action taken an esthetic quality.

Orem speaks of the art of nursing as being "expressed by the individual nurse through her creativity and style in designing and providing nursing that is effective and satisfying."[10(p155)] The art of nursing is creative in that it requires development of the ability to "envision valid modes of helping in relation to 'results' which are appropriate."[10(p69)] This again invokes Dewey's sense of a perceived unity between an action taken and its result—a perception of the means of the end as an organic whole.[9] The experience of helping must be perceived and designed as an integral component of its desired result rather than conceived separately as an independent action imposed on an independent subject. Perhaps this is what is meant by the concept of nursing the whole patient or total patient care. If so, what are the qualities that enable the creation of a design for nursing care that eliminate or would minimize the fragmentation of means and ends?

Esthetic Pattern of Knowing

Empathy—that is, the capacity for participating in or vicariously experiencing another's feelings—is an important mode in the esthetic pattern of knowing. One gains knowledge of another person's singular, particular, felt experience through empathic acquaintance.[11,12] Empathy is controlled or moderated by psychic distance or detachment in order to apprehend and abstract what we are attending to, and in this sense is objective. The more skilled the nurse becomes in perceiving and empathizing with the lives of others, the more knowledge or understanding will be gained of alternate modes of perceiving reality. The nurse will thereby have available a larger repertoire of choices in designing and providing nursing care that is effective and satisfying. At the same time, increased awareness of the variety of subjective experiences will heighten the complexity and difficulty of the decision making involved.

The design of nursing care must be accompanied by what Langer refers to as sense of form, the sense of "structure, articulation, a whole resulting from the relation of mutually dependent factors, or more precisely, the way the whole is put together."[7(p16)] The design, if it is to be esthetic, must be controlled by the perception of the balance, rhythm, proportion, and unity of what is done in relation to the dynamic integration and articulation of the whole. "The doing may be energetic, and the undergoing may be acute and intense," Dewey says, but "unless they are related to each other to form a whole," what is done becomes merely a matter of mechanical routine or of caprice.[9]

The esthetic pattern of knowing in nursing involves the perception of abstracted particulars as distinguished from the recognition of abstracted universals. It is the knowing of a unique particular rather than an exemplary class.

The Component of Personal Knowledge

Personal knowledge as a fundamental pattern of knowing in nursing is the most problematic, the most difficult to master and to teach. At the same time, it is perhaps the pattern most essential to understanding the meaning of health in terms of individual well-being. Nursing considered as an interpersonal process involves interactions, relationships, and transactions between the nurse and the patient-client. Mitchell points out that "there is growing evidence that the quality of interpersonal contacts has an influence on a person's becoming ill, coping with illness and becoming well."[13(p4950)] Certainly the phrase "therapeutic use of self" which has become increasingly prominent in the literature implies that the way in which nurses view their own selves and the client is of primary concern in any therapeutic relationship.

Personal knowledge is concerned with the knowing, encountering, and actualizing of the concrete, individual self. One does not know *about* the self; one strives simply to *know* the self. This knowing is a standing in relation to another human being and confronting that human being as a person. This "I-Thou" encounter is unmediated by conceptual categories or particulars abstracted from complex organic wholes.[14] The relation is one of reciprocity, a state of being that cannot be described or even experienced—it can only be actualized. Such personal knowing extends not only to other selves but also to relations with one's own self.

It requires what Buber refers to as the sacrifice of form, i.e., categories or classifications, for a knowing of infinite possibilities, as well as the risk of total commitment.

> Even as a melody is not composed of tones, nor a verse of words, nor a statue of lines—one must pull and tear to turn a unity into a multiplicity—so it is with the human being to whom I say You. . . . I have to do this again and again; but immediately he is no longer You.[14(p59)]

Maslow refers to this sacrifice of form as embodying a more efficient perception of reality in that reality is not generalized nor predetermined by a complex of concepts, expectations, beliefs, and stereotypes.[15] This results in a greater willingness to accept ambiguity, vagueness, and discrepancy of oneself and others. The risk of commitment involved in personal knowledge is what Polanyi calls the "passionate participation in the act of knowing."[16(p17)]

The nurse in the therapeutic use of self rejects approaching the patient-client as an object and strives instead to actualize an authentic personal relationship between two persons. The individual is considered as an integrated, open system incorporating movement toward growth and fulfillment of human potential. An authentic personal relation requires the acceptance of others in their freedom to create themselves and the recognition that each person is not a fixed entity, but constantly engaged in the process of becoming. How then should the nurse reconcile this with the social and/or professional responsibility to control and manipulate the environmental variables and even the behavior of the person who is a patient in order to maintain or restore a steady state? If a human being is assumed to be free to choose and chooses behavior outside of accepted norms, how will this affect the action taken in the therapeutic use of self by the nurse? What choices must the nurse make in order to know another self in an authentic relation apart from the category of patient, even when categorizing for the purpose of treatment is essential to the process of nursing?

Assumptions regarding human nature, McKay observes, "range from the existentialist to the cybernetic, from the idea of an information processing machine to one of a many splendored being."[17(p399)] Many of these assumptions incorporate in one form or another the notion that there is, for all individuals, a characteristic state which they, by virtue of membership in the species, must strive to assume or achieve. Empirical descriptions and classifications reflect the assumption that being human allows for prediction of basic biological, psychological, and social behaviors that will be encountered in any given individual.

Certainly empirical knowledge is essential to the purposes of nursing. But nursing also requires that we be alert to the fact that models of human nature and their abstract and generalized categories refer to and describe behaviors and traits that groups have in common. However, none of these categories can ever encompass or express the uniqueness of the individual encountered as a person, as a "self." These and many other similar considerations are involved in the realm of personal knowledge, which can be broadly characterized as subjective, concrete, and existential. It is concerned with the kind of knowing that promotes wholeness and integrity in the personal encounter, the achievement of engagement rather than detachment; and it denies the manipulative, impersonal orientation.

Ethics: The Moral Component

Teachers and individual practitioners are becoming increasingly sensitive to the difficult personal choices that must be made within the complex context of modern health care. These choices raise fundamental questions about morally right and wrong action in connection with the care and treatment of illness and the promotion of health. Moral dilemmas arise in situations of ambiguity and uncertainty, when the consequences of one's actions are difficult to predict and traditional principles and ethical codes offer no help or seem to result in contradiction. The moral code which guides the ethical conduct of nurses is based on the primary principle of obligation embodied in the concepts of service to people and respect for human life. The discipline of nursing is held to be a valuable and essential social service responsible for conserving life, alleviating suffering, and promoting health. But appeal to the ethical "rule book" fails to provide answers in terms of difficult individual moral choices, which must be made in the teaching and practice of nursing.

The fundamental pattern of knowing identified here as the ethical component of nursing is focused on matters of obligation or what ought to be done. Knowledge of morality goes beyond simply knowing the norms or ethical codes of the discipline. It includes all voluntary actions that are deliberate and subject to the judgment of right and wrong—including judgments of moral value in relation to motives, intentions, and traits of character. Nursing is deliberate action, or a series of actions, planned and implemented to accomplish defined goals. Both goals and actions involve choices made, in part, on the basis of normative judgments, both particular and general. On occasion, the principles and norms by which such choices are made may be in conflict.

According to Berthold, "goals are, of course, value judgments not amenable to scientific inquiry and validation."[18(p196)] Dickoff, James, and Wiedenbach also call attention to the need to be aware that the specification of goals serves as "a norm or standard by which to evaluate activity . . . [and] . . . entails taking them as values—that is, signifies conceiving these goal contents as situations worthy to be brought about."[19(p422)]

For example, a common goal of nursing care in relation to the maintenance or restoration of health is to assist patients to achieve a state in which they are independent. Much of the current practice reflects an attitude of value attached to the goal of independence, and indicates nursing actions to assist patients in assuming full responsibility for themselves at the earliest possible moment or to enable them to retain responsibility to the last possible moment. However, valuing independence and attempting to maintain it may be at the expense of the patient's learning how to live with physical or social dependence when necessary—for example, in instances when prognosis indicates that independence cannot be regained.

Differences in normative judgments may have more to do with disagreements as to what constitutes a "healthy" state of being than lack of empirical evidence or ambiguity in the application of the term. Slote suggests that the persistence of disputes, or lack of uniformity in the application of cluster terms, such as *health*, is due to "the difficulty of decisively resolving certain sorts of value questions about what is and is not important." This leads him to conclude "that value judgment is far more involved in the making of what are commonly thought to be factual statements than has been imagined."[20(p220)]

The ethical pattern of knowing in nursing requires an understanding of different philosophical positions regarding what is good, what ought to be desired, what is right; of different ethical frameworks devised for dealing with the complexities of moral judgments; and of various orientations to the notion of obligation. Moral choices to be made must then be considered in terms of specific actions to be taken in specific, concrete situations. The examination of the standards, codes, and values by which we decide what is morally right should result in a greater awareness of what is involved in making moral choices and being responsible for the choices made. The knowledge of ethical codes will not provide answers to the moral questions involved in nursing, nor will it eliminate the necessity for having to make moral choices. But it can be hoped that:

> The more sensitive teachers and practitioners are to the demands of the process of justification, the more explicit they are about the norms that govern their actions, the more personally engaged they are in assessing surrounding circumstances and potential consequences, the

more "ethical" they will be; and we cannot ask much more.[21(p221)]

USING PATTERNS OF KNOWING

A philosophical discussion of patterns of knowing may appear to some as a somewhat idle, if not arbitrary and artificial, undertaking having little or no connection with the practical concerns and difficulties encountered in the day-to-day doing and teaching of nursing. But it represents a personal conviction that there is a need to examine the kinds of knowing that provide the discipline with its particular perspectives and significance. Understanding four fundamental patterns of knowing makes possible an increased awareness of the complexity and diversity of nursing knowledge.

Each pattern may be conceived as necessary for achieving mastery in the discipline, but none of them alone should be considered sufficient. Neither are they mutually exclusive. The teaching and learning of one pattern do not require the rejection or neglect of any of the others. Caring for another requires the achievements of nursing science, that is, the knowledge of empirical facts systematically organized into theoretical explanations regarding the phenomena of health and illness. But creative imagination also plays its part in the syntax of discovery in science, as well as in developing the ability to imagine the consequences of alternative moral choices.

Personal knowledge is essential for ethical choices in that moral action presupposes personal maturity and freedom. If the goals of nursing are to be more than conformance to unexamined norms, if the "ought" is not to be determined simply on the basis of what is possible, then the obligation to care for another human being involves becoming a certain kind of person—and not merely doing certain kinds of things. If the design of nursing care is to be more than habitual or mechanical, the capacity to perceive and interpret the subjective experiences of others and to imaginatively project the effects of nursing actions on their lives becomes a necessary skill.

Nursing thus depends on the scientific knowledge of human behavior in health and in illness, the esthetic perception of significant human experiences, a personal understanding of the unique individuality of the self, and the capacity to make choices within concrete situations involving particular moral judgments. Each of these separate but interrelated and interdependent fundamental patterns of knowing should be taught and understood according to its distinctive logic, the restricted circumstances in which it is valid, the kinds of data it subsumes, and the methods by which each particular kind of truth is distinguished and warranted.

The major significances to the discipline of nursing in distinguishing patterns of knowing are summarized as (1) the conclusions of the discipline conceived as subject matter cannot be taught or learned without reference to the structure of the discipline— the representative concepts and methods of inquiry that determine the kind of knowledge gained and limit its meaning, scope, and validity; (2) each of the fundamental patterns of knowing represents a necessary but not complete approach to the problems and questions in the discipline; and (3) all knowledge is subject to change and revision. Every solution of an existing problem raises new and unsolved questions. These new and as yet unsolved problems require, at times, new methods of inquiry and different conceptual structures; they change the shape and patterns of knowing. With each change in the shape of knowledge, teaching and learning require looking for different points of contact and connection among ideas and things. This clarifies the effect of each new thing known

on other things known and the discovery of new patterns by which each connection modifies the whole.

REFERENCES

1. Carper, B. A. "Fundamental Patterns of Knowing in Nursing." PhD dissertation, Teachers College, Columbia University, 1975.
2. Kuhn, T. *The Structure of Scientific Revolutions* (Chicago: University of Chicago Press 1962).
3. Northrop, F. S. C. *The Logic of the Sciences and the Humanities* (New York: The World Publishing Co. 1959).
4. Nagel, E. *The Structure of Science* (New York: Harcourt, Brace and World, Inc. 1961).
5. Weitz, M. "The Role of Theory in Aesthetics" in Rader, M., ed. *A Modern Book of Esthetics* 3rd ed. (New York: Holt, Rinehart and Winston 1960).
6. Rader, M. "Introduction: The Meaning of Art" in Rader, M., ed. *A Modern Book of Esthetics* 3rd ed. (New York: Holt, Rinehart and Winston 1960).
7. Langer, S. K. *Problems of Art* (New York: Charles Scribner and Sons 1957).
8. Wiedenbach, E. *Clinical Nursing: A Helping Art* (New York: Springer Publishing Co., Inc. 1964).
9. Dewey, J. *Art as Experience* (New York: Capricorn Books 1958).
10. Orem, D. E. *Nursing: Concepts of Practice* (New York: McGraw-Hill Book Co. 1971).
11. Lee, V. "Empathy" in Rader, M., ed. *A Modern Book of Esthetics*, 3rd ed. (New York: Holt, Rinehart and Winston 1960).
12. Lippo. T. "Empathy, Inner Imitation and Sense-Feeling" in Rader, M., ed. *A Modern Book of Esthetics* 3rd ed. (New York: Holt, Rinehart and Winston 1960.)
13. Mitchell, P. H. *Concepts Basic to Nursing* (New York: McGraw-Hill Book Co. 1973).
14. Buber, M. *I and Thou*. Translated by Walter Kaufman (New York: Charles Scribner and Sons 1970).
15. Maslow, A. H. "Self-Actualizing People: A Study of Psychological Health" in Moustakas, C. E., ed. *The Self* (New York: Harper and Row 1956).
16. Polanyi, M. *Personal Knowledge* (New York: Harper and Row 1964).

17. McKay, R. "Theories, Models and Systems for Nursing." *Nurs Res* 18:5 (September-October 1969).

18. Berthold, J. S. "Symposium on Theory Development in Nursing: Prologue." *Nurs Res* 17:3 (May-June 1968).

19. Dickoff, J., James P., and Wiedenbach, E. "Theory in a Practice Discipline: Part I." *Nurs Res* 17 (September-October 1968).

20. Slote, M. A. "The Theory of Important Criteria." *J Philosophy* 63 (April 14 1966).

21. Greene, M. *Teacher as Stronger* (Belmont, Calif.: Wadsworth Publishing Co., Inc. 1973).

4

Multiple Paradigms of Nursing Science

ELIZABETH J. MONTI, MSN, CRNA

MARTHA S. TINGEN, PHD, RN, ANP, CS

Of the many controversies that have accompanied the growth of nursing as a discipline, few have been debated as long and as vigorously as the question of which paradigm should guide nursing science. Despite more than 20 years of discussion, the question remains unresolved. This article discusses the concept of paradigm, explores the paradigms that influence nursing science, and presents a comparison of the advantages and disadvantages of theoretical unification and mutiparadigmism. Additionally, the implications and consequences of multiparadigmism for the present and future development of nursing as a science within a practice discipline are presented. Key words: empirical methods, interpretative methods, multiple paradigms, nursing science, practice discipline

A discipline is a community of interest that is organized around the accumulated knowledge of an academic or professional group.[1] The discipline of nursing represents the body of knowledge related to the study of caring in human health that encompasses both the science and art of nursing.[1,2] Within the discipline, nursing science is devoted to answering questions of interest to the profession and adding to the body of knowledge. Nursing practice represents the art of the discipline.

The unique perspective of the discipline is exemplified by the metaparadigm, which describes, from a global perspective, the concepts and themes chosen as the focus of the discipline and those that differentiate it from others.[3] The metaparadigm concepts of nursing generally are agreed to be person, environment, nursing, and health; however, these are not exclusive.[2-5] The metaparadigm also reflects the shared values and beliefs of the discipline. For example, nurses subscribe to common values and beliefs including respect for persons, caring, autonomy of persons, health promotion, illness prevention, professional competence, and ethical conduct.[1,6]

While nursing scientists are in general agreement about the metaparadigm, they often are in disagreement about the paradigms of the discipline. This disagreement stems in part from failure to agree on a single definition of the term; as a result, writers often are describing different concepts. However, the debate also stems from the idea that the discipline must have a predominant paradigm in order to demonstrate progress as a legitimate science. Because primary paradigms in nursing are considered to represent fundamentally different patterns of knowing and perspectives

Source: Monti, E. J., & Tingen, M. S. (1999). Multiple paradigms of nursing science. *ANS*, 21 (4): 64 – 80. Reprinted with permission from and copyright © 1999 Aspen Publishers, Inc of reality,[3] these disagreements also focus on the ability of paradigms to answer questions and to explore reality in different ways, the relevance of different types of knowledge for the discipline, and the congruence between paradigm and metaparadigm concepts.

Of the many controversies that have accompanied the growth of nursing as a discipline, few have been debated as long or as vigorously as the question of which paradigm should guide nursing science. Despite more than 20 years of discussion, the question remains unresolved. This article discusses the concept of paradigm, explores the paradigms that influence nursing science, and compares and contrasts the advantages and disadvantages of theoretical unification and multiparadigmism. In addition, the implications and consequences of multiparadigmism for the present and future development of nursing as a science within a practice discipline are presented.

THE NATURE OF PARADIGMS

Many definitions of the word "paradigm" exist. Webster defines it first as "a pattern, example, or model" and secondarily as "an overall concept accepted by most people in an intellectual community, as a science, because of its effectiveness in explaining a complex process, idea, or set of data."[7(p979)] A paradigm also has been described as an abstract view or perspective of a discipline, a set of systematic beliefs, a world view, and a theory.[8] Kuhn,[8] who popularized the term, provided multiple descriptions of a paradigm in the first edition of his book, yet failed to precisely define it. In an effort to resolve the confusion that arose from his varying uses of the term, Kuhn later provided two definitions for a paradigm. In the primary sense of the word, a paradigm is a "disciplinary matrix," the ordered elements of

which are held by the practitioners of a discipline. According to this definition, a paradigm includes symbolic generalizations (laws and definitions), shared beliefs, and shared values. In an alternate use, Kuhn defines paradigms in a more circumscribed manner as exemplars or shared examples. Exemplars are a part of the disciplinary matrix by which students learn to solve problems through the application of concrete solutions.

Nursing authors also have contributed to a lack of coherence about paradigms. Fawcett stated that ". . . paradigms are represented by diverse conceptual models of nursing that provide distinctive contexts for the metaparadigm concepts and themes."[4(p2)] Newman[9] states that paradigms are pervasive in nature and that a paradigm's values are deeply imbedded in its followers. Kim defines paradigms as ". . . general scientific perspectives and traditions," because nursing science is developing from various research traditions and the discipline's problems require different perspectives. Lincoln and Guba define a paradigm as ". . . a systematic set of beliefs, together with their accompanying methods."[11(p15)] Hardy,[12] citing Kuhn, defines the paradigm as a gestalt or world view, a metaparadigm that is broader than theory and precedes it. The definition of paradigm as a world view or philosophy that reflects the values and beliefs embraced by a segment of the discipline does not seem useful for the development of nursing science because values and beliefs seldom are amenable to change and the nature of science is about change. The authors of this article prefer Kim's definition because it infers methodologies that scientists apply to solve problems regardless of their philosophy and perspective or lens through which phenomena can be viewed. Kim's definition of paradigm is used throughout this article.

Paradigms are important to scientific communities because they not only answer the discipline's most important questions—or puzzles, as Kuhn[8] called them—but also shape the way scientists "do" research. The ontological and epistemological assumptions of a paradigm drive its methodologies. Scientists who share a paradigm ". . . are committed to the same rules and standards for scientific practice."[8(p11)] A paradigm is useful in that it provides scientists with a general orientation to phenomena, a way of organizing perceptions, criteria for selecting problems, guidelines for investigations and methods, and limitations on possible solutions. Thus, a paradigm provides a guiding framework for resolving problems, conducting research, and deriving theories and laws. For nursing scientists, paradigms direct the perspective from which research questions are asked, problems are investigated, research is designed as well as what methods are used and how data are collected, analyzed, and interpreted.[2]

PARADIGMS IN NURSING

Nursing science is characterized by two predominant paradigms that are broadly classified as the empiricist and the interpretative. These two paradigms represent fundamentally opposing views of knowledge development and reality. Several conceptual frameworks of nursing depict the metaparadigm concepts from the perspective of the different paradigms. The contribution of the primary paradigms to nursing science will be discussed and examples of conceptual frameworks that are derived from them will be presented. The cardinal features of the two paradigms are presented in Table 4.1.

Empiricism is based on the assumption that what is known can be verified through the senses.[5] The ontological assumption of empiricism is that there is one reality, which is out there somewhere and can be validated through the senses. In the empiricist paradigm, knowledge is developed through sense observation of the natural world in order to verify and justify theories that describe, predict, and prescribe. Research studies in this tradition focus on the context of justification. Theories depicting reality are reduced into components that can be either validated or disproved empirically in order to justify the relationships set forth. Empiricism also has been described as reductionistic because parts rather than the whole of phenomena are examined and because of the positivistic emphasis on theory reduction.

TABLE 4.1. A comparison of the empiricist and interpretative paradigms

	EMPIRICISM	INTERPRETATIVE
Alternative names	Mechanistic Positivism	Organismic
Nursing	Particulate-deterministic	Unitary-transformative
Paradigms	Totality	Simultaneity
Ontology	One reality Reality is independent of context	Multiple realities Composite reality
	Truth can be determined	Meaning is grounded in experience
	Certainty is possible	Truth can never be determined

cont. on page 34

Table 4.1 cont.

	EMPIRICISM	**INTERPRETATIVE**
Epistemology	Reality can be verified by the senses Value-free observations Cognition and perception are separate entities	Knowledge is derived from experience, art, ethics Value-laden observations Cognition, perception and experience affect what is seen or conceptualized Shared meaning
Purpose	Verification and justification Theory testing Identify cause and effect	Discovery and meaning Theory generating Increase understanding and knowledge of lived reality
Human beings are:	Machines The sum of their parts Closed systems	Living organisms Holistic beings Greater than the sum of their parts Open systems
Researcher is	Observer Objective Uninvolved	The instrument Co-creating Involved in the process
Phenomena	Can be reduced to parts	Holistic view Irreducible Context dependent
Behavior	Predictable, linear	Probabilistic Unpredictable
Movement	Organism is passive or at rest Exterior forces cause movement	Active From within organism
Methodologies	Quantitative Observation Control	Qualitative Attention to context and interpretation Interview, observation
Research question	What is the relationship? of A and B What is the effect of A on B? Hypothesis testing	What is the meaning of . . .? What is the structure of the lived experience?
Designs	Experimental Quasi-experimental	Emergent Phenomenology Grounded theory
Sample	Random selection Random assignment Convenience	Purposive Theoretical Volunteer
Data collection techniques	Instrumentation Observation	Interviews Observation Analysis of art, literature, documents
Data analysis	Deductive Statistical analysis	Inductive Interpretation Constant comparative method

The ontological assumption of empiricism is that there is one reality, which is out there somewhere, which can be validated through the senses.

Empiricism has its roots in the logical positivist school of philosophy. Logical positivism, also called logical empiricism and the received view, was espoused by a group of philosophers known as the Vienna school.[11,13-14] Positivists disavowed religious and metaphysical explanations of reality and analyzed theories for logical patterns of reasoning that could be verified in reality.[14] Logical positivism, however, was an extremist variant of empiricism because it espoused the idea that the only reality was that which could be observed in the world.[13,15] Thus, the mind was not an object of study unless the mind could be associated with a physical reality, a position reminiscent of Descartes' theory of mind-body dualism. Positivism also was associated with an antiquated view of the universe that equated it with a machine operated by laws understood only by God.[13] The purpose of science was to discover these laws, or products, in order to be able to explain and predict events in the world. Theories describing reality in formal language either could be verified or disproved by observation of objects in the world. Thus, science resulted in a product, a theory, that could be used to describe, predict, and prescribe.

Positivism fell into disfavor in the 1960s when it was criticized for using defective methods of analysis and having little to do with actual science.[14] Although discredited and recognized as a dead movement since the 1960s,[6,16] many nursing scientists continue to react to contemporary empiricism as though positivism were flourishing. Gortner feels that empiricism has been given short shrift in nursing, because of ". . . continued fallacious identification with logical positivism."[6(p482)] Modern empiricism, also called post-positivism, incorporates a historical approach to science along with empirical methods.[6]

Historicism is concerned with the values and beliefs of scientists as well as the sociological and historical context in which decisions regarding scientific research are made.[16] Historical approaches incorporate the ideas of philosophers such as Laudan, who thought that science should be judged by the number of problems it solved rather than whether or not theories were verified.[16] Thus, post-positivist empirical research retains the empiricist elements of precision, deductive reasoning, objectivity, theory testing, and substantiation of theoretical claims with valid data,[17] while recognizing the impossibility of verification and the value-laden qualities of theory and observation.[6,15] However, post-positivists also recognize that the purpose of scientific investigation in nursing is patient care; that the meaning of relationships can be clarified: that generalizable patterns can be ascertained without full prediction and control; that the conditions or context in which the phenomenon occurs is important; and that the researcher must prevent personal biases from influencing the outcomes of research.[17]

The methodology associated with empiricism is the scientific method. This method focuses on the experiment, control, objectivity, precise measurement, quantification of data, and description of results in statistical terms. Because empiricists believe that the senses can be used to verify reality, observation is the preferred method of data collection. The scientist uses tools and instruments to measure the phenomenon of concern while remaining a detached observer in order to prevent personal biases from influencing the study results.[18] Numerical values are assigned to data in order to test relationships using statistical methods.

The empiricist paradigm is necessary if nursing science is to substantiate claims regarding nursing care and the responses of persons in health and illness situations, provide explanatory models, and test and generate theory.[6,17] The value of the empirical approach to knowledge development lies in its ability to test hypotheses, compare interventions, produce generalizations, and generate confidence intervals that uncover influences.[15] The ability to test hypotheses allows the relationships in theories to be tested and validated.[18] Although no one study ever can verify a relationship, the data collected can offer strong support for the presence of a relationship. Establishment of valid relationships enables theories to be used to explain, predict, and prescribe notions that are essential and relevant for clinical practice.[19] Control limits the problem being researched and attempts to limit extraneous factors so that relationships can be examined more precisely. Random assignment of subjects or treatments also allows factors that may affect the variable of interest to be equally distributed.[15] Generalizability is an important goal of empirical research, as it allows relationships to be extrapolated to a larger population or different situation, a factor that is advantageous in nursing practice.[18] Statistical methods allow for both exploratory and confirmatory analyses of data to describe the data and search for potential relationships.[18] However, discovery of statistical significance does not indicate necessarily clinical significance.[15]

CRITICISMS OF EMPIRICISM

Objectivity and control are aspects of empiricism that have been criticized severely by many nursing researchers. In empirical investigations, researchers control extraneous or confounding variables in order to increase the validity of study results. However, when studying humans, it is impossible to control many factors that might affect the outcome of a study. In addition, excessive control of variables in human studies can remove important contexts that influence a situation and contribute to its meaning. Excessive control pro-

duces an artificial situation that bears no resemblance to reality and thus decreases generalizability. Objectivity is also seen as preventing ". . . full recognition of the other as a person"[20] while experimental conditions can decontextualize the human experience. Thus, the traditional experimental method, in which persons respond to the environment like a machine rather than interacting with the environment, is seen as having a dehumanizing effect.[20]

Some nursing scientists criticize positivism because it does not recognize other forms of knowing besides that which can be verified. Nurses always have recognized the knowledge embedded in practice. Carper[21] identified four fundamental patterns of knowing in nursing: empirics, ethics, esthetics, and personal knowledge. Empirics, or the science of nursing, is concerned with describing, explaining, and predicting phenomena of concern. Esthetics, or the art of nursing, is the expressive and perceptive aspect of nursing that can defy expression. Ethics focuses on moral questions of right and wrong and what ought to be done. Personal knowledge ". . . is concerned with the knowing, encountering, and actualizing of the concrete, individual self."[21(p251)] The four are not isolated entities but interrelate to form a whole that is greater than the sum of the parts. Thus, knowledge acquisition does not occur as a result of one isolated way of viewing the world but through the simultaneous interaction of the four patterns. Logical positivism ignored aspects of nursing knowledge that were acquired through means other than empirical methods and thus negated a rich source of nursing knowledge.

Prior to the 1950s, nursing research activities were limited.[18] In the 1950s and 1960s, empiricism was the predominant approach to developing nursing knowledge. Strongly influenced by the medical model and education in other disciplines, early nursing scientists favored the empiricist paradigm because they were eager to establish the scientific basis of the profession and demonstrate that nursing was a unique, professional discipline.[22] However, many nursing scientists became frustrated with the positivistic approach and began questioning its use because it often did not reflect the values and beliefs of nursing nor the discipline's focus on holism, person-centered care, and understanding of human experiences in health and disease. Desiring a more humanistic approach that could address the concerns of nurses and their patients, many researchers turned to the methods proposed by phenomenological and existential schools of philosophy that are concerned with the meaning of human experience and understanding the day-to-day experience of individuals.[20]

THE INTERPRETATIVE PARADIGM

The interpretative paradigm in nursing science evolved for several reasons. First, many early nurse scientists were educated in disciplines such as philosophy, sociology, and anthropology that exposed them to alternate ways of viewing the world and the methodologies associated with those paradigms. Second, to some nurse scientists, empiricism did not recognize the esthetic, ethical, and personal knowledge inherent in nursing. Interpretative traditions acknowledge that reality has multiple meanings and that knowledge can be derived from sources other than the senses. Thus, other patterns of knowing important to nursing are given credence by interpretative approaches. Third, the interpretative approach was seen as more congruent with the language and beliefs of nursing. Where nursing spoke of holism, individualism, autonomy, and self determination, the dominating scientific/medical model spoke of reductionism, objectivity, manipulation, prediction, and con-

trol.[22] A fourth reason for embracing the interpretative paradigm is that nursing wished to establish a theoretical base for the discipline. The interpretative paradigm provided methods for generating theory that are representative of nursing views rather than borrowed from other professions.[22] Finally, a qualitative approach offers new perspectives and methodologies for answering the questions of the discipline.[23]

The interpretative paradigm is characterized by the ontological assumptions that reality is complex, holistic, and context-dependent.[11,24] The focus of investigation is on human experience: thus, subjectivity rather than objectivity is emphasized.[12] Because reality and human experience are variable, multiple ways of knowing are valued to uncover the knowledge that is embedded in human experience. Tacit or intuitive knowledge is recognized in addition to that which is expressed in language or can be observed.[11] Therefore, the methodology includes techniques that result in extended contact of the researcher with the participant and in mutual interaction. A natural setting is selected because ". . . wholes cannot be understood in isolation from their contexts . . ."[11(p39)] nor can they be separated into parts for study. Inductive reasoning is used to identify patterns of meaning in the data.[11]

Broadly grouped under the term qualitative research, interpretative methods include phenomenology, hermeneutics, grounded theory, ethnography, and others. The general goal of interpretative methods is to understand and derive meaning from the human experience; however, instrumentation and conceptualization are other identified purposes.[24] Common features of these research traditions are a holistic approach to questioning, a focus on human experience, purposive sampling, sustained contact with participants, the involvement of the researcher in the process, emergent design, negotiated outcomes, and special criteria for trustworthiness.[11] In-depth interviews with open-ended questions and participant observations are used for data collection. Data analysis proceeds through analysis of written narratives to extract the meaning of the experience.[24]

A strength of the interpretative paradigm is the usefulness of this approach for generating theories. When little is known about a subject, qualitative methods are useful in identifying patterns of experiences and the relationships between them. Relational statements reflecting these relationships can be written and used to develop new theories.[18] For example, grounded theory methods can identify basic social structures or processes (BSP) through the method of constant comparative analysis. These BSPs are then linked into a theory.[24]

CRITICISMS OF THE INTERPRETATIVE PARADIGM

Although anti-positivist perspectives have been embraced by many nursing researchers, they are not without their limitations for developing knowledge in nursing. While the interpretative paradigm emphasizes humanistic approaches, it ignores the reality of physiological problems that are an integral part of a discipline that deals with health and disease.[6,25] Nursing is not a social science and must acknowledge that physiological and psychosocial phenomena are at the core of the discipline. Nursing science must address the complex clinical problems that practicing nurses deal with daily. Research traditions that rely solely on interpretation and gaining understanding are not amenable to testing theory.[6] Practitioners need theories that help guide their practice and answer questions posed by clinical situations. Although qualitative methodologies such as grounded theory can present theories

describing the knowledge embedded in practice, testing of these nascent theories by empirical methods is required.

Interpretative methodologies have been criticized for a lack of rigor, primarily on the basis of criteria used to judge quantitative studies.[18] However, quantitative criteria are inappropriate for evaluating the rigor of qualitative studies.[11,18] Issues that have been cited as reflecting a lack of rigor include failure to adhere to the philosophy of the method being used, inadequate time spent collecting data, failure to identify values and beliefs that may impinge on the study, and poorly developed methods.[18] Credibility, transferability, dependability, and confirmability are the appropriate criteria for judging qualitative methodologies.[11]

> Credibility, transferability, dependability, and confirmability are the appropriate criteria for judging qualitative methodologies.

The results of qualitative studies have been characterized as ". . . a set of interesting stories" that result in isolated findings that do not advance the discipline because they do not form the basis for further work.[25] Although nursing is concerned with the uniqueness of individuals, in daily practice, nurses must identify patterns, look for commonalities, and establish priorities. While the results of qualitative research may serve to uncover some of the aesthetic, ethical, and personal knowledge of nurses, practice demands that this knowledge also be put to use. Knowledge that does not help nurses meet society's needs, understand and explain the concepts and relationships of the metaparadigm and conceptual models, and predict events and effects does not contribute to the discipline.

Various writers have suggested other names for the empiricist and interpretative world views in nursing. Parse characterized the world views of the empiricist and interpretative paradigms as the totality and simultaneity paradigms.[3,26] The simultaneity world view regards the person as more and different than the sum of its parts, an open being, free to choose, in rhythmic interaction with the environment.[3,26] In the totality paradigm the person is the sum of bio-psycho-social-spiritual parts, and interacts with the environment in a linear manner.[26] Newman[9] proposed the particulate-deterministic, interactive-integrative, and unitary-transformative perspectives. In the first world view, phenomena can be viewed as isolated, reducible entities with measurable properties that have an orderly relationship. The second paradigm is related to the first except that the context of phenomena is considered and reality is understood to be multidimensional. In the third paradigm, human beings are considered to be evolving as unitary self-organizing fields.[9] Fawcett,[26] attempting to integrate these different models, coined the reaction, reciprocal interaction, and simultaneous action world views. Despite the differences in names, the totality, particulate-deterministic, interactive-integrative, and reaction world views are representations of the empiricist or mechanistic paradigm, while the others are derived from the interpretative or organismic tradition.

IS NURSING SCIENCE A MATURE SCIENCE?

Does the fact that nursing science lacks a predominant paradigm mean that nursing is not a mature science? Nurses too often attempt to measure the success of the discipline with criteria proposed by others that only serve to highlight the limitations of nursing science and fail to acknowledge its successes.[27] Zbilut states that "perhaps nursing has become a full-fledged professional discipline inasmuch as it succumbs to academic fashion."[28(p.188)] Many nursing scientists subscribe to Kuhn's[8] depiction of a mature science. Kuhn characterized science as having three distinct phases: pre-paradigmatic, normal science or post-paradig-matic, and transformative periods that he calls "revolutions." The pre-paradigmatic stage is characterized by ". . . debates over legitimate methods, problems and standards of solution" . . .[8(p.48)] and the lack of primacy of a particular world view. Change from pre-to post-paradigm science is characterized by multiple schools of thought giving way to one and science finding a more satisfactory method of "solving puzzles." A period of "normal science" exists when one paradigm emerges as the predominant way of solving problems, members of a scientific community accept the paradigm as foundational, and use the world view espoused by the predominant paradigm to solve problems. Debates about methods, questions for study, and ways of answering questions disappear during periods of normal science. Revolutions occur following a crisis, when scientists begin to see the world differently and debates emerge about the paradigm. Gradually, one paradigm supplants that previously in favor and a new period of normal science begins.

Mature science develops through revolutions that provide a transition from one paradigm to another.[8] According to Kuhn.[8] a mature science is characterized by

1. the scientific community's acceptance of a paradigm.

2. approaches to solving the discipline's problems that are driven by the paradigm.

3. the presentation of knowledge as research articles in scientific journals rather than books, and

4. the development of a language that is unintelligible to the uninitiated.

A predominant paradigm is the most important criterion.

Using these criteria, nursing science is at a pre-paradigmatic stage, because several paradigms are extant. There is vigorous, ongoing debate within the nursing scientific community about the appropriateness of philosophies and methodologies for directing and conducting research as well as about the questions of relevance to the discipline. However, nursing does meet Kuhn's requirements for shared values, a unique language, scientific journals, and reporting of research findings in articles. A review of the numerous scientific nursing journals indicates that nursing has developed a language of its own and that a significant body of scholarly activity has been accumulated. However, Kuhn,[8] a physicist by training, has been criticized as providing an inaccurate account of the history of science and evaluating science from a positivist perspective due to his emphasis on facts, empiricism, experimentation, and natural science. This positivist perspective is inappropriate and too narrow for a human science such as nursing that confronts a variety of problems.[27,29] Other ways of evaluating scientific progress may be more useful to nursing science.

Meleis[27] proposed a theory of integration for evaluation of progress in nursing science that is more congruent with the tortuous path by which the discipline has developed. Diversity, theory development, competition, creativity, innovation, openness, flexibility, and change are characteristics of a mature discipline according to Meleis. She states nursing has achieved disciplinary status when evaluated by these criteria.[27]

Fawcett[4] identified three areas of success in nursing research and suggested yard-sticks for measuring future progress in nursing science. She recognized "hallmarks of success" that nursing has achieved as identification of the boundaries of research, the types of research required by the discipline, and the types of research activities appropriate for nurses with different educational preparation.

Goals for the 21st century are elimination of obstacles to nursing research, acceptance of multiple methods of inquiry, and utilization of research findings in practice. Whether or not nursing science achieves these goals or nursing scientists are in agreement about these criteria, they are important because they provide a nursing perspective of what is important to the discipline rather than applying qualifications developed by those unfamiliar with the history and advances of nursing science.

SINGLE OR MULTIPLE PARADIGMS?

Kuhn's[8] conceptualization of an overarching paradigm that directs the scientific endeavors of a discipline is the basis for the idea of theoretical unification in nursing. This idea is reminiscent of the positivist philosophy of theoretical reduction and reflects his philosophical underpinnings. Paradigmatic supremacy represents the outmoded positivist viewpoint that considers theory reduction an important goal of science.[16] This philosophy assumes that there is one inclusive theory that can reveal the characteristics of reality.[16] However, the concept of unification suggests the mingling of paradigms rather than the dominance of one over the other. Given that the empiricist and interpretative paradigms represent opposing ontological and epistemological views, it is impossible to reconcile the differences underlying the two paradigms to form a unified paradigm.

Several authors suggest that theoretical unification is beneficial to the profession. The advantage of one paradigm lies in its simplicity and parsimony, as there are fewer concepts and relationships to be examined.[16] Hardy suggests that one possible reason for adopting a predominant paradigm is to define the boundaries of the profession or "turf."[12(p92)] Others believe that a unified focus ". . . has the potential for claiming the shared vision of nursing."[2(p5)] Reed believes that accepting multiple paradigms is contrary to the idea of holism and ". . . nursing may be sacrificing coherence for diversity."[30(p78)] Reed[30] advocates a "meta-narrative" or overarching ideal of nursing to direct knowledge development in the profession. While a metanarrative offers potential for discourse and reflection, it does not offer resolution for the differences between the interpretative and empiricist paradigms.

A disadvantage of theoretical unification or the ascendancy of one world view is the narrowness of vision afforded by such a perspective. Kuhn describes the paradigm as an "inflexible box,"[8(p24)] which directs periods of normal science. In this respect, the purpose of normal science is not to examine new phenomena; rather, the aim of normal science is to articulate ". . . the phenomena and theories that the paradigm already supplies."[8(p24)] Because a paradigm directs the work of a community of scientists, selection of one perspective narrows the focus of vision to examining in detail only those phenomena it recognizes. However, when the paradigm becomes too restrictive, scientists "behave differently" and change the nature of their research problems. Thus, theoretical unification can be likened to the idea of the young child who enthusiastically scribbles in a coloring book, only to be told to stay within the lines. Initial enthusiasm for the task quickly becomes discouragement. The challenges confronting practitioners of nursing art and science are too numerous and pressing to permit disenchantment for change or challenge to occur by the unqualified acceptance of a single paradigm.

The existence of multiple paradigms in nursing science indicates a strong and flourishing science. Multiple paradigms are indicative of a "healthy" scientific community because they encourage creativity, stimulate debate and the exchange of ideas, provide diversity of views,[10,31] promote productivity,[1] and keep open avenues of inquiry.[31]

Creativity is a vital and necessary source of ideas in science. Multiple paradigms stimulate creativity by providing different points of view from which to examine a problem or question.[13] Because nursing deals with human behavior, one viewpoint is not sufficient to explain the variety of phenomena and relationships nurses encounter.[27] Theoretical unification focuses vision in one plane, like a microscope, but multiple paradigms expand vision, like a wide-angle lens. Because the goal of nursing science is not simply to add to the discipline's knowledge base, but to develop theories that explain, predict, and prescribe numerous ways of conceptualizing ideas and examining phenomena are beneficial. Multiple paradigms encourage "thinking outside the box" rather than in the box like theoretical unification.

Debate is stimulated by the existence of multiple paradigms. According to the theory of integration, it is debate and competition of theories and ideas that make a discipline scholarly.[27] Compendiums of articles such as Perspectives in Nursing Theory[32] offer a window through which to view debate within the discipline. A review of these articles reveals the intensity with which authors have supported and defended their particular world view, resulting in clarification, codification, and modification of views. The active exchange of opinions and ideas through discourse stimulates growth and development.[31] Just as a growing organism achieves maturity through rapidly dividing and multiplying, so can a discipline grow through a multiplicity of paradigms. Selection of one world view can be considered analogous to the loss of variability that accompanies aging and death in complex physiological systems.[33]

Diversity of view points has been likened to a cable that is strengthened by multiple strands.[34] Nursing is a complex profession with many providers with differing educational preparation and areas of specialization caring for many types of clients in varying situations. How can one paradigm for nursing science possibly reflect this diversity? Just as people have been urged to celebrate their differences, so should nursing science rejoice in the fact that within nursing is a rich and varied assortment of threads that, when woven together, draw a strong, resilient, whole tapestry. The problems of nursing are so diverse that multiple answers and solutions to a question can be appropriate. Multiple perspectives encourage appreciation of the uniqueness of individual nurses and patients by finding multiple answers to common problems. Problems may be erroneously considered solved and questions answered if one perspective for developing knowledge is selected.

Different paradigmatic views may increase productivity. Reliance on one perspective may limit a scientist to repeatedly investigating the same problem from the same approach in different populations. However, applying different viewpoints provides new insights to formulate new ideas to old questions. For example, the continual use of a phenomenological approach will result in many studies about the meaning of an experience. However, for both the discipline and the investigator to advance in knowledge, those studies must be used as a foundation on which to build others that generate and test theory. Other perspectives are needed to channel these initial findings into further studies. In addition to maximizing the strengths and minimizing the weakness of each method, combining or triangulating methods can involve more than one investigator in a research project, resulting in more discussion, more ideas, and more projects.[35]

> Different paradigmatic views may increase productivity.

Premature closure also may result from the selection of one paradigm. Cognitive dissonance may not be noted if only those phenomena that are congruent with a single perspective are examined.[3] In other words, a single perspective is similar to wearing blinders: phenomena that might attract attention are not seen, as they are outside the field of vision. Thus, opportunities to go somewhere more interesting or follow a different path are thwarted.

Multiple paradigms also have disadvantages for nursing science in that practitioners may become confused and divided over the conflicting claims of different view points.[30] Many in the profession find continuing debate over such matters inconclusive, frustrating, and not germane to the business of nursing. Students can become confused if exposed to new, untested ideas, and even experienced practitioners may find the seemingly never-ending debate mystifying.[28] For example, it is difficult to reconcile the pragmatic aspects of everyday nursing with ideas espoused by interpretative paradigms. If each individual is unique, why are standard care plans devised? What does it mean for a person to be an open system and how can this be evaluated? Why do nurses assess patients systematically if they are holistic beings? How can the accomplishments of empiricism be accepted while its methods are condemned as controlling and dehumanizing? If empiricism is abandoned, what will replace it?

IMPLICATIONS OF MULTIPARADIGMISM FOR NURSING SCIENCE

A change of perspective is required for nursing science to reconcile the philosophical differences between the two extant paradigms. A perspective that emphasizes inquiry rather than paradigmatic supremacy or unification is more advantageous to nursing as a discipline. Dzurec and Abraham[36] noted that there were few real differences between quantitative and qualitative methods of research. Although specific techniques may vary between methods. ". . . the findings generated by both . . . are based on description, probability, and inference."[36] [(p74)] The results of both empirical and interpretative studies are due to interpretation of raw data by the investigator.[36] The authors argue that neither method is more scientific than the other and that the process of inquiry is the same despite the methods used to acquire knowledge. Therefore, nursing scientists can take heart in the thought that careful adherence to the principles and philosophy of the method they chose will result in valid and reliable findings that will add to the body of knowledge of the discipline.

Integration of qualitative and quantitative methods has been suggested as advancing nursing science.[20,35,36] Research traditions from the empirical and interpretative paradigms are complementary as each presents a different approach.[15] Qualitative methods can describe phenomenon of interest in nursing and generate theories that propose relationships between identified concepts. Quantitative methods can test the relationships of qualitatively developed theories and suggest whether the theory should be accepted or revised. The different perspectives presented by the empiricist and interpretative paradigms can examine different dimensions of a phenomenon.

Collaboration towards solving problems is more beneficial for the discipline than acrimony and competition over which tradition is most useful.[16] Collaboration will result in increased opportunities for all nursing scientists. For example, critical multiplism, a strategy similar to triangulation, has been recommended as an approach for nursing research.[34] This strategy is ". . . based on the premise that . . . thoughtful choices are the approach most likely to yield an objective body of knowledge."[34] Multiple-multiples are involved: of researchers, institutions, frameworks, research

questions, issues, methods, and data collection and analysis modes. The approach increases efficiency by spreading the workload and increases utility by studying more than one question at a time.[34] Methods such as this offer greater opportunities for collaboration and discourse than traditional, single-investigator approaches.

When paradigms are associated with values and beliefs, polarization occurs between different views, with little hope of bridging the gulf between the sides. Acceptance of multiple paradigms as perspectives and research traditions rather than as values has the potential to lessen the division between the academic and scientific communities. Practicing nurses often are blind to the relevance of theoretical arguments for the everyday practice of nursing. However, clinicians readily understand that there are many ways to accomplish the same goal and that a nurse uses whatever method he or she is most comfortable with or whatever works best in a particular situation.

Presenting research as a system of inquiry that can be accomplished in several ways may also improve the palatability of research in educational programs. Both baccalaureate and masters students often are overwhelmed by research courses and rate their usefulness to practice as low. However, student interest in research may be spurred by courses that emphasize principles of sound inquiry rather than the vagaries and quirks of different paradigmatic approaches. Just as students learn sound principles of nursing care on which to build their nursing practice, so must they learn basic principles of inquiry that recognize the equality of all methods. Presenting a system of inquiry rather than a philosophy also will require that instructors provide a more balanced view of different research traditions.

A variety of paradigms allows the development of more theories for nursing. Different perspectives of nursing practice enhance the ability to understand and interpret the meaning in different practice situations, identify relationships, and develop theories. Laudan[37] recommends a process of integration of different research traditions with the goal of expanding the number of theories in order to solve the problems of the discipline.

The feasibility and importance of a multiparadigmatic approach ultimately will be established through its usefulness in practice. If differing perspectives can generate and test theories that provide faithful representations of practice and are useful in practice settings, they will flourish. As a pragmatic profession, nurses choose the method that works best to provide the critical services clients require. Practice will indicate those aspects of a perspective that are not useful and discard or revamp them into a new variant. Applying different paradigms together in practice situations can help to determine whether the perspective offered by opposing perspectives results in different nursing actions. According to history, often that which is not useful does not survive. If the multiparadigmatic approach is not congruent with practice, it too, may become obsolete or extinct.

SUMMARY

The discussion about theoretical unification or multiparadigmism is reminiscent of the debate over single or multiple conceptual frameworks for nursing. Interestingly, that debate has been abandoned as the discussion shifts to paradigms. The war of words over single or multiple paradigms cannot be won easily. However, multiparadigmism is an approach to the development of nursing knowledge that offers greater promise for the discipline than theoretical unification. Multiparadigmism recognizes the differences inherent in opposing world views while celebrating the possibilities that each offers and the way that each complements the other. Downplaying paradigmatic differences while enhancing the value of scholarly inquiry through multiple approaches is paramount for the advancement of nursing science.

REFERENCES

1. Donaldson SK, Crowley DM. The discipline of nursing. In: Nicoll LH, ed. *Perspectives on Nursing Theory*. 3rd ed. Philadelphia. PA: Lippincott; 1997.
2. Newman MA, Sime AM. Corcoran-Perry SA. The focus of the discipline of nursing. ANS. 1991;14:1–6.
3. Fawcett J. *Analysis and Evaluation of Conceptual Models of Nursing*. 2nd ed. Philadelphia. PA: F.A Davis Company; 1989.
4. Fawcett J. Hallmarks of success in nursing research. ANS. 1984;8:1–11.
5. Chinn PL, Kramer MK. *Theory and Nursing: A Systematic Approach*. 4th ed. St. Louis. MO: Mosby; 1995.
6. Gortner SR. Nursing's syntax revisited: a critique of philosophies said to influence nursing theories. *Int J Nurs Studies*. 1990;30:477–488.
7. *Webster's New World Dictionary*. 3rd. College ed. New York: Webster's New World; 1988.
8. Kuhn TS. *The Structure of Scientific Revolutions*. 2nd ed. Chicago: The University of Chicago Press; 1970.
9. Newman MA. Prevailing paradigms in nursing. *Nurs Outlook*. 1992;40:10–13.
10. Kim HS. Theoretical thinking in nursing: Problems and prospects. In: Nicoll LH. ed. *Perspectives on Nursing Theory*. 3rd ed. Philadelphia. PA: Lippincott; 1997.
11. Lincoln YS, Guba EG. *Naturalistic Inquiry*. Newbury Park, CA: Sage; 1985.
12. Hardy ME. Perspectives on nursing theory. In: Nicoll LH. ed. *Perspectives on Nursing Theory*. 3rd ed. Philadelphia. PA: Lippincott; 1997.
13. Jacox AK, Webster G. Competing theories of science. In: Nicoll LH. ed. *Perspectives on Nursing Science*. 3rd ed. Philadelphia. PA: Lippincott; 1997.
14. Suppe F, Jacox AK. Philosophy of science and the development of nursing theory. In. Werley H, Fitzpatrick J. eds. *Annual Review of Nursing Research*. New York: Springer; 1985.
15. Poole K, Jones A. A re-examination of the experimental design for nursing research. *J. Adv. Nurs*. 1996;24:108–114.

16. Silva MC, Rothbart D. An analysis of changing trends in philosophies of science on nursing theory development and testing. In: Nicoll LH. ed. *Perspectives on Nursing Theory* 3rd ed. Philadelphia. PA: Lippincott; 1997.

17. Weiss SJ. Contemporary empiricism. In: Omery A, Kasper CE. Page GG, eds. *In Search of Nursing Science*. Thousand Oaks, CA: Sage; 1995.

18. Burns N, Grove SK. *The Practice of Nursing Research: Conduct, Critique, & Utilization*. 3rd ed. Philadelphia. PA: W. B. Saunders; 1997.

19. Schumacher KL, Gortner SR. (Mis)conceptions and reconceptions about traditional science. *ANS*. 1992;14:1–11.

20. Holmes CA. Alternatives to natural science foundations for nursing. *Int J Nurs Studies*. 1990;27:187–198.

21. Carper BA. Fundamental patterns of knowing in nursing. In: Nicoll LH. ed. *Perspectives on Nursing Theory*. 3rd ed. Philadelphia. PA: Lippincott; 1997.

22. Munhall PL. Language and nursing research. In: Munhall PL, Boyd CO, eds. *Nursing Research: A Qualitative Perspective*. 2nd ed. New York: National League for Nursing; 1993.

23. Bramlett MH, Gueldner SH, Boettcher JH. Reflections on the science of unitary human beings in terms of Kuhn's requirement for explanatory power. *Visions*. 1993;1:22–35.

24. Boyd CO. Philosophical foundations of qualitative research. In: Munhall PL. Boyd CO. eds. *Nursing Research: A Qualitative Perspective*. 2nd ed. New York: National League for Nursing; 1993.

25. Downs FS. New questions and new answers. *Nurs Res*. 1989;38:323.

26. Fawcett J. From a plethora of paradigms to parsimony in world views. *Nurs Sci Q*. 1993;6(2):56–58.

27. Meleis AI. *Theoretical Nursing: Development & Progress*. 3rd ed. Philadelphia. PA: Lippincott: 1997.

28. Zbilut JP. Contradictions of nursing in a postmodern world. *Image*. 1997;38:188–189.

29. Fry ST. Science as problem solving. In: Omery A. Kasper CE. Page GG. eds. *In Search of Nursing Science*. Thousand Oaks. CA: Sage; 1995.

30. Reed PG. A treatise on nursing knowledge development for the 21st century: beyond postmodernism. *ANS*. 1995;17:70–84.

31. Ramos MC. Adopting an evolutionary lens: an optimistic approach to discovering strength in Nursing. In: Nicoll LH. ed. *Perspectives on Nursing Theory*. 3rd ed. Philadelphia. PA: Lippincott; 1997.

32. Nicoll LH. *Perspectives on Nursing Theory*. 3rd ed. Philadelphia, PA: Lippincott; 1997.

33 Lipsitz LA, Goldberger AL. Loss of "complexity" and aging: potential application of fractals and chaos theory to senescence. JAMA. 1992; 267:1806-1809.

35. Knaft KA, Pettengill MM, Bevis ME, Kirchhoff KT. Blending qualitative and quantitative approaches to instrument development and data collection. *J Prof Nurs*. 1988;4:30-37.

36. Dzurec LC, Abraham IL. The nature of inquiry: linking quantitative and qualitative research. *ANS*. 1993;16:73–79.

37. Laudan L. *Progress and Its Problems: Towards a Theory of Scientific Growth*. Berkeley, CA: University of CA Press; 1977.

38. Kim HS, Holter IM. Critical theory for science of nursing practice. In: Omery A, Kasper CE, Page GG, eds. *In Search of Nursing Science*. Thousand Oaks, CA: Sage; 1995.

5

Aspects of "Reality" and Ways of Knowing in Nursing: In Search of an Integrating Paradigm

JOHN WOLFER, RN, PhD

Types of knowledge, theory and research needed in a practice-oriented discipline are considered in relation to different "aspects of reality." Major changes in nursing epistemology are reviewed to show an expanding model of inquiry. It is argued that a paradigm which recognizes a spectrum of reality from "body" through "mind" to "spirit" provides a philosophical basis for understanding the necessity of multiple modes of inquiry and multiple types of knowledge and theory. From this perspective, fundamentally different modes of inquiry are seen as complementary rather than competitive or inherently superior or inferior. [Keywords: epistemology, theory construction]

One way to approach the question of what types of knowledge, theory and research a practice-oriented discipline such as nursing needs is to ask with what "aspects" of "reality" is the discipline concerned? "Reality" here refers to what people experience and more or less share as "real," that is, consensual reality. A familiar way of conceptualizing reality or existence in Western culture has been to identify three fundamental aspects: body, mind and spirit. Body refers to the material world. Mind refers to the "mental" world and spirit refers to the "transcendental" world. The material refers to all we know about the physical world as experienced through the senses and organized by rational thought. The mental refers to all we know about the "human world" primarily through conceptual/symbolic processes. The transcendental refers to all we directly experience of the world through contemplative modes. Metaphorically speaking, the way we know and experience these aspects of reality is through the "eye of flesh" (sensory based), the "eye of mind" (cognitively based) and the "eye of contemplation" (non-cognitively mediated direct experience) (Wilber, 1990).

A central point of this paper is that the distinction between aspects of reality which require fundamentally different ways of knowing to access and understand phenomena within the domains has not been recognized or made explicit in the nursing literature. The arguments for the need for, or the superiority of, some methodologies over others (usually cast as quantitative vs. qualitative approaches) have essentially boiled down to a recognition that basically different types of "problems" require different methods (the "problem-method fit" issue). Recog-

Source: Wolfer, J. (1993) Aspects of "Reality" and Ways of Knowing in Nursing: In Search of an Integrating Paradigm. IMAGE: *Journal of Nursing Scholarship* 25 (2):141–146. Reprinted with permission from Sigma Theta Tau International.

nition that fundamentally different types of problems require very different types of methods has been necessary and extremely helpful in our evolving understanding of the nature and process of knowledge development especially in liberating us from the early constraint of trying to force all problems into a positivistic straight-jacket. The claim here is that the recognition of the necessity of a proper problem-method fit can be strengthened by also recognizing the ontological differences underlying basically different types of problems (e.g., "body" problems vs. "mind" problems) which lead to different epistemologies and hence general methodologies and specific methods.

The intent of this paper is to review the ontological and epistemological arguments for an "aspects of reality" approach in the nursing literature for critical discussion, not as a competing or merely semantic alternative to the problem-method-fit approach, but as an additional way of understanding why we need multiple ways of knowing and multiple types of knowledge. This additional way of understanding has emerged as an explicit and formally developed philosophical perspective in the relatively new field of transpersonal psychology as represented in the work of one of its leading theorists, Ken Wilber (1977, 1984). Wilber has synthesized a vast amount of knowledge from both Eastern and Western traditions along with the work of many recent scholars in philosophy and the social and behavioral sciences. The present paper is based primarily on the paradigm developed in *Eye to Eye*, (Wilber, 1990).

If we can tentatively accept an "aspects of reality" paradigm as a "map" for representing part of the broad spectrum of human experience that nurses work with at one time or another, then we can examine the relationship between this paradigm and the major forms of knowledge, theory and research ("ways of knowing") identified in nursing literature.

Table 5-1 presents the paradigm. The main focus of this paper will be on the first two aspects, body and mind. That is not to imply the spiritual aspect is not relevant and important, even central from some perspectives (e.g., Watson, 1975).

SCIENCE OF BODY AND MIND

The primary academic model for knowledge generation in nursing has been the familiar analytic/empirical model of the traditional "hard" or "basic" sciences that provides knowledge of physical reality. Empirical data are obtained through the senses (the "eye of the flesh") and organized through rational thinking into theories about structures, processes, mechanisms and relationships that lead to causal explanations about "natural" phenomena. The investigator's primary purpose is to produce accurate descriptions, explanations and predictions in the interest of understanding for its own sake (satisfaction of curiosity, so-called "pure" science) and/or for a "technical" interest (Allen, 1985) in controlling the physical world. The theories can be characterized as relatively objective, deterministic, reductionistic, mechanistic, universal, quantitative and relatively "value-free." They are free in this context because scientific theories survive in the long run primarily on the basis of how well they work in solving scientific problems and not primarily on the basis of the investigator's personal moral/ethical values. (The choice of problem, the allocation of scarce resources for certain research, the social problems created by science and the applications of knowledge are not, of course, value-free. The "value problem" in science is also beyond the scope of this paper.) The "truth value" of any theory is determined through the "canons of science" which incorporate the methodological

TABLE 5.1.   A Spectrum of Reality and Modes of Inquiry

	Aspects of Reality		
	Body----------------------	**Mind**-------------------	**Spirit**
Type of Phenomena	material/physical	mental/symbolic	transcendental transcognitive
Type of Data	sensory-based	language-based	trans-data
Type of Knowledge	theories about structures functions relationships cause/effect	theories of processes relationships experience meaning	direct, non-cognitive experience
Knowledge Characteristics	objective deterministic reductionistic mechanistic universal quantitative less value oriented	interpretive indeterminate holistic dynamic/organic historical/contextual qualitative value-oriented	non-cognitive, immediate experience
Interest/Purpose	technical description explanation prediction control/ application	understanding description explanation empowerment emancipation justice	salvation/ enlighten- ment peace
Validation/Credibility	precision prediction replication serve purpose	relevance persuasive expert consensus serve purpose	experiential confirmation
Types of Discource	linear-discursive rational-analytic mathematical	linear-discursive rational-analytic narrative	paradoxical negation mythical
Methods/Ways of Knowing	observation classification measurement experiment quantitative- analysis	observation phenomenology ethnography grounded theory critical/feminist inquiry philosophical inquiry hermeneutical analysis	contemplate prayer/ mediation
Examples	physiological- nursing physics biology behavioral- psychology astronomy etc.	transcultural- nursing transpersonal- psychology sociology history philosophy etc.	spiritually supportive care

principles and specific methods and objective observation/description, accurate measurement, quantification of variables whenever possible, mathematical and statistical analysis, experimental methods and verification through replication. Validation/verification of theoretical propositions comes through precision of observation and measurement, successful prediction, replication, and in the final analysis, the theory works to solve the problems scientists are interested in (Lauden, 1977). That is, the theory serves its intended purpose. The main types of discourse in this area are linear-discursive, rational-analytic and mathematical.

For the material world, this model or paradigm has worked well. In accordance with the nature of physical reality, the world view and methods of the traditional physical sciences have served their intended purposes in extraordinary ways. In spite of the inhumane uses of scientific methods and knowledge at times, the physical sciences have been fantastically successful in describing, explaining, predicting and controlling many facets of biophysical reality. This obvious point is often overlooked in most of the recent criticisms of traditional scientific methodology. Characteristics of scientific theory about the physical world, such as reductionism, universality and quantification are positive attributes that are crucial for the intended purposes of the physical sciences (causal explanation, prediction and control). Reducing certain physical wholes to their parts (e.g., in molecular biology) in order to describe and understand how the parts determine, at least to a large extent, what is going on with the whole, has resulted in accurate prediction and control in the biophysical world. Reductionism works for much of physical reality even though complex wholes such as human bodies cannot be totally explained and controlled by knowing and manipulating the physical parts only. Nursing investigations related primarily to as-

pects of physical care fall into this part of the spectrum. Other obvious examples of "basic" sciences are listed in Table 5.1.

Jumping across the continuum to a clearly different aspect level of reality is the domain or realm of "mind." Everything individual and collective minds do and produce as part of human experience falls within this area of the continuum. Roughly speaking, we are moving from the physical sciences to the "interpretative sciences" (Allen, 1985) and "human sciences" (Watson, 1985). The phenomena are "mental" and symbolic, not merely material or physical. Something new has been added that is distinctly human, namely the creation of intersubjective "meaning." To describe, understand and participate in this realm of meaning, one must engage the phenomena with some form of language. Hence the "data" are language-based where language is used in a very broad way to include not only rational, linear, discursive language, but also nondiscursive, metaphoric language as well as non-verbal forms of communicating meaning. In other words, this is primarily the domain of the "qualitative." The primary modes of knowing here are experiential in addition to "empirical" in the more limited physical sense, participatory, intersubjective, rational, analytic and for certain phenomena, intuitive-empathic. These modes of knowing result in understanding the meaning and intent of individual and collective human experience. Systematic knowledge here takes the form of descriptive theories regarding structures, processes, relationships, and traditions that underlie psychological, social, and cultural aspects of reality. In order to make sense, that is, derive meaning and understanding of individual and collective human experience, the raw data must be *interpreted* within the appropriate context (Allen, 1985; Allen, Benner, & Diekelmann, 1986; Lincoln & Guba, 1985). Interpretation leads to generalization in the form of theories that describe and elucidate structures, processes, and relationships within a limited historical and social-cultural context. Hence the theories can be characterized as interpretive, indeterminate, holistic, dynamic/organic, historical/contextual, qualitative, and for some types of inquiry toward the right side of this part of the spectrum such as feminist and critical theory, strongly value-oriented. The theories are value-oriented in the sense that humanistic values are often central at this level of investigation. Typically but not exclusively, the primary purpose of the investigator is producing descriptions and interpretations that, in addition to satisfying curiosity, result in understanding the nature of human experience in the interest of freeing people from unnecessary suffering, ignorance, constraint and oppression. Procedures for strengthening the "trustworthiness" and "credibility" of the more empirical types of research in this domain have been worked out and articulated (Lincoln & Guba, 1985). For the less strictly "empirical" forms of inquiry such as critical theory, consensual agreement among qualified investigators over time plays a very important role for establishing "truth" where truth is taken as "useful" for understanding certain human phenomena in such a way as to lead to the possibility of liberation, empowerment and justice. In other words, in addition to whether the theory serves its knowledge development purpose, there may be an additional criterion regarding the degree to which the theoretical understanding is embodied in practice and leads to relief from suffering, ignorance, constraint and oppression.

Nursing literature regarding the evolving self-understanding of theory and knowledge development in the discipline shows a shift from thinking about theory primarily in terms of traditional "hard" scientific theory with a positivistic bias (Jacox, 1974; Fawcett, 1978) to the recognition of the legitimacy and neces-

sity of "soft" or "interpretative," or "phenomenological" or "human" sciences (Allen 1985; Allen et al. 1986; Silva & Rothbart, 1984). This distinction has often been oversimplified as "quantitative vs. qualitative" research. Much necessary effort has been expended to justify theory based on a post-positivistic model of theory and research which a practice profession especially needs. As a result, the methods and principles of "qualitative research" have been clarified and well articulated (Lincoln & Guba, 1986; Sandelowski, 1986). In effect, the definition or model of what is considered legitimate science has been expanded from a narrow, essentially positivistic one, more appropriate for the physical and behavioristic sciences, to a much broader and more appropriate one for many aspects of the reality in nursing.

VALUE THEORY

While the model of science has been expanding, there also has been an increasing recognition of the need for some other forms of theory and knowledge which are not "scientific" in either the strict, traditional sense or the liberal, expanded sense of the human sciences. One of the first milestones of this trend was the work of Dickoff, James, and Wiedenbach (1968) which developed the understanding that a practice profession such as nursing needs something more than, and different from, "mere" scientific theory, namely, "practice" or "prescriptive" theory. The significant addition here was the explicit recognition that scientific theory from any level of investigation must be organized at a "higher" level of theory which is grounded in practice and incorporates *goals* based on *values*. Most of nursing practice is directed towards the achievement of outcomes that are held to be desirable and valuable. The choice of, and prioritization of goals in a clinical setting is not itself a "scientific" activity or product of scientific research in the usual sense and is based (often implicitly) on beliefs and feelings about what is valuable and right for people needing nursing care.

Although Dickoff et al. (1968) did not emphasize or expand the need for, and nature of, normative/ethical theory, this type of theory would seem to be an inherent and necessary part of theory at the prescriptive level. By implication then, the systematic explication and clarification of the values and ethics underlying nursing care goals, and how they lead to what are primarily nursing goals, should be an integral part of nursing practice theory. Therefore, practice theory requires the development and articulation of relevant normative and ethical theory. Systematic theory which articulates the normative/ethical rationale for goals and priorities in practice is not based on empirical fact *per se* and does not involve the empirical methods of either quantitative or qualitative research. Depending on one's definition of "science," such theory, although the work of the trained and qualified "mind's eye," is not the direct product of scientific research in either the traditional or expanded sense. Methods of inquiry for the development of value theory as an intrinsic part of practice theory are referred to as philosophical, intellectual, or scholarly research (Donaldson & Crowley, 1978; Ellis, 1984). Risking social stigma for advocating what some might call "non-scientific" research and theory development in an age of scientism, the new paradigm in concert with the "realities" of nursing as a practice and professional discipline calls for and justifies it. Within this paradigm human values are seen as real and as important as empirical aspects of reality. Accordingly, a practice discipline needs "researchers" articulating normative and ethical theory in nursing through the appropriate "methods" of scholarly, philosophical and hermeneutical inquiry. The new paradigm

recognizes and makes legitimate these modes of inquiry as absolutely essential for developing knowledge regarding these aspects of human reality. It should not be necessary to call this type of systematic inquiry "science" (Watson, 1985) in order to justify it.

Another landmark in the nursing literature which added something significantly new to our understanding of the types of knowledge and theory needed in a practice oriented discipline was Carper's (1978) paper on "patterns of knowledge." Although other authors in nursing have recognized the need for theory and knowledge which is not strictly scientific according to either positivistic or postpositivistic definitions (Donaldson & Crowley, 1978; Ellis, 1984; Schultz & Meleis, 1988), Carper's epistemological study of nursing knowledge as an example of philosophical inquiry, identified three patterns of nursing knowledge in addition to empirical knowledge. Ethical, esthetic and "personal" knowledge were seen as part of, and required in, nursing's "body of knowledge" or theoretical base. By implication this requires "investigators" reporting the "results" of their "research" where the "methods" and principles of "intellectual inquiry" involve the "mind's eye" at the mental/symbolic level of human experience and understanding.

Failure to clearly distinguish the fundamental difference between phenomena at the physical level and phenomena at the mental/symbolic level runs to the core of the limited view of reality expressed in a positivistic model of analytic/empiric science. The early positivistic model held, in effect, that any proposition about reality which could not be expressed in strictly empirical terms was either meaningless or unimportant. When the goal is to explain physical reality, this position might not be so absurd. But as it happened, the positivistic view was overgeneralized in such a way as to claim, in effect, that there was no other reality, at least one that could be known "scientifically." What was in the beginning a narrow and inaccurate philosophy of science (Webster & Jacox, 1981) became a cultural bias now known as "scientism." The fallacy of scientism went from saying, "That which cannot be seen by the eye of flesh cannot be empirically verified" to "That which cannot be seen by the eye of flesh does not exist." It went from saying, "There is an excellent method for gaining knowledge in the realm of the five senses" to "Thus the knowledge gained by mind and contemplation is invalid" (Wilber, 1990, p. 23). Scientism is the world view that holds only the physical is real and the "true" business of science is to learn about this reality through the strict methods of traditional science. In other words, scientism became an ideology with a very limited view of reality and how it is known. But when we turn to the mental/symbolic realm of human discourse, the epistemology and methods of the physical sciences are inappropriate. No amount of scientific rigor and quantification can discover the meaning, intention and value of human interaction at the symbolic level. ". . . values, life meanings, purposes and qualities slip through physical science like sea slips through the nets of fishermen" (Smith, 1976, p. 16).

To assume that the symbolic world can be known through the methods of physical science is to commit a "category error." A category error is made when the modes of knowing in one domain (e.g., the physical with the eye of the flesh) are used in an attempt to "see" in a different domain (symbolic) which requires different modes of knowing (the eye of the mind) or vice versa (attempting to know the physical realm through rational thought without an empirical data base). To hold that nursing research should only use the eye of the flesh (so called quantitative research) or only the eye of the mind (so called qualitative research) is a form of category error in that either position categorically negates the reality and importance of the other. Much of the recent criticism of the epis-

temology and methodology of traditional hard science concerns their inappropriate application to mental/symbolic phenomena of the social sciences which it can not access. This criticism usually does not make the ontological distinction between physical and mental/symbolic aspects of reality. Consequently, it fails to acknowledge the necessity and effectiveness of the physical sciences for solving problems in their proper domain.

A NEW PARADIGM

In order to avoid category errors in any direction and at any level, the new paradigm holds that there are three fundamental components or strands of valid knowledge attainment for all three aspects of reality (Wilber, 1990).

(1) The "instrumental" strand is a set of instructions which tell the "investigator" what must be done in order to know something at any level. These are the specific methods and general principles of inquiry for physical science, interpretative/phenomenological science, all types of intellectual/philosophical inquiry, and contemplative/spiritual experience. One must know and follow the methods correctly (i.e., be properly "trained" and "disciplined") in a domain in order to arrive at the "truth" in that domain. No proper training and discipline, no valid knowing.

(2) The "illuminative" strand refers to what is experientially known when one has followed the methods and principles correctly. Examples would be confirmation of an hypothesis from a replicated experiment on pain reduction in patients with AIDS, a shared understanding of what it "means" and "feels like" subjectively phenomenologically for people who are dying of AIDS, the clarification of patient care goals for patients with AIDS reached by logically, dialogically and empathetically working through relevant normative and ethical understandings, or the direct, non-cogni-

tively mediated experience of a spiritual "truth" after following the "methods" of a given spiritual tradition.

(3) The "communal" strand is the confirmation of (or lack of) what is known by checking it out with others who have adequately completed the injunctive and illuminative strands in a given domain. This is the "public" confirmation of a "truth" through the community of "experts" who arrive at consensual agreement through systematic and shared experience within a domain. The specific methods of confirmation/validation differ across the domains, but the principle of systematic consensual confirmation holds. The major category error of our time has been for the strict empiricists to claim that only their methods of consensual validation were valid. The consensual agreements reached by experts over time after systematic study about truths at the mental/symbolic level in the interpretative sciences and scholarly disciplines, or at the transcendental level in the spiritual/contemplative traditions, were meaningless and invalid from that restricted world view. The scholastics and churchmen of the early 1600s refused to look through Galileo's telescope on the grounds that pure rational thought had already arrived at the "truth" about the earth and celestial bodies (Wilber, 1990).

Recognition that there are different but systematic and legitimate ways of knowing (methods and principles) for different aspects of reality which lead to publicly validated theories or knowledge or direct experience of the phenomena in a given realm is consistent with the full spectrum of human experience. This full spectrum, including the transcendental or spiritual is what nursing practice engages (or desires to engage) in the course of providing "holistic" care. Presently, this "new" paradigm, as an epistemological map of the types of possible knowledge and the multiple ways of producing or engaging that knowledge, is rough and incomplete. Many types of research and

theory do not fall neatly into any one of the three aspects and there are many intriguing questions in the intersections and across areas of the spectrum. For example mind-body interaction research obviously spans the physical and mental and critical social and feminist inquiry or "critical scholarship" in nursing (Thompson, 1987) will at times span large areas of the spectrum from the physical to the spiritual. The real territories are multidimensional continua which can be mapped many different ways for many different purposes. The different maps are tools for achieving different ends. No single map depicts the one and absolute "truth" about the territory. For our purposes we seek maps that will enable us to develop and use theory and knowledge that is appropriate and useful for understanding the full multidimensional continuum of nursing practice, education and research.

This map enables us to see that different research methodologies must be different to address the fundamental differences in the nature of the phenomena being investigated. To say different investigators use different methods simply because they address different problems and questions is only partially correct. They *must* use different methods because fundamentally different phenomena (aspects of reality) *require it*. Methods strictly from the eye of flesh will not permit "seeing" the *meaning* of dying from AIDS or what the ethical and empathetical rationale is for changing care priorities. These aims require methods from the eye of the mind (and heart). Methods from the eye of the mind will not "see" whether one physical care procedure is more effective than another which requires methods from the eye of the flesh. Minds eye methods will not give the bedside nurse the transcendental "knowledge" to "be there" for the patient in a "spiritual" way. All of these modes of knowing will be needed to improve the quality of caring for the whole patient (and the whole nurse). In other words, this map offers a way of looking at the reality of nursing which "sees" different types of knowledge, theory and research as complementary rather than competitive or exclusionary. To nurse the whole patient (or educate the whole student) we must have knowledge about the whole spectrum of the patient's (and student's) reality in the nursing care (education) situation. From this perspective so called qualitative compared to quantitative approaches do not have to be seen in opposition (Munhall, 1982) or seen as one inherently better than the other (Moccia, 1988; Tinkle & Beaton, 1983) without taking into account the fundamental differences in the nature of the phenomena or part of the spectrum under investigation. To advocate the exclusive or primary justification for one set of approaches over another is a form of category error which negates one aspect or the other of the full spectrum of the nurse's and patient's body-mind-spirit reality. This is not to say that in a given clinical area at a given time there may be normative and ethical arguments for doing one kind of research rather than another because of scarce resources and compelling human needs. That is a value decision, not strictly an ontological or epistemological one. When the motivating interest of nursing inquiry is to help make things "better" for patients and clients (or staff or students), this interest can lead to any type of research at any level of investigation for any aspect of reality. Although the interpretative sciences in general, and critical and feminist theory in particular, begin with an explicit interest in making things better for people (e.g., freedom from ignorance and oppression), this does not mean that a nurse researcher cannot use the methods of biological science to find more effective nursing techniques for reducing pain in the interest of "making things better," humanly speaking.

REFERENCES

Allen, D. (1985). Nursing research and social control: Alternative models of science that emphasize understanding and emancipation. *Image, 17,* 58–64.

Allen, D., Benner P. & Dielkelmann, N.L. (1986). Three paradigms for nursing research: Methodological implications. In P.L. Chinn (Ed.), *Nursing research methodology: Issue and implementation,* (23–37). Rockford, MD: Aspen.

Carper, B. (1978). Fundamental patterns of knowing in nursing. *Advances in Nursing Science, 1,* 13–23.

Dickoff, J., James, P. & Wiedenbach, E. (1968). Theory in a practice discipline: Part 1. *Nursing Research, 17,* 415–435.

Donaldson, S.K. & Crowley, D.M. (1978). The discipline of nursing. *Nursing Outlook, 26,* 113–120.

Ellis, R. (June, 1984). Nursing knowledge development. Paper presented at the National Forum on Doctoral Education in Nursing. Denver, CO.

Fawcett, J. (1978). The relationship between theory and research: A double helix. *Advances in Nursing Science, 1,* 49–62.

Jacox, A. (1974). Theory construction in nursing. *Nursing Research, 23,* 4–13.

Laudan, L. (1977). *Progress and its problems: Towards a theory of scientific growth.* Berkeley: University of California Press.

Lincoln, Y.S. & Guba, E.G. (1985). *Naturalistic inquiry.* Beverly Hills: Sage Publications.

Moccia, P. (1988). A critique of compromise: Beyond the methods debate. *Advances in Nursing Science, 10,* 1–9.

Munhall, P.L. (1982). Nursing philosophy and nursing research: In apposition or opposition? *Nursing Research, 31,* 176–181.

Sandelowski, M. (1986). The problem of rigor in qualitative research. *Advances in Nursing Science, 8,* 27–37.

Schultz, P.R. & Meleis, A.I. (1988). Nursing epistemology: Traditions, insights, questions. *Image, 20,* 217–221.

Silva, M.C. & Rothbart, D. (1983). An analysis of changing trends in philosophies of science on nursing theory development and testing. *Advances in Nursing Science, 1,* 1–13.

Smith, H. (1976). *Forgotten truth.* New York: Harper & Row.

Thompson, J. (1987). Critical scholarship: The critique of domination in nursing. *Advances in Nursing Science, 10,* 17–37.

Tinkle, M.B. & Beaton, J.L. (1983). Toward a new view of science: Implications for nursing research. *Advances in Nursing Science, 5,* 27–36.

Watson, J. (1985). *Nursing: Human science and*

human care. Norwalk, CT: Appleton-Century-Crofts.

Webster, G. & Jacox, A. (1981). Nursing theory and the ghost of the received view. In J.C. McCloskey & H.K. Grace (Eds.) *Current issues in nursing* (26–35). Boston: Blackwell Scientific Publications.

Wilber, K. (1977). *The spectrum of consciousness.* Wheaton, IL: Theosophical Publishing House.

Wilber, K. (1984). *Quantum questions.* Boston: Shambhala.

Wilber, K. (1990). *Eye to eye: The quest for the new paradigm.* Boston: Shambhala.

Part II

HISTORY AND EVOLUTION OF NURSING SCIENCE

Historically, nursing practice was initially learned by performing care activities during a hospital apprenticeship. Gradually, nursing education moved from hospital-based programs to academic institutions, and students were taught an abbreviated form of medical sciences, with a focus on understanding pathophysiology and treatment protocols. In their search for recognition as a profession, nurses adopted the nursing process, which exemplifies the medical model, and began conducting empirical research to establish a scientific base for practice. Graduate nurses sought doctoral degrees in other disciplines, and learned non-nursing methods for developing new knowledge. Many nurse scholars designed nursing theories and conceptual models based on their philosophy of nursing. Thus, the evolution of nursing science has been influenced by numerous factors. These factors include nurse scholars' education in other disciplines, belief in the supremacy of empiricism to determine the 'truth,' support of empirical research by funding and publication, a dogmatic belief that nursing paradigms must be rigorously 'tested' before they are applied in practice, and the research-practice gap.

The following four chapters explore different authors' views of factors that have influenced and continue to influence the development of nursing science. In her chapter on the evolution of nursing as a discipline, Judith Wuest compares the historical development of nursing with changes in the women's movement and feminist perspectives. She believes, as do others, that nurses were overly influenced by male-dominated values and beliefs about the criteria for a profession, and the need for empirical research to achieve recognition as a discipline. Her chapter provides an excellent history lesson, along with information about how society's values have shaped nursing's evolution.

In an effort to diminish the importance of empirical research in nursing, Peggy Chinn wrote the classical article, "Debunking Myths in Nursing Theory and Research." Dr. Chinn examines the underlying assumptions of empirically based knowledge, and logically explains their fallacies. She explains how myths represented by empirical science as the ultimate 'truth' are unfounded because their research is not unbiased, objective, nor value-free. In her analysis, Dr. Chinn identifies the limitations of male-dominated empirical science, and levels the playing field for recognizing that all four patterns of knowing are relevant in nursing. She encourages nurses to design new research methods essential to advancing nursing science.

In the nursing literature, nurse scholars have debated for years their different perspectives about the scope and nature of nursing science. In his brief article, "What Constitutes Nursing Science?," John Phillips describes the shifting perspectives about nursing research by recognized scholars in the field. He advocates that nurses design new research methods through creative synthesis to enhance our understanding of human processes and nursing, and thus expand the science of nursing.

Looking toward the future, Drs. Shaké Ketefian and Richard Redman challenge nurse leaders to expand nursing knowledge beyond their parochial and ethnocentric boundaries. In their article, "Nursing Science in the Global Community," the authors describe the historical influence of contextual, quantitative, and qualitative perspectives on shaping the development of nursing theory. They explain how Western values and our social environment have led to assumptions that theories developed by American nurse scholars are universal and acultural, yet these theories are often not applicable in other countries. The authors offer suggestions on how to address internationally relevant nursing concerns and test nursing theories and models in other geographical locations. Collectively, these chapters reflect many factors that continue to influence the evolution of nursing science today.

6

Professionalism and the Evolution of Nursing as a Discipline: A Feminist Perspective

JUDITH WUEST, RN, MN

The evolution of nursing knowledge and nursing as a practice discipline has been stunted by the quest for professionalism. Liberal and socialist feminist theory clarifies the hazards inherent in the masculine institution of professionalism for a predominately female discipline. Socialist feminist theoretical perspectives facilitate a vision of nursing that includes altering social structure such that caring is valued. (Index words: Feminism; Knowledge development; Nursing discipline; Theory) J Prof Nursing 10:357–367, 1994. *W.B. Saunders Copyright © 1994*

The development of nursing as a discipline has been dominated by the hegemony of the patriarchal institutions of professionalism. Feminism can broadly be defined as seeking to end the domination of women (Jaggar, 1983). Nursing, historically a women's occupation, has been a vehicle of both liberation and oppression. The lens of liberal and socialist feminist theory provides a perspective for examining the evolution of nursing as a discipline. Professionalism has played a key role in marginalizing nursing and in constraining knowledge development. Feminism with its emphasis on praxis illuminates possible future directions in knowledge development for nursing as a practice discipline.

FEMINIST THEORETICAL PERSPECTIVES

Feminist theories have defined the causes of women's oppression and offer a means for

Source: Wuest, J. (1994) Professionalism and the Evolution of Nursing as a Discipline: A Feminist Perspective. *Journal of Professional Nursing*, 10(6):357–367. Reprinted with permission from W.B. Saunders. Copyright© 1994.

eliminating it (MacPherson, 1991). Alison Jaggar (1983) clearly distinguished between liberal and socialist feminism.

Liberal Feminist Theory

"Liberal feminism rests on a conception of human nature that is radically individualistic" (Jaggar, 1983, p 355). Impartiality is a key tenet of liberal feminism. Thus, all individuals should be treated equally, and women should receive no special privileges. The focus of liberal feminism is on eliminating oppression by seeking equal opportunity for women, not on determining the factors that lead to women's oppression (MacPherson, 1991). The major approach to knowledge development is logical positivism, a legacy of Cartesian dualism. Adequacy of scientific theory is based on objectivity, scientific method, and value-free criterion. Within the liberal tradition, judgments must be impartial to the perspective of a particular group or individual.

Socialist Feminist Theory

Socialist feminism adopts the Marxist view that individual existence requires interaction with other humans and the non-human world. Knowledge development occurs in the process of human activity that is influenced by society. Knowledge is not value free and is always shaped by the perspective of the class from which the knowledge emerges. In contrast to the Marxist view that the perspective of the working class is most adequate, socialist feminism asserts that the standpoint of women is most valid because women's social position gives them access to a reality not accessible to men, and because women have no vested interest in maintaining the status quo of a patriarchal society. Although this is a similar position to that of radical feminists, the difference lies in how the knowledge is acquired. Socialist feminists do not accept that the standpoint of women is expressed in "women's naive and unreflective worldview" (Jaggar, 1983, p 371) because this is distorted by male-dominated structure and ideology. Instead, women's standpoint is continually evolving through scientific and political struggle. Jaggar acknowledged that individual women's standpoints may differ especially by race and class but suggested that this diversity contributes to a representation of reality that is continuously unfolding. Women's standpoint evolves in a matrix operation in which women's distinctive social experience guides the pattern of research in a particular discipline and the outcomes of the research are then tested within the social reality of women. Knowledge is deemed useful if it helps to reconstruct a world in which women's interests are not subordinate to those of men.

FEMINISM, PROFESSIONALISM, AND NURSING

Until recently, nursing links with feminism have been tenuous. A brief historical look at both the women's movement and the growth of professionalism in North America will shed light on the development of the discipline of nursing. From a socialist feminist perspective, examining historical context is essential; however, this examination reveals that any links between nursing and feminism have largely been in the liberal feminist tradition of seeking equality.

Early Women's Movement

Cott (1987) identified three foci in the women's movement of the nineteenth century: service and social action performed by charitable, altruistic women who felt their gender gave them a special mandate and who found new strength in their collectivity and self-assertion; women's rights action performed by individually motivated women who wanted "rights equivalent to those men enjoyed on legal, political, economic, and civic grounds" (p 16); and action for self-determination through "emancipation from structures, conventions and attitudes enforced by law and custom" (p 16). Regardless of specific beliefs, "the spectrum of ideology in the women's movement had a see-saw quality" (Cott, 1987, p 19). At one end was elimination of limitations and the attainment of equal rights, a liberalist perspective. At the other was the desire to value the unique qualities and abilities that women had to offer society. This valuing resulted either in acceptance of the unique but subservient status of women's existing social order or in adoption of a socialist feminist approach to change the existing social order to one that valued women in different ways. "No collective resolution of these tensions occurred and seldom even did individuals resolve them in their own minds" (Cott, 1987, p 20).

Nursing's Early Development in North America

The three positions of maintaining the status quo, seeking equality, and seeking to change the social order can be seen in nursing's development. "Nursing's identity has been inextricably bound to the very word and notion of nurturance as well as to the *myth* that women exist to be mothers" (Church, 1990, p 7). Initially, nursing was simply one of the many domestic roles that women were expected to fulfill on the basis of love and obligation (Reverby, 1987). "To practice it [nursing] at home was to fulfil the true calling of womanhood" (O'Brien, 1986, p 14). By the mid-1800s in North America, despite the desire of middle class women to be ladies, many found themselves economically in need of work. The affluent could afford to hire others to take on many of their domestic responsibilities. Hence, the emergence of the professed nurse.

> They brought to the bedside only the authority their personalities and community stature could command. Neither credentials nor a professional identity gave weight to their efforts. Their womanhood and the experience it gave them, defined their authority and taught them to nurse. (Reverby, 1987, p. 6).

In contrast to factory work, "the nature of nursing with its roots deep in the domestic world of the family, muted the dramatic shift in self-perception that women in factory work experienced" (O'Brien, 1986, p 13).

Reverby (1987) noted that within the hospital setting, working class women attempted to exert control on working conditions and relationships with physicians, despite their lack of formal training and subservient class position.

> The sense of rights of working class womanhood gave them authority to press their demands. The necessity to care, and their perception of its importance to patient outcome also structured their belief that demanding the right to be relatively autonomous was possible. (Reverby, 1987, pp 6–7).

Nevertheless, these women were unsuccessful largely because of class differences between nurses and hospital administrators, paternalism, and very demanding work.

Few nurses at this time were engaged in trying to change the social order. Lavinia Dock was a pioneer in nursing history who was labeled a suffragist, a pacifist, and a Marxist. Her overriding concern was self-determination for women, nurses, and nursing (Church, 1990). Throughout her life, she challenged nurses to fight against male dominance but was considered by the majority of nurses as deviant. Dock urged nursing leaders to involve public and political activism (Ashley, 1976). A more widely known nurse feminist was Margaret Sanger, birth control agitator, who championed women's rights to control their sexuality regardless of church or state (Cott, 1987). These nurses made a significant contribution to the development of nursing but were representative of a minority view within nursing.

During this time period, Nightingale's philosophy of nursing education, legitimated by her successes in the Crimea, was developing a following in North America. Her intentions were to establish autonomous schools of nursing, under the control of nurses who would ultimately share power with physicians in the health care setting. Although this approach was admirable from the liberalist feminist perspective, her intended hierarchy within the nursing school eliminated the possibility of equality among nurses (Reverby, 1987). Nightingale's vision was distorted in its implementation by the physicians and hospital superintendents in North America who viewed schools of nursing as vehicles for obtaining cheap labor. They supported the establishment of apprenticeship schools and in doing so gained control over nurse's labor (Melosh, 1982). Nightingale indicated that nurses were prepared by developing womanly virtue. Thus, she legitimized paid work by embodying in it nineteenth century social values and needs (O'Brien, 1986). From a socialist feminist perspective, nursing is an example of household work shifted to the outside world of production. Because this work was not valued when it took place within the home, it similarly received little economic or status reward when practiced publicly (Miller, 1991). Coburn (1987) noted that despite the desire of upper-class Nightingale nurses to attract refined women to nursing, the difficult working conditions and unpleasant work deterred many. The majority of recruits were working-class women whose only other option was factory work.

> The school's emphasis on high moral character constituted an imposition of upper-class values on working-class women. The socialization process during training rested largely in the hands of middle- and upper-class nursing educators—women whose financial and social position allowed them to receive the necessary qualifications to teach. (Coburn, 1987, p 447)

This was the beginning of a class system within nursing: the elite educators and administrators versus the bedside practicing nurses. From a socialist feminist perspective, many of the decisions made from this point forward ensured the continuation of this division.

Ashley (1976) suggested that the apprenticeship system of nursing educations entrenched the dominations of nurses by physicians and hospital administrators.

> Convinced of their inferiority and of the need for their subordination to the medical profession, many nurses identified with the system that oppressed them and worked to support its continuing existence. Nurses learned to believe in the virtues of hospital training. Early conditioning within these institutions intensified the capacity of women to aid the

cause of their oppressors. (Ashley, 1976, p 32)

Nursing training was rigid, orderly, and disciplined and students were overworked. Nevertheless, standards of care were established, nurses developed pride in their skills, had their idealism nurtured, and felt empowered to care (Reverby, 1987).

> . . . nurses have emphasized perceived womanly qualities and differences from men by stressing a role complementary to that performed by men. This position, often labelled anti-feminist, has led present-day feminists to disregard nursing because it tends to epitomize a set of characteristics and problems from which women are attempting to distance themselves. (Kirkwood, 1991, p 53)

In this sense, nursing embodies the dilemma of early (and present day) feminists who, by seeking equality, deny the very uniqueness of their contribution to society. But nursing was being controlled by forces beyond simply their desire to care.

> . . . caring was shaped not simply by women's psychological identity but by the social and political context in which nursing developed. It was a duty to care directed by a male medical hierarchy, not an ethic of care in which nurses would be able to make more autonomous judgments about the kind of care patients should receive. (Baines, 1991, p 63)

Nurses and Physicians

At the turn of the century, the medical profession was not well established in North America and was open to competition from nurses, pharmacists, and other allied occupations

(Torrance, 1987). Medical students had no internship and nursing students in training schools had greater opportunity to observe and to care for the sick. Although the training system had established physicians as dominant, their position was not secure. In 1904 through 1905, Abraham Flexner, a sociologist, visited and assessed Canadian and American medical schools. His report, published in 1910, was highly critical of schools that lacked the facilities to teach laboratory-based scientific medicine and resulted in the closure or reorganization of 92 medical schools. "The Flexner Report . . . helped to consolidate the dominance of the allophatic practitioners and to establish laboratory-based scientific medical education and practice. This mechanistic-individualistic conception is currently pervasive in medical practice and research" (Bolaria, 1988, p 3). The alliance of medicine with science and the subsequent entrenchment of medical education in the university resulted in the definition and domination of the health care field by the physicians. Flexner's study led also to a definition of "profession" and that had significant implications for the future of nursing.

Professionalism

In 1915, Flexner presented a paper that identified the criteria for characterizing professions from an analysis of the universally acknowledged professions of law, medicine, and clergy (Parsons, 1986).

> Professions involve essentially intellectual operations; they derive their raw materials from science and learning; this material they work up into a practical and definite end; they possess an educationally communicable technique; they tend to self-organization; they are becoming in-

creasingly altruistic in motivation. (Flexner, 1915, p 904)

This definition stressed rationalism, scientific standards, and objectivity, all characteristics that embodied the masculine ethos. His masculine, sociological view was never questioned and the criteria became the sociological standard for distinguishing professions (Parsons, 1986). Professions were dominated by men and "a culture developed that affirmed male-centered values of order, efficiency, and hierarchical division of labour" (Baines, 1991). Flexner's paper also suggested that occupations could alter their status and become professions by developing the traits that were lacking.

Professions, reinforced by their scientific credibility became sources of power and prestige. Professionalization offered white, middle-class men a means of carving out new roles and obtaining monopoly on their services (Baines, 1991). Women who entered women-dominated professions were more motivated by an ethic of service or care than by a desire for power (Baines, 1991). "The bases for women's special expertise and place within the professions continued to rest on an ideology of service that lionized caring as a virtue particular to women" (Baines, p 55). The norm of professionalism is historically and socially unacceptable to women because of their exclusion from its conception (Parsons, 1986). Cott (1987) noted that although women professionals were seen as leaders before obtaining the vote, once the vote was attained, the bond that held them together was gone. A barrier developed between women professionals and nonprofessionals. To progress within the professions, and hold the tenets of non-bias, objectivity, and impersonality, women were required to abandon allegiance to feminism and create a community of interest with professional men rather than nonprofessional women (Cott, 1987). Glazer and Slater (1987) noted that professionals scorned nurturant, expressive, and familial interaction, valuing expertise and monopoly over an ethic of service.

Nursing and Professionalism

"Prior to Flexner, American nurses . . . were secure in their identity as professionals" (Parsons, 1986, p 273). However, nursing did not measure up to Flexner's criteria. By 1936 there were articles in nursing journals that indicated nursing was a developing profession (Parsons, 1986). Nursing had a limited body of scientific knowledge defined as nursing and exclusive of other disciplines. Because the phenomena unique to nursing had not been articulated and studied, nursing lacked control over practice and was subordinate to the medical profession (Lyon, 1990). Varying levels of educational preparation resulted in the absence of pervasive ideology and monopoly over work. Roberts (1984) asserted that nurses, once autonomous, became oppressed through societal forces and now exhibit the characteristics of an oppressed group. "Nurses have also accepted the fact that if they could only attain the characteristics of the powerful, or professional status, they too would be powerful" (Roberts, 1984, p 26).

In the early twentieth century, women who wanted recognition for nurses as significant health care providers readily accepted Flexner's assertion that an occupation could become a profession. Acceptance of professional ideology can be viewed as a strength from a liberal feminist perspective. It pushed nurses to sever the link with domestic labor and establish standards of paid work, to refuse the limitations of gender in their own lives and in goals for nursing profession, and to challenge the traditional constraints on women in the workforce (Melosh, 1982). Because nursing was a women's profession, women had the potential monopoly and

power to effect change. What nurses and other women striving for more traditional professions failed to recognize was that the criteria that they were trying to meet were established by men. The rightness of these criteria was not questioned. In fact, by accepting these criteria, and striving to meet them, nursing was supporting the existing patriarchal order. This decision resulted in securing privileges for few nurses at the expense of many (Melosh, 1982).

KNOWLEDGE DEVELOPMENT

Professionalism and Knowledge Development

When nursing leaders decided to respond to the Flexner report by seeking to meet his criteria of profession, they recognized that nursing had to establish a scientific knowledge base. Because professionals had to be scientific, and the only academic preparation for nurses at that time was at the Columbia Teacher's College, most study and research related to education and administration and not to clinical practice (Baer, 1987). Thus, academically prepared nurses were further divided from those practicing at the bedside, and there was much debate about whose work was the most meaningful. This divisiveness is characteristic of the horizontal violence of oppressed groups. Roberts (1984) noted that whether nurses were in the hospital or the academic setting they were (and are) rewarded for being marginal and taking on the characteristics of the dominant groups. As nursing programs opened up in universities in Canada and the United States, nurses struggled to have their knowledge and experience validated as scholarship. "A knowledge base for nursing stemming from women's private, domestic sphere was suspect within the male-dominated culture of the university, which took pride in intellectual scientific achievements" (Kirkwood, 1991, p 54).

World War II opened opportunities for nurses to expand their practice roles and to have advanced university study in post-war years; however, Baer (1987) noted that all nurses were not enthusiastic about these openings. Nurses seeking professionalization were anxious to upgrade their educational preparation, but this was very threatening to nurses who had trained under the hospital system. Hospital educators, anxious to support apprenticeship, failed to grasp post-war opportunities for upgrading. This further developed the class system in nursing.

Research became an issue for nurses as they attempted to establish a scientific knowledge base. Nurses ignored gender issues and moved away from its domestic heritage. "Nurses believed that, if they met university demands to demonstrate nursing was a scholarly discipline with a unique scientific base, nurses would be accorded the same professional respect as others in the university" (Kirkwood, 1991, p 61). Hughes (1990, p 31) noted that the development of nursing as a discipline is often equated with its evolution as a profession but history "suggests that professional status is not likely to evolve passively from nursing's recognition as a scholarly discipline." However, it is significant that "by successfully developing and maintaining university nursing education, nurses have to some extent undermined the patriarchal structure of the university by locating work, traditionally assigned to women in the public sphere of higher education dominated by men" (Kirkwood, 1991, p 62).

In November 1951, the *American Journal of Nursing* announced the publication of *Nursing Research*, noting that research was essential for knowledge development in nursing (Baer,

1987). It was 1976 before over half the articles published focused on clinical practice rather than education, because most of the researchers were nursing faculty whose higher education had been in education. Whereas their institutions required that they participate in scholarly activity to meet criteria for tenure and promotion, service agencies and hospitals did not encourage such activity from practicing nurses (Baer, 1987). Hence, the gap widened with practitioners viewing educators as more and more removed from the real world of nursing.

> Nursing's major goal in fostering research was to achieve recognition of its professional status. Some individual nurses certainly saw research as a means, a method through which they could answer questions and expand their ideas. But for most nurses, it was an end, a criterion of professionalism they yearned to attain. (Baer, 1987, p 24)

Research and Theory Development

Early approaches to research followed the reductionistic methods of the biomedical model as the surest way to be credible as scientists (Nagle & Mitchell, 1991). Nursing adopted the empirical ethic of science through a research tradition "that concentrates on objectivity, facts, measurement of smaller and smaller parts, and issues of instrumentality, reliability, validity, and operationalization to the point that nursing is in danger of exhausting the meaning, relevance, and understanding of the values, goals, and actions that it espouses in its heritage and ideals" (Watson, 1988, p. 17). Researchers have only recently begun to recognize that the scientific method is insufficient for addressing many of nursing's concerns and are beginning to embrace more diverse, qualitative approaches to research.

Concern for nursing's lack of theory base developed in the 1960s when nurses began to study at a doctoral level in other disciplines. The embryonic nursing science was attached to other sciences and fed on their theories, methods, and instruments (Stainton, 1982). Much debate developed surrounding such issues as whether nursing theory should be borrowed from other disciplines, single versus multiple theories, and whether theories should influence or be influenced by practice.

At early nursing theory conferences, the views of theory development expressed by such leaders as Dickoff and James and Abdellah supported the logical empiricist tradition for the development of nursing science (Silva & Rothbart, 1983). "Early nurse theorists such as Roy and Orem maintained the status quo of objective reductionism by focusing on problems and defining health according to medical and/or societal norms" (Nagle & Mitchell, 1991, p 18). Although nurses were strongly supporting this approach, the philosophers of science from where this tradition stemmed were seriously questioning the limitations of this approach (Silva & Rothbart, 1983; Webster & Jacox, 1985). Nurse researchers and theorists recognized the limitations of the received view in theorizing about people's experiences with health and illness; however, the drive for professionalism and scientific legitimacy resulted in nursing, as an emerging discipline, holding on to this respectable approach.

> In the 1960s the unity and political and academic power of the received view theorists was sufficiently great that lip service had to be paid to their basic beliefs. Now we are free to choose among the insights of the received view and select only those which we find useful and sound for our purposes in constructing nursing theory. (Webster & Jacox, 1985, p 27)

These authors suggest that nursing is free to develop its own philosophy of science. Evidence of changing views about the philosophy of science is in the works of such theorists as Watson (1988) and Parse (1981).

Theory and Nursing Practice

Theory is argued to be important in the establishment of the unique body of knowledge essential for nursing to be recognized as a profession and as a means of fostering communication and improving patient care. Theory development through creative conceptualization expanded nursing knowledge. However, the language of theory is frequently abstract and there is much discussion among theorists and those attempting to understand and apply nursing theories to practice. "There are serious credibility gaps between the ideal prescriptive theory that is taught and the practical knowledge used by practitioners" (Aydelotte, 1990, p 10).

> Resultant debates have tended to develop into a vicious circle, with theorists berating practitioners for their lack of concern with the conceptual basis for their actions, whilst practitioners bemoan theoretical approaches which are seen as having little or no relevance to their daily work. (Nolan & Grant, 1992)

Fawcett (1992) asserted the existence of a reciprocal relationship between conceptual models and nursing practice, but she was adamant that the models come first and are tested for their credibility and refined in the field of clinical practice. This position fails to consider the fact that many practitioners find the conceptual model too obscure to enter into that reciprocity.

Nagle & Mitchell (1991) noted that nursing is being driven by professional licensing bodies and accreditation bodies to adopt a single theory as a base for practice within their agency. They suggested that this is a paternalistic action that denies nurses the autonomy of choosing their own theoretic base for practice consistent with their unique worldview. This suggestion assumes that most practicing nurses have articulated a worldview and is further evidence of the rift between practitioners and those nurses with advanced education. This imposition may give practicing nurses a means for voicing what they do and do not like about practicing within a specific, theoretical framework. This may be the key to Fawcett's reciprocity.

FEMINISM: LOOKING TO THE FUTURE FOR NURSING

The acceptance of patriarchal professionalism has resulted in nursing adopting liberalist traditions for the development of research and practice. "Feminism, in its liberal form, appears to give nursing a political language that argues for equality and rights within the given order of things" (Reverby, 1987, p 10). Nurses have often been criticized for rejecting liberal feminism.

> From a feminist perspective, the individualism and autonomy promised by this rights framework often fails to acknowledge collective social need, to provide a way for adjudicating conflict over rights, or to address the reasons for the devaluing of female activity. (MacPherson, 1991, p 30).

Reverby (1987) suggested that nursing will have to create the social climate that values caring. This implies the need for a socialist feminist approach in which nursing takes a more active role in altering social structure.

Professionalization has objectified those for whom nurses care. "A feminist ethos of professionalism needs to be based on an ideology that integrates an ethic of care and forms a more equal partnership with the cared for" (Baines, 1991, p 67). Feminism offers some revolutionary ideas for nursing (Chinn, 1987). "Feminism values and endorses women, critiques male thinking, challenges patriarchal systems, and focuses on creating self-love and respect for all others and all forms of life" (Chinn, 1987, p 23).

Knowledge Development

Dorothy Smith (1990) addressed the impact that hegemony has on knowledge development by influencing the issues that are valued and by dictating an approach to those issues based on the conceptual view of those institutions rather than the lived experienced of the people involved. As people are educated to take up roles within institutions, they are exposed to a "conceptual imperialism" (Smith, 1990, p 15) that ensures a perpetuation of the worldview of the institution under the guise of objectivity. People have two ways of knowing, experiencing and doing: one on a local, immediate, bodily level, and one that is at an objective, conceptual level. The objective account, giving the appearance of neutrality and impartiality in fact conceals class, gender, and race and puts forward the ideology of the governing groups. The objectified text has power because of the way it organizes social relations. People read the objectified text as fact and repress their own lived experience. Thus, people begin to see things the same way. "Objectified knowledge, as we engage with it, subdues, discounts, and disqualifies our various interests, perspectives, angles, and experience, and what we might have to say speaking from them" (Smith, 1990, p 80).

Smith's account sheds some light on the current division that exists between nursing theory and practice. Nursing theory has been developed by the elite and educated, the nurses who have wielded power in the development of nursing as a profession. The separation of these nurses from those at the bedside has been well documented. These nurses identified a professional route for the development of nursing knowledge and endorsed the patriarchal structure. Hence, the approaches to nursing theory reflect the dominant culture rather than the lived experience of nurses at the bedside.

Smith (1990) argued that women must create a reflexive critique through investigation that is grounded in the lives of women and people. This requires an exploration of women's everyday experience with socially organized practices and an examination of how women's practices contribute to and are articulated with the relations that rule our lives. This emphasis on praxis is most consistent for the development of nursing knowledge that reflects the human experience of nursing. However, a major barrier exists. Many nurses who wield educational and administrative power within nursing have a vested interest in maintaining their current positions of power and this is readily accomplished through Smith's "conceptual imperialism." For a significant change to occur nurse leaders and educators must be conscious of this oppression.

There is evidence that nursing is beginning to consider some more revolutionary approaches to knowledge development. Critical scholarship, a pattern of thought and action that challenges institutionalized power relations in the social reality of nursing has been suggested by Thompson (1987) as one means of addressing the issues that nursing faces. She urged nurses to question the assumption that underlie our liberal undergraduate education such as the logical positivist approach to science, the functionalist framework of the social world, and professional ideology because

these assumptions foster acceptance of the status quo. "Critical scholarship in nursing can speak about the process of reweaving, regaining confidence in new reality, regaining a commitment to new definitions of nursing practice, and feeling grounded in new value orientations" (Thompson, 1987, p 37). Anderson (1991, p 2) noted that feminism and poststructuralist perspectives

> challenge us to extend our analysis of phenomena relating to the lives of clients or patients beyond the micro level of analysis to an examination of the broader social processes that influence health and illness behaviour. This has the potential for the development of nursing science that will be inclusive of the complex socioeconomic, historical, and political nexus in which human experience is embedded.

Silva and Rothbart (1983), drawing on the work of Laudan, suggested that nursing theory development is currently in a state of transition, that it will never result in a static set of truths but will always be evolving.

> Data for nursing theory development and testing will include the common practices of nurse clinicians, the social and psychological factors affecting the profession of nursing, the widely held beliefs of the community of nurses, and the reasoning patterns of individual nurse theorists. A result of integrating these data will be a nursing theory that more explicitly addresses the human dimension of nursing (Silva & Rothbart, 1983, p 11).

The test for adequacy of theory will be more focused on solution of nursing care problems than on truth and error. This is very consistent with socialist feminist theory for which the criteria of adequacy is usefulness. These approaches hold promise for future development of nursing research and theory development.

Feminist Epistemology and Research Methodology

Jaggar and Bordo (1989, p 4) indicated that feminist epistemology shares the critique of many philosophers that "the Cartesian framework is fundamentally inadequate, an obsolete and self-deluded world view badly in need of reconstruction and revisioning" borrowing from other traditions such as Marxist historicism, psychoanalytic theory, literary theory, and sociology of knowledge to support its claim. Contemporary feminism's arguments differ from others in the assertion that the Cartesian framework is not gender neutral. Feminist epistemology is not about women being able to conduct science in its current form as well as men can. "Rather its position is that women who have come to recognize and accept feminist assumptions about the world will practice science differently in a world that legitimates these assumptions . . ." (Farganis, 1989, p 208). Belenky, Clinchy, Goldberger, and Tarule (1986) have identified that the epistemological perspectives that influence how women see and know the world are different from those of men.

Farganis (1989) suggested that feminism acknowledges that each person has a different position from which they view the world but does not accept that each view is equally good. Feminism has a moral dimension that opposes normative relativism. Because of their experiences as marginal persons and their experiences of care and concern, "women can offer an epistemically sounder and politically and morally better position" (p 217). Rose (1986) supported this view urging that knowledge gained through the practice of caring be a base for a science that values people. Harding (1986) went one step further and suggested that the hierarchy of positivism should be re-versed with studies directed by such moral emancipatory interests as the elimination of sexist, racist, and classist understandings of social life being most valued.

In the health care field, patriarchal standards have reigned and the personal experience of professional caregiving has been devalued. "Feminist ideology holds that marginal persons in society are those whose roles threaten those in power" (Miller, 1991, p 49). Nursing can be considered marginal and this results in "the development of care modalities that are unspoken, unrecognized, and unappreciated by the dominant groups and, therefore, by society at large" (Miller, 1991, p 49). Feminist approaches to science support the development of a nursing science based on the knowledge that nurses have gained through practice.

A further contribution that feminism makes to nursing knowledge development is direction for research. Fonow and Cook (1991) distilled four common, interdisciplinary themes of feminist epistemology and methodology that are helpful for nursing research.

Reflexivity

This is the practice of reflecting on, examining critically, and exploring analytically the research process and using it to understand the underlying assumptions about gender relations. Consciousness raising is one method of reflexivity that is reflected in the increased consciousness of the researcher of the effects of the research process on the researcher's identity, the impact of the research on the subjects, and finally as a feminist research method. Collaboration between women researchers is another focus of reflexivity: ". . . there is also the expectation among some scholars that feminist collaboration will bring about a deeper intellectual analysis, an original approach to framing questions, with a mind-set of innovation to deal with the gendered context of research" (Fonow & Cook, 1991, p 5).

Action Orientation

The orientation of feminist research is toward social change. This can be accomplished by participating with people in an examination of positions and options, by historically analyzing the past for the purpose of future social change, or by focusing on the policy implications of research findings. "A personal commitment to feminism and to caring as a standard for professional nursing practice can only lead to the demand for major changes in the structure and provision of health care service to all human beings" (Gaut, 1991, p 6). This change can be accomplished by attention to research with an action orientation.

Attention to the Affective Components of the Research Act

Feminist research recognizes the affective dimension and sees emotion as a source of insight. This can be connected to the notion of reciprocity between researcher and the researched manifested either in friendship or in negative interactions.

Use of the Situation at Hand

This use of everyday, existing situations is particularly important for nursing research because nursing's major interest is the experiences of people in health and illness situations.

CONCLUSION

Professionalism has failed to bring nursing the power and prestige that were anticipated by nursing's early leaders. Professionalism is a patriarchal invention and by its very nature is alienating to women. By accepting the liberal tradition of knowledge development embodied in professionalism, nurses have not appreciated their own knowledge acquired through their caring experience. Rather than joining with other women to change the dominant social order to one that values women's unique differences, nurses have focused primarily on attaining professional status. Only recently have nurses begun to recognize that the received view of knowledge development is not sufficient for addressing the complex concerns of nursing as a human science. This realization has resulted in nursing seeking alternate approaches.

Feminism offers much to nursing through its focus on praxis. The liberalist feminist tradition of seeking equality is not sufficient to meet the challenges facing nursing. The socialist feminist perspective offers more direction. It suggests that nursing knowledge development should be directed toward creating a social order in which women are not subordinate to men. This means that our efforts should not be geared to maintaining the status quo within our field of practice but rather should be focusing on ways to alter public policy. Socialist feminism suggests that women as a social group have the more valid perspective because they have no vested interest in maintaining the status quo in society. Applying this view to nursing, nurses in practice have a more legitimate perspective of nursing than nurse leaders and educators. Thus, the distinctive experience of nursing practice should guide nursing research and the outcomes of research should be tested within the reality of practicing nurses because that reality may be quite different to that of the nurse researcher. The actual process of research should itself be dialectical, thus effecting some change in those participating. This approach may help to reduce the current chasm between nursing practice and research. Jean Watson urged nursing to "question its old dogmas, transcend its existing paradigms, and refocus its scientific attention to human phenomena that are consistent with the nature of nursing and preservation of humanity" (1988, p 22). Feminism, particularly socialist feminism, has the potential to help nurses to meet this challenge and to make a significant contribution to changing the existing social order of health care and gender relations.

REFERENCES

Anderson, J. (1991). Current directions in nursing research: Toward a poststructuralist and feminist epistemology. *The Canadian Journal of Nursing Research*, 23(3), 1–3.

Ashley, J. (1976). *Hospitals, paternalism, and the role of the nurse*. New York: Teachers College Press.

Aydelotte, M. (1990). The evolving profession: The role of the professional organization. In N. Chaska (Ed.) *The Nursing Profession: Turning Points*. (pp. 9–15) St. Louis, MO: Mosby.

Baer, E. (1987). 'A cooperative venture' in pursuit of professional nursing status: A research journal for nursing. *Nursing Research*, 36, 18–25.

Baines, C. (1991). The professions and the ethic of care. In C. Baines, P. Evans, and S. Neysmith (Eds.) *Women's caring: Feminist perspectives on social welfare*. (pp. 36–72) Toronto, Canada: McClelland & Stewart.

Belenky, M., Clinchy, B., Goldberger, N., & Tarule, J. (1986). *Women's ways of knowing*. New York: Basic Books.

Bolaria, B. S. (1988). Sociology, medicine, health, and illness: An overview. In B. S. Bolaria & H. Dickinson (Ed.). *Sociology of health care in Canada* (pp. 1–14). Toronto, Canada: Harcourt Brace Jovanovich.

Chinn, P. (1987). Response: Revision and passion. *Scholarly Inquiry for Nursing Practice*, 1(1): 21–24.

Church, O. (1990). Nursing's history: What it was and what it was not. In N. Chaska (Ed.). *The nursing profession: Turning points*. (pp. 3–8). St. Louis, MO: Mosby.

Coburn, J. (1987). I see and am silent. In D. Coburn, C. D'Arcy, G. Torrance, & P. New (Eds.). *Health care and Canadian Society: Sociological perspectives*. (pp. 441–462) Markham: Fitzhenry and Whiteside.

Cott, N. (1987). *The grounding of modern feminism*. New Haven, CT: Yale University Press.

Farganis, S. (1989). Feminism and the reconstruction of social science. In A. Jaggar & S. Bordo (Eds.). *Gender/Body/Knowledge: Feminist reconstructions of being and knowing*. (pp. 207–223). New Brunswick, NJ: Rutgers.

Fawcett, J. (1992). Conceptual models and nursing practice: The reciprocal relationship. *Journal of Advanced Nursing*, 17, 224–228.

Flexner, A. (1915). Is social work a profession? *School Soc*, 1, 901–911.

Fonow, M., & Cook, J. (1991). Back to the future: A look at the second wave of feminist epistemology and methodology. In M. Fonow & J. Cook (Eds.). *Beyond method: Feminist scholarship as lived research*. (pp. 1–15) Bloomington, IN: Indiana University Press.

Glazer, P., & Slater, M. (1987). *Unequal colleagues*. New Brunswick, NJ: Rutgers.

Gaut, D. (1991). Caring and nursing: Explorations in feminist perspectives-Introductory remarks. In R. Neil & R. Watts (Eds.). *Caring and nursing: Explorations in feminist perspectives*. (pp. 5–8). New York: National League of Nursing.

Harding, S. (1986). *The science question in feminism*. Ithaca, NY: Cornell University Press.

Hughes, L. (1990). Professionalizing domesticity: A selected synthesis of nursing historiography. *Advances in Nursing Science*, 12(4), 25–31.

Jaggar, A. (1983). *Feminist politics and human nature*. Totowa, NJ: Rowman & Allenhead.

Jaggar, A., & Bordo, S. (1989). *Gender/body/knowledge: Feminist reconstructions of being and knowing*. New Brunswick, NJ: Rutgers.

Kirkwood, R. (1991). Discipline discrimination and gender discrimination: The case of nursing in Canadian universities, 1920–1950. *Atlantis*. 16(2), 52–63.

Lyon, B. (1990). Getting back on track: Nursing's autonomous scope of practice. In N. Chaska (Ed.). *The nursing profession: Turning points*. (pp. 267–274). St. Louis, MO: Mosby.

MacPherson, K. (1991). Looking at caring and nursing through a feminist lens. In R. Neil & R. Watts (Eds.). *Caring and nursing: Explorations in feminist perspectives*. (pp. 25–43). New York: NLN.

Melosh, B. (1982). *The physician's hand: Work culture and conflict in American Nursing*. Philadelphia, PA: Temple University Press.

Miller, K. (1991). A study of nursing's feminist ideology. In R. Neil & R. Watts (Eds.). *Caring and nursing: Explorations in feminist perspectives*. (pp. 43–56). New York: NLN.

Nagle, L. & Mitchell, G. (1991). Paradigmatic issues in research and practice. *Advances in Nursing Science*, 14(1), 17–25.

Nolan, M., & Grant, G. (1992). Mid-range theory building and the nursing theory-practice gap: A respite care case study. *Journal of Advanced Nursing*, 17, 217–223.

O'Brien, P. (1986). 'All a woman's life can bring': The domestic roots of nursing in Philadelphia, 1830–1885. *Nursing Research*, 36, 12–17.

Parse, R. (1981). *Man-living-health: A theory of nursing*. New York: Wiley.

Parsons, M. (1986). The profession in a class by itself. *Nursing Outlook*, 34, 270–275.

Reverby, S. (1987). A caring dilemma: Womanhood and nursing in historical perspective. *Nursing Research*, 36, 5–11.

Roberts, S. J. (1984). Oppressed group behavior: Implications for nursing. *Advances in Nursing Science*, 5(4), 21–30.

Rose, H. (1988). Beyond masculine realities. In R. Bleier (Ed.). *Feminist approaches to science*. (pp. 57–76). New York: Pergammon.

Silva, M. C., & Rothbart, D. (1983). An analysis of changing trends in philosophies of science on nursing theory development and testing. *Advances in Nursing Science*, 6(3), 1–13.

Smith, D. (1990). *The conceptual practices of power: A feminist sociology of knowledge*. Toronto, Canada: University of Toronto Press.

Stainton, M. C. (1982). The birth of nursing science. *Canadian Nurse*, 78, 24–28.

Thompson, J. (1987). Critical scholarship: The critique of domination in nursing. *Advances in Nursing Science*, 10(1), 27–38.

Torrance, G. (1987). Socio-historical overview. In D. Coburn, C. D'Archy, G. Torrance, & P. New (Eds.). *Health care and Canadian Society: Sociological perspectives*. (pp. 6–32) Markham: Fitzhenry and Whiteside.

Watson, J. (1988). *Nursing: Human science and human care: A theory of nursing*. USA: National League of Nursing.

Webster, G., & Jacox, A. (1985). The liberation of nursing theory. In J. McCloskey & H. Grace (Eds.). *Current issues in nursing*. pp. 20–29. Boston, MA: Blackwell.

7

Debunking Myths in Nursing Theory and Research

PEGGY L. CHINN, RN, PhD, FAAN

This chapter examines myths that persist in the traditional male-defined scientific enterprise. Science per se is not rejected, but specific ways of confronting the myths are explored. The methods for debunking the myths derive from the concept of future search, wherein health and the values of nursing for the future direct the discovery of knowledge. The alternatives include a more ethical and responsible use of the methods of science as well as specific alternatives to science derived from Carper's (1978) patterns of knowing in nursing.

The nursing literature has reflected growing recognition of the limitations of the scientific method in addressing problems in nursing (Gorenberg, 1983; Munhall, 1982; Newman, 1979; Smith, M. C., 1984; Vredevoe, 1984; Webster, Jacox, & Baldwin, 1981). Taken together, the literature leaves the impression that we should perhaps forsake the scientific method; alternatives for acquiring knowledge in nursing are not adequately described, and the alternatives that are suggested are not clearly alternatives to the scientific method.

A fundamental issue that is lacking in most critiques of the scientific method is recognition that science is based on a male worldview and that the myths sustained by this partial worldview have perpetuated erroneous knowledge about the world. The purposes of this chapter are (a) to present an analysis of myths of science that arise from the partial male worldview, (b) to propose methods for debunking

these myths to attain a more whole science consistent with the essence of nursing, and (c) to propose alternative approaches to science where an alternative is indicated.

MYTHS

The concept of "myth" carries many meanings. Two dictionary definitions focus attention on the meanings that are relevant to the focus of this article: "a traditional story of ostensibly historical events that serves to unfold part of the worldview of a people, or explain a practice, belief, or natural phenomenon. . . ." and "an ill-founded belief held uncritically, especially by an interested group" (*Webster's New Collegiate Dictionary*, 1981).

Myths remain a powerful force in the creation of sociocultural patterns, and science and scientists are equally subject to their influence. Myths are not entirely false and in fact contain an element of reality. This is why they are so seductive and difficult to recognize. Since myths are based on a particular world-

Source: Chinn, P. L. (1985). Debunking myths in nursing theory and research. *IMAGE: Journal of Nurse Scholarship, 17* (2): 45–49. Reprinted with permission from Sigma Theta Tau International.

view, they function actually to shape and create reality. Until we examine myths critically, we are not able to sort out what is ill founded from that which is well founded, or whose interests are served.

Traditional science has created beliefs about reality that are taken to be "true." Science, for all practical purposes, rests on a white, upper-class, male view of the world (Spender, 1981). This view is not necessarily wrong or bad, but it is not universal. Regardless of the actual origins of the prevailing worldview or whether it arose from the maleness per se of its originators, the traits of this worldview are characterized as being male because of the remarkable consistency with such masculine concepts as power, control, instrumentation, technology, competition, rationality, logic, objectivity, hard data. Not only does this view rest on the superiority of male-assigned traits but it also disdains concepts that are consistent with that which is assigned as being "feminine"—soft data, subjectivity, feeling, emotion, intuition, and so forth. This arbitrary value assignment clearly does not serve the interests of nursing or the best interest of humanity. Spender (1980) spoke of the myth of the superiority of that which is masculine in language:

> The myth was made a long time ago and for centuries it has been fostered by women and men so that now it is deeply embedded in virtually every aspect of our existence. It is a myth which may be attacked but one which is not easy to eradicate, for all myths still have a hold over us long after they have been intellectually repudiated, and this one, which is fundamental to our social order, is particularly pervasive and particularly hard to dislodge. The fabric of our social organization has been woven to support and substantiate it and nothing less than a restructuring of our beliefs and values is necessary, if it is to be laid to rest. (pp. 1-2)

FUTURE SEARCH

Just as language is a powerful tool for conveying the prevailing worldview, an examination of new meanings for language can be used to create a shift. The word *research* is a useful starting point. The activities that happen under the name of research are often literally re-searching what has been done over and over again. Usually the hypotheses shift from project to project, but there is seldom any creativity in the conceptualizations or methods used primarily because credibility depends on doing the same thing (or close to it) in the same way. What this does is perpetuate the status quo—a past-oriented perspective.

Heide (1982) proposes that we shift our focus to future search. Future search requires that we envision the world as it could be, or as we want it to be—a healthy, productive, peaceful, enduring, nurturing environment and society. Once we have this vision, we can begin to discover knowledge that is required to create this world. As nursing scholars, we can end the perpetuation of a status quo that values illness more than health; we can enact what we know in our practice by focusing our scholarly energies in the direction of health for all. In short, we can be change agents (Smith, M. J., 1984).

Future-search methods that serve to debunk myths in nursing science rest on the following assumptions:

- Nursing's worldview is both reasonable and valuable. This worldview focuses on health, life, human interaction, and environmental integrity. Further, nursing values are intimately related to that which has been assigned a feminine value and as such contradicts many values of traditional science.
- The scientific method is useful for some questions but not for all questions.
- In conceptualizing methods of generating knowledge, it is not useful to think in terms

of dichotomies of "scientific" or "nonscientific." Other analogous concepts include "the received view" versus the "nonreceived view" (Webster, Jacox, & Baldwin, 1981) and "paradigm I logic" versus "paradigm II logic" (Tinkle & Beaton, 1983). These dichotomies imply that science remains the standard for judging all methods. Future search views science as one method, but not the standard for judging all methods.

- The appeal in the literature for alternative methods and logical systems are valid, and the types of knowledge that are required in nursing have been described (Carper, 1978). However, the methods are yet to be created, described and demonstrated to be useful.

THE MYTHS OF RE-SEARCH

There are several ways to approach a movement toward future search. The movement begins with debunking myths of the scientific enterprise. In considering the myths, I am not suggesting that we eliminate the concepts entirely; I am suggesting that we debunk these ideas as sacred truths, examine the dimensions of the idea that are partial or false, and move in a direction of wholeness consistent with our worldview.

Myth 1: The Myth of the Ultimate Truth

The myth of the ultimate truth leads us to think that truth is true because it is true. Scientific theory is supposed to represent reality, and reality is supposed to be truth. Truth, as it is conceptualized in the traditional scientific enterprise, is represented in the assumptions of theories and research. For the most part the assumptions are rarely recognized much less questioned. By subscribing to the assumptions

as "truth," we seek data that conform to our view and ignore contrary evidence that does not support the underlying assumption of what is true. We ignore as being idiosyncratic (insignificant) data that do not conform to our preconceived beliefs.

The method for debunking this myth is to identify and reverse existing assumptions. Once existing assumptions are reversed, contrary evidence can be sought that debunks the original assumption. In a world that is whole, with established scientific "truths" based on universal experience, all the evidence would be valued and integrated into our knowing. However, we do not live in such a world, and for now it is essential that we work diligently and deliberately to produce the evidence that we know contradicts much of what passes for truth about the world.

The work of Gilligan (1982) demonstrates the importance of questioning underlying "truths" and unstated assumptions. She studied with Kohlberg and learned his theory of moral development. Later, she realized there was important information that had not been disclosed in final reports of the research or integrated into the theory. Kohlberg's theory is based on all-male research. When the theory and tools derived from it were used with women, women were found not to achieve development beyond the third stage of a 10-stage process and were assumed to be inferior to men. Gilligan reexamined the theory and reversed the assumption that failing to be a "10" represents an inferiority. Using methods of traditional science but simply reversing the assumption of universality of the theory, she demonstrated contrary evidence required to debunk the myth of the universality of Kohlberg's theory, revealing that women are not inferior; the theory is inferior. In a very fundamental way, Kohlberg's theory does not withstand the test of universality, as Kohlberg has claimed. In the process of discovering contrary evidence, Gilligan also contributed knowledge that has begun to change how women are viewed—a hallmark of the future-search enterprise (see also Munhall, 1983).

Myth 2: The Myth of Objectivity

Traditional science prides itself on being "value free" and therefore objective and not subjective. Intellectually, some traditional scientists recognize that no science is value free; neither is it free from subjective influence. However, it is not the value-laden bias of the scientific enterprise that is the problem; it is the continuing failure to acknowledge and take seriously the nature of the values and subjective interpretations that are imposed on the so-called objective ideas, methods, and designs.

One of the dictionary meanings given for the word *objective* is particularly enlightening: "methods that eliminate the subjective by limiting choices to fixed alternatives requiring a minimum of creative interpretation (eg, tests of personality)" (*Webster's New Collegiate Dictionary*, 1981). Of course, the dictionary does not ask, Who determined the alternatives? What values influenced their choice of the "fixed alternatives?" Who decided that it was desirable to eliminate the "subjective" and "creative" in the testing of personality?

The most insidious technique used to perpetrate the myth of objectivity is the erasure, abdication, and obfuscation of responsibility, thereby obscuring the subjective influence. The scientific literature, including that in nursing, is abundant with such phrases as "research results show" (what research, what kind of research, by whom?), or "it is generally known that" (by whom?). This is a tradition that works well to obscure responsibility and should be a major ethical concern for all scientists of our day. It is both an individual and a collective problem.

The method for debunking the myth of objectivity is to name the responsible agent, to demystify the assumptions, the motives, the values, the processes that were used to arrive at the definition of what purported to be objective. We have a wonderful example in our own history of a nursing scholar who recognized this problem and took a strong stand opposing it. Writing in the *American Journal of Nursing* in 1915, Lavinia Dock stated:

> As a result of the European war, there are reappearances of ailments that were practically nonexistent. Gaseous gangrene, never seen in surgery now-a-days, has come again. . . . When we know how surely and certainly these diseases are caused by men's own acts and deeds, does it not seem as if we should say, "Man's actions have produced gas-gangrene and typhus;" instead of the flabby statement, "Typhus is prevalent; gas-gangrene is developing." Seeing such ruthless and dastardly energies at work, does one not understand Florence Nightingale's impatient contempt for the germ theory, and comprehend her insistence that it was the things people did that caused disease? (p. 666)

Exposing explicit responsibility exposes underlying assumptions and myths and creates a new view of reality. For example, Florence Nightingale experienced the horrors of war and the destruction of human life and health; she refused to accept that the unsanitary conditions that she witnessed were "natural." Her personal and subjective response to these conditions created an awareness of reality that was not generally accessible to other scholars of her day. Margaret Sanger grieved for the waste of human life and human potential that was created by the uncontrolled frequency of pregnancy, and she refused to assume that this condition was "natural." Her subjective, self-acknowledged response created the motive to seek the knowledge that would create health.

Myth 3: The Myth of the Perfect Method

The myth of the perfect method results in compulsive orderliness, repetitiveness, and a fixation on minute details. It encourages us toward mental laziness in envisioning alternative methods, alternative approaches, and alternative assumptions. We re-search and re-search to the point that we know less and less about more and more, failing to recognize the relevance or irrelevance of what we are studying. The perfect method, by definition, leads us on a path of examining small segments and parts of reality apart from the whole and is based on the assumption that a segmented analysis of the parts will yield knowledge of the whole.

The method for debunking this myth begins with the recognition that there is no one perfect method and that various methods must be used in relation to each question that is asked. Most important, this shift requires valuing alternative methods in a fundamental way. It requires refusing to apologize for what is presumed to be inadequate when contrasted with the "perfect method." It also requires that we cease to view alternative methods as merely a stepping stone to the "perfect method." The alternative methods, whether they are variations on the theme of the "'perfect method" or an entirely different approach (such as those I will describe in the following section), are to be used and developed for their own worth and value.

Nursing is faced with what might be called an imperative to debunk this myth arising from the nature of the work we do, what we have identified as important, and how we view our goals. In conceptualizing health, the client, the environment, and the nurse-client interactions, a clear holistic view has emerged. If we remain committed to this foundational view, then the traditional method, which requires studying parts or segments of things or people, is simply not adequate (Newman,

1979). A segmented, partial approach might serve to enlighten or might serve some limited pragmatic purpose; it might be preferable to adapt the traditional methods to complex problems rather than to do nothing; however, as new methods emerge, their future viability will depend on our conscious valuing of them, free from false judgment against the "standard" of the perfect method.

Myth 4: The Myth of Scientific Supremacy

The myth of scientific supremacy focuses on the religious-like quality of science as the means for delineating truth, knowledge, and reality—and as an end in and of itself. A critical component of this myth is the rejection of any other possibility for creating knowledge. Science, which is based on the notion of empirical validation, is thought to result in true knowledge; all other forms of knowledge are judged as being merely speculation, opinion, or not what can be conceptualized as knowledge. If this myth did not have a strong hold on us, we would long ago have begun serious work to develop other ways of knowing.

Science has served well to debunk myths perpetuated by the ancient philosophies and religions, and it is undoubtedly an effective way to obtain knowledge. However, science as the supreme end in and of itself has produced knowledge that has not turned out to be in the best human interest; indeed it has been used to create planetwide contamination and has brought us to the brink of worldwide destruction.

The method for debunking the myth of scientific supremacy is to insist on the integration of all patterns of knowing into the whole of knowing. The patterns of knowing described by Carper (see Chapter 1) derive from our own nursing literature and serve well as a basis for envisioning that which is possible. Any one patten of knowing used in isolation of the others is an incomplete, partial form of knowing. All patterns must be integrated to create what I would call Knowledge. Each pattern requires its own process of discovery and its own method for determining what is credible, as distinguished from isolated fantasy:

- Empirical knowledge is determined to be credible using empirical validation. This process requires verification—agreement that what is observed by one person in one situation is replicable in other instances by other observers. The evidence used to judge credibility is what we know as reliability and validity.
- Ethical knowledge is determined to be credible by the method of justification. The philosophic and logical premises surrounding an ethical dilemma are stated explicitly, and from these are derived logical evidence that justifies a decision, or a conclusion. Other observers do not have to agree with the decision, but the decision, the evidence that produces the decision, and the logic used must be judged to be responsible and just.
- Esthetics is judged to be credible through the method of criticism. Criticism as used in the arts is directed toward knowing, making explicit, exposing the meaning of the creative process/product. Consensus, or agreement between observers, related to meaning is not required but, for the criticism to function as a method for revealing credible esthetic meaning, consistency must exist between the expressions of the esthetic process and the criticism of it.
- Personal knowledge is determined to be credible through introspection. Introspection makes it possible to integrate and actualize that which is experienced in relation to others and the self. As introspection occurs, the authenticity of the self is revealed, and personal knowledge is actualized.

Myth 5: The Myth of Empirical Evidence

The myth of empirical evidence is the belief that "what is" is that which is observable through sensory experience, and whatever is not observable through sensory experience does not exist. Furthermore, whatever is observable is measurable; it is quantifiable. The fundamental usefulness of empirical validation of phenomena is not to be rejected, but the myth represents a good idea gone wild. The myth extends the value of empirical validation of phenomena to encompass the belief that, if something cannot be empirically validated, it does not exist or is not worth pursuing. Further, the myth sustains the tendency to proclaim that something either is or is not empirically accessible when in reality phenomena are relatively accessible to empirical knowing. Science has stimulated ideas that give rise to possibilities for empirical validation long before empirical validation is possible; we call this the discovery of instrumentation, or methods for empirical observation. As we have moved into areas of knowledge that are relatively inaccessible, we create methods that are increasingly indirect in relation to the phenomena, still naming the indirect measure "empirical evidence" to justify the scientific nature of our enterprise. Once this is done, we call the phenomenon empirically validated: It exists.

As we leap through these mental exercises, we fail to seriously confront the artifacts that are created in the process of "empirical validation." I am not arguing that highly abstract phenomena (eg, health or motive) cannot and should not be empirically validated; nor do I reject scholarly work in this direction; but I reject the assumption that empirical tools or observations are adequate to create comprehensive knowledge about these phenomena. I also question the assumption that empirical evidence itself will produce accurate knowledge.

The method for confronting the myth of empirical evidence is to recognize the limitations of empirical evidence in relation to developing knowledge and to value other ways of knowing related to the phenomena that we are exploring. As we recognize the limitations of empirical evidence, we can begin to untangle distortions that are created by artifacts of empirical validation. The untangling process will include improvements in our approaches to obtain empirical evidence as well as open possibilities for knowledge that do not derive from empirical evidence. I submit that our body of knowledge about a phenomenon such as "motive" in relation to health will ultimately require strong, sound empirical evidence free of artifacts. But the complex keys to understanding this and other phenomena do not reside solely within the scope of empirical validation. The key to understanding these complex phenomena requires integration of the methods of justification, criticism, and introspection as well.

Myth 6: The Myth of Higher Authority

The myth of higher authority governs the scientific enterprise in a number of ways. It perpetuates ethical, empirical, and moral dishonesty. Most scholarly work begins with a review of "authoritative" literature, and we use the authority of existing literature to justify everything we do. The halo effect that an idea or a belief acquires by being published is a remarkable transition that I can only perceive as being magic.

The very fact of being engaged in the academic/scientific enterprise confers a societally sanctioned myth of authority. We are in a position to give or withhold information at will, to use, coerce, and manipulate people with little if any challenge to our authority. Even the language we use in research communicates authority—control, manipulation (of variables, conditions, numbers, people), inference, standardization, operationalization, subjects, instruments.

Being a scientist also confers the authority to assign value judgments and worth to phenomena, ideas, or things. The act of measuring produces dichotomous thinking, or hierarchical assignment of value. We speak of high and low, we rank order things and assign values to those things without questioning the meaning of the valuing or the contextual possibilities that might exist or be created by our valuing. This myth has made it possible for male scientists to assign the value of "the norm" to maleness. Simply assigning a value does not make a thing true or right, but assigning a value often creates the illusion of truth or rightness.

The method for debunking the myth of higher authority is to place ourselves in the position of the grassroots people with whom we work, or for whom our knowledge might have the most direct effect. In essence, this strategy is one of ethical justification, esthetic criticism, and personal introspection. We must reverse the myth that the scientific enterprise is by definition a higher authority and that the scientist by definition has rights or authorities that are different from those of any other individual. Once we make this shift in our thinking, we can examine how well our approaches, our methods, our conclusions are consistent with experiential reality.

Myth 7: The Myth of Significance

The myth of significance is most clearly recognized by examining the statistical concept of significance. When we are told that something is significant at the .01 level of probability, it assumes a halo effect of significance far beyond the strictly technical and statistical meaning of the term. The statistician and the researcher (we hope) know the limitations and restrictive meanings of the term *significance* in a statistical sense. However, scientists rarely adhere to the strict statistical meaning in interpreting their results. As long as the results reach statistical significance, the findings have meaning. If the results do not reach statistical significance, the findings must be explained and have little meaning. The "significance" of the results of studies is used to imply not the statistical concept but the more common language understanding of the term: that it is important. Rarely does anyone ask, Significant for what, for whom, in what context? We seldom ask for what purpose, or in whose interest, the scientific enterprise has been directed. These factors are critical in determining how much importance we attach to the results of our research—those that are statistically significant as well as those that are not.

The method for debunking the myth of significance is to apply the test of importance in relation to future-search purposes and goals regardless of the statistical findings. By shifting our attention to the importance of the research, we can detect ways in which the research may or may not contribute to knowledge that can create the kind of world in which we wish to live and work.

We will dis-cover many subtle ways in which our scientific enterprise limits the universality of the theories and the generalizability of the research. A statistically significant study that is based on white, male, middle-class values, that draws on a white, male, middle-class population (as in much nursing research), probably has little or no meaning, much less importance, for the majority of people in this world who are not white, middle-class, or male.

WHY DEBUNK MYTHS?

In conclusion, I want to acknowledge that there are pitfalls in taking a skeptical view of the status quo, even though scientists are by definition supposed to be skeptical. My interpretations of the myths of the scientific enterprise are deliberately severe to stimulate awareness of the actual behavioral practices of many scientists and

the flaws in that which we take to be truth. I have not recommended the abandonment of science, but I do recommend that we equally credit the limitations of this method. By debunking the myths of science, we will find critical areas for new applications of that which is valuable in the scientific method and ways of integrating other patterns of knowing.

The fundamental question is not why we should question and challenge the myths of the scientific enterprise but why not? Why not conceptualize the purposes and the goals of our research and theory in terms of the world that we want to create? Why not seriously value other ways of knowing? Why not value nursing and health? Why not identify actions, behaviors, and assumptions that we know to be consistent with health and behave as scientists in ways that are consistent with our vision? I believe that we are already beginning to do this; and if we choose to, we will increasingly focus our energies in this direction.

Acknowledgments

This article was adapted from a presentation given at the Research Day sponsored by Sigma Theta Tau Alpha Nu Chapter, Villanova University, Villanova, Pennsylvania, November 2, 1984. The author wishes to acknowledge the contributions of Charlene Eldridge Wheeler in conceptualizing the myths; of Barbara Carper in critiquing the methods for determining credibility of ethical, esthetic, and personal knowledge; and of the members of the Nursing Theory Think Tank for discussion that prompted the development of this article.

REFERENCES

Carper, B. (1978). Fundamental patterns of knowing in nursing. *Advances in Nursing Science, 1*(1), 13-23. [Chapter 4 of this book]

Dock, L. (1915). Foreign department. *American Journal of Nursing, 15*(8), 666.

Gilligan, C. (1982). *In a different voice: Psychological theory and women's development.* Cambridge, MA: Harvard University Press.

Gorenberg, B. (1983). The research tradition of nursing: An emerging issue. *Nursing Research, 32*(6), 347-349.

Heide, W. S. (1982). *Feminism for the health of it.* Ann Arbor, Michigan, University Microfilms International, 1982. Also in preparation for publication (revised) by Margaretdaughters, Inc., P.O. Box 70, Buffalo, NY, 14222.

Munhall. P. L. (1982). Nursing philosophy and nursing research: In apposition or opposition? *Nursing Research, 31*(3), 176-177.

———. (1983). Methodological fallacies: A critical self-appraisal. *Advances in Nursing Science, 5*(4). 41-50.

Newman, M. (1979). *Theory development in nursing.* Philadelphia: F. A. Davis.

Smith, M. C. (1984). Research methodology: Epistemologic considerations. *Image: The Journal of Nursing Scholarship, 16*(2), 42-46.

Smith, M. J. (1984). Transformation: A key to shaping nursing. *Image: The Journal of Nursing Scholarship. 16*(1), 28-30.

Spender, D. (1980). *Man made language.* Boston: Routledge and Kegan Paul.

———. (1981). *Men's studies modified.* New York: Pergamon Press.

Tinkle, M. B., & Beaton, J. L. (1983). Toward a new view of Science: Implications for nursing research. *Advances in Nursing Science, 5*(2), 27-36.

Vredevoe, D. L. (1984). Curology: A basic science related to nursing. *Image: The Journal of Nursing Scholarship. 16*(3), 89-92.

Webster, G., Jacox, A. & Baldwin, B. (1981). Nursing theory and the ghost of the received view. In H. K. Grace & J. C. McCloskey (Eds.), *Current Issues in Nursing.* Boston: Blackwell Scientific Publications.

Webster's New Collegiate Dictionary. (1981). Springfield. MA: G.C. Merriam Co.

8

What Constitutes Nursing Science?

JOHN R. PHILLIPS, RN, PhD

Science is an organized body of knowledge concerning human beings and their worlds; it encompasses "the attitudes and methods through which this body of knowledge is formed" (Chernow & Vallasi, 1993, p. 2452). Chernow and Vallasi (1993) also state that since scientific methods do not always guarantee scientific discovery, other factors such as intuition, experience, and good judgment "contribute to new developments in science" (p. 2452). In addition, a survey of the evolution of knowledge shows that abstract thinking is integral to the advancement of science. This broad view of science is essential in understanding the development of any particular science and its phenomena of concern.

This is especially true for nursing science with its unique body of knowledge. Controversy arises, however, when attempts are made to identify this body of knowledge, where some nurses make little distinction between nursing knowledge and the knowledge of other sciences, such as medicine. Too, some nursing models and theories still include knowledge from other sciences that has not been transposed into a nursing perspective. Furthermore, it must be determined how or if these nursing models and theories can be used to generate *nursing* knowledge that constitutes nursing science.

Some nurses may say this is a moot point, and probably not worthy of further pursuit. However, one needs to realize that it is nursing science that gives direction to the further generation of nursing knowledge, and it is nursing science that provides the knowledge for all aspects of nursing. Moreover, it is through the art of nursing, "the imaginative and creative use of knowledge" (Rogers, 1988, p. 100), that nurses can know and understand the health care needs of people. How adequately can this be achieved if nursing science is not constituted with nursing knowledge?

Fawcett (1993, 1995) in her metaparadigm of nursing has helped to provide an understanding of what constitutes nursing science. Her analysis and evaluation of nursing models and theories make it clear that there is a particular perspective of the metaparadigm concepts for each of the nursing models and theories. For example, the definitions of person, environment, health, and nursing are different for each model and theory. Since each nursing model and theory has a different philosophical and theoretical foundation, nurses who use them have different realities of nursing. How are these differences related to what constitutes nursing science?

Parse (1987) and Newman (1992) in their paradigms of nursing and Fawcett (1993) in her worldviews of nursing address these differences and provide for further understanding of what constitutes nursing science. The

Source: Phillips, J. R. (1996) What Constitutes Nursing Science? *Nursing Science Quarterly*. 9(2):48–49. Reprinted by permission of and copyright © 2002 Sage Publications, Inc.

use of these paradigms and worldviews reveals that some nursing models and theories are composed of conflicting philosophical and theoretical foundations. Too, some nursing models and theories overlap more than one paradigm or worldview. If a nursing model or theory lacks coherence within its philosophical and theoretical foundation and overlaps more than one paradigm or worldview, then a close examination of it is needed to determine whether it constitutes nursing science. Will a time come when particular nursing models or theories will no longer be appropriate to constitute nursing science?

Nursing models and theories provide multiple diverse and divergent nursing realities. These realities foster creative ideas and insights that are essential to the methods that are used to discover knowledge. It is time, however, to evaluate how the various scientific methods contribute to the development of nursing science. Realizing, for example, that statistics is only one language of science, nurses can no longer be satisfied with only the traditional scientific methods that often give a cloudy vision of what nursing science is. Nurses must emerge from the womb of other sciences so as to give birth to scientific methods that give a clear vision of what nursing is and can be, knowing that today there is only an inkling of the future of nursing science.

Nurses can design these new methods through a creative synthesis of the various aspects of science and the human processes such as intuition and lived experiences. Some of our current nursing scientific methods already provide for imaginative, abstract, and logical reasoning processes that are required to discover knowledge to develop nursing science. Such scientific methods will give unity to nursing science through the diversity of nursing models and theories. This assumption is acceptable when Moody's (1990) quote of Bronowski is considered: "Science is nothing else than the search to discover unity in the wild variety of nature or . . . in the variety of our experiences" (p. 18).

A cumulative body of knowledge that is flexible and open to change flows from the unitary nature of nursing science. The wholeness of this knowledge provides further understanding of the ambiguity and uncertainty found in the multiple realities of nursing models and theories. This understanding will reveal the rigid and static nature of knowledge from other sciences, which in many instances is outdated and not from a nursing perspective. However, as nurses develop knowledge through the use of nursing models and theories, they must remain in doubt and be open to changes in it (Wilson, 1985). This is essential if nurses are to advance a nursing science that provides the knowledge for the changing art of nursing, where there is concern for the wholeness of people.

Questions of what constitutes nursing science have revealed an evolving phenomenon in nursing. The revelation is that facts alone do not constitute nursing science, however important they may be; it is the pattern of knowledge that gives unity to nursing science. As the pattern is revealed, nurses are being challenged to relook at what constitutes nursing science. Needless to say, the focus on the pattern of knowledge brings a profound provocation to create a new vision of nursing science, a vision that will eventually sever the umbilical cord of subjugation to the knowledge of other sciences. This new vision may save some of the nursing models and theories from becoming obsolete, even extinct.

The recognition and use of the pattern of knowledge is moving nursing science to the forefront of science in general. This new, prominent position enables nurses to respond to the public's desire for quality health care, where the concern is the healing of the whole person. In such an arena of health care, nurses will not compete with other health care providers since they will be using nursing knowledge for the practice of nursing, rather than knowledge from other sciences, particularly medicine. Can we say that the "gap" between theory and practice will disappear as nurses continue to use nursing models and theories that constitute the nursing science for their practice?

Yes, nursing models and theories do constitute nursing science. Nurses must not accept the perennial denigration of nursing models and theories and the call to abandon them for the knowledge from other sciences. If nurses do, nursing will become a wasteland filled with "illiterate nurses" where all of humanity will suffer in immeasurable ways.

Nursing models and theories are the savior of nursing science, and nurses' ravenous use of them will bring redemption from a wasteland composed of knowledge from other sciences. This is the power that nursing models and theories give nurses in determining what constitutes nursing science, its knowledge, and its scientific methods. As nurses continue to use nursing models and theories, nursing science will no longer be invisible in the world of science.

REFERENCES

Chernow, B. A., & Vallasi, G. A. (1993). *The Columbia encyclopedia* (5th ed.). New York: Columbia University Press.

Fawcett, J. (1993). *Analysis and evaluation of nursing theories*. Philadelphia: Davis.

Fawcett, J. (1995). *Analysis and evaluation of conceptual models of nursing* (3rd ed.). Philadelphia: Davis.

Moody, L. E. (1990). *Advancing nursing science through research, volume 1*. Newbury Park, CA: Sage.

Newman, M. A. (1992). Prevailing paradigms in nursing. *Nursing Outlook, 40*, 10–13, 32.

Parse, R. R. (1987). *Nursing science: Major paradigms, theories, and critiques*. Philadelphia: Saunders.

Rogers, M. E. (1988). Nursing science and art: A prospective. *Nursing Science Quarterly, 1*, 99–102.

Wilson, H. S. (1985). *Research in nursing*. Menlo Park, CA: Addison-Wesley.

9

Nursing Science in the Global Community

SHAKÉ KETEFIAN, RN, EdD, FAAN
RICHARD W. REDMAN, RN, PhD

Knowledge development and research are generally embedded in cultural values and perspectives. This article examines the development of knowledge in nursing in a global context and addresses the degree to which Western values and the social environment in the United States shape nursing theory development. Three perspectives illustrate the influence of U.S. values and contextual factors. Questions are raised about the relevance of knowledge to other cultural or national contexts. Recommendations are made for nursing inquiry that makes knowledge more applicable to the global community. [Keywords: Knowledge development; International nursing]

For many years, nurses from other countries have been enrolled in U.S. graduate programs. Colling and Liu (1995) report a 10% increase in international students attending U.S. graduate programs in nursing in the past decade. In their survey of international students, these authors identified 239 students from 49 countries. In many parts of the world, U.S. nursing appears to be highly regarded.

As the diversity and ethnic mix of the U.S. population has increased, global awareness has also increased. In the past decade, many institutions and nurses have become involved in international activities such as consultation, collaborative research, and exchange visitor arrangements.

Yet, despite the increase in international activities, the nature of nursing theory, research, education, and practice has not changed appreciably to be globally relevant.

The degree to which parochialism may have played a role in explaining the slow pace of change in this regard has not been fully examined.

Boyacigiller and Adler (1991) examined the degree to which Western parochialism and ethnocentrism are embedded in the concepts of organizational theory. These authors reviewed the research literature in management science from three perspectives: (a) the influence of post World War II America and its environment on organizational theory development; (b) the volume of international articles published in American management journals; and (c) the degree to which American beliefs and values have shaped organizational theory development. Their assessment, overall, was that organizational theories are parochial and many do not acknowledge awareness of non-U.S. contexts, models, or values. Many Americans have shaped theories central to organizational and human behavior with the assumption that these beliefs have universal applicability. Free will (versus deter-

Source: Ketefian, S., Redman, R. (1997) Nursing Science in the Global Community. IMAGE: *Journal of Nursing Scholarship* 29(1):11–15. Reprinted with permission by Sigma Theta Tau International minism) and individualism (versus collectivism) are just two examples of how Western values have shaped research and theory in organizational science. The authors call for the development of organizational sciences in which universal, intercultural theories are clearly explicit.

Following the approach taken by Boyacigiller and Adler (1991), we describe three perspectives in our examination: (a) contextual—the influence of the U.S. social environment on nursing theory development; (b) quantitative—the rapid expansion of U.S. doctoral programs in nursing, the shaping of nursing journals by U.S. nurse scientists, and the degree of international scientific representation in these journals; and (c) qualitative—the degree to which U.S. values have shaped nursing theory development. The status of multicultural knowledge development in the United States is then presented followed by selected recommendations. Given the magnitude of the topic, no attempt is made to be comprehensive. Rather, the ideas presented represent select perspectives and observations of the authors who are educators in the United States, but who have had extensive international experience. The views presented here are intended to serve as catalysts for further discussion.

PERSPECTIVES

Contextual Perspective

The influence of social forces on American nursing can be examined from several perspectives. These include (a) social trends and values and how they shape nursing knowledge development, (b) the influence of technology and reimbursement systems on nomenclature in nursing, and (c) the development of nursing education and research infrastructures as social phenomena. Each is described briefly to illustrate the contextual influences.

Many recent U.S. social movements have had considerable effect on nursing theory. One example is the emphasis on health promotion and risk reduction. The social emphasis on behavior related to diet, exercise, and other types of health-promoting behaviors have influenced the shaping of public policy as well as the education of health professionals. To a considerable degree, they have also shaped the direction of nursing science and research. Another example is the way in which the emergence of the women's movement has shaped the thinking of a whole generation of women and has led to the development of new public policies in education, employment, health, and other domains. Recognition that women's health problems should be given priority has led to research by health professionals, including nurses, resulting in a body of scientific knowledge in this domain.

The Nursing Interventions Classification (NIC) work at Iowa (McCloskey & Bulechek, 1994) is another example of a social force influencing nursing knowledge development. NIC has been developed as a comprehensive classification of treatments that nurses perform in an attempt to create a standardized language of both nurse- and physician-initiated nursing interventions. Interest in developing this taxonomy can be traced in part to the need for nurses to develop a universal language. Catalytic social forces such as the rapid technologic development of literature data bases, clinical information systems in practice settings, and the need for taxonomies that are compatible with reimbursement systems have resulted in the need for standardized nursing nomenclature. This development has profound implications for nursing practice and knowledge development internationally. The degree to which U.S. nursing interventions are shaping the rapid development of "universal" taxonomies and languages that reflect nursing practice throughout the world is a pressing question. In addition, there is considerable interest in using taxonomies such as NIC to redefine nursing knowledge inductively. Again, the degree to which U.S. nursing interventions and practices reflect nursing practice in other countries is a question of critical importance internationally.

Social values and contextual influence also relate to the quality of nursing care. Definitions of nursing care quality vary, ranging from using the proper amount of resources to accomplish nursing goals to meeting patients' requirements. Assessing the quality of nursing care, whether focused on the appropriateness of a given intervention to a patient's needs or the selection of alternatives as a function of resources available illustrates how context-dependent quality can be. The expectations of a client, the socially defined role of the nurse, and the technology available can vary considerably. Furthermore, the importance of each of these variables in the quality equation can vary, depending on the context, and in turn drive the research questions and methodologies. Thus, the manner in which the pressing questions of the discipline are framed are very likely to reflect the values, philosophy, and practices of the culture and society in which they are asked.

Explorations of theory in nursing began in the 1960s. Since then, in an effort to define what is distinctive about nursing science and theory, nurse scholars and theorists have widely debated their ideas. Many of these ideas have been characterized as metatheories or conceptual frameworks. In the past decade, the nursing literature has reflected a shift in thinking. Now many investigators favor working with propositions and theories characterized as middle-range theories rather than with conceptual frameworks because middle-range theories provide the basis for generating testable hypotheses related to particular nursing phenomena and to particular patient populations.

Expansion of doctoral programs along with the magnitude and refinement of nursing research over the past several decades has been impressive. Thus, it can be argued that such advances in U.S. nursing have rightfully placed it in an enviable position vis-à-vis international peers.

The scope and orientation of much of nursing research is American without global characteristics. Frequently, research findings are presented and received by international colleagues as though the work is applicable to other national and cultural contexts. In addressing such issues, Zwanger (1987) states that American nurses are recognized as leaders in doctoral education in the world and that,

> They are . . . the oracles of the international academic nursing community. As a consequence, in many instances, their ambiguous tendencies, unclarified ideas, and conceptions are accepted as bona fide facts (pp. 33–34).

Zwanger draws on the Israeli experience in stating that some of those who complete their degree in the United States wish to transplant American ideas to their native land. She then describes the inappropriateness of doing so, which in some cases results in failure to function effectively in one's home settings. She makes a case for U.S. doctoral faculty to "pay attention to global content and international nursing issues," emphasize comparative studies, and assist international students to gear their doctoral research to problems in their own countries.

Quantitative Perspective

The International Council of Nurses now represents 110 national associations as members, with a total of 1 million nurses (Splane & Splane, 1994). Of 110 schools worldwide offering doctoral degrees in nursing, 62 are in the United States and 48 in all other countries combined. Moreover, according to anecdotal data, an indeterminate number of non-U.S. educational programs are programs where nurses have the opportunity to obtain doctoral degrees in fields other than nursing.

A limited number of international exchanges of students and faculty has occurred over the years (Fenton, 1994), although exchange has gained momentum recently. Yet, such opportunities are not made available to students by many institutions; further, international exchanges typically occur during undergraduate study rather than graduate study. At the doctoral level, during the 1970s, many institutions either abandoned a second language requirement altogether or began accepting a computer language in its stead. A recent American Academy of Nursing publication (1995) identifies five graduate programs in nursing in the United States with a cross-cultural focus, some of which include international nursing. Thus, in most cases, doctoral students' exposure to the world beyond the United States might come when they have the opportunity to study with international students as peers.

Examination of the growth in journal publication and in doctoral education gives readers another perspective on the growth in nursing knowledge and science. The major journal for reporting research in nursing, *Nursing Research*, was established in 1952 by the *American Journal of Nursing* Company; later it was followed by the publication of *Research in Nursing and Health* in 1977, and *Advances in Nursing Science* in 1978. Since that time, many journals have been established that report research in nursing, nursing theory, and nursing practice. As specialty organizations grew, so did journals concerned with the practice and research of their clinical area of practice. In the early days of *Nursing Research*, it was not uncommon to see papers authored by social scientists, reporting on studies concerned with *nurses* rather than with *nursing*.

Ketefian and Redman (1994) reported that the first doctoral programs in nursing were established in 1933 (Teachers College, Columbia University), and 1934 (New York University), both offering the Doctor of Education degree. In the next 25 years, only two more programs were established. Growth in doctoral programs since then has been exponential. Of the 62 institutions in the United States offering doctoral degrees in nursing 75% offer the PhD, the remainder offer a DNS, DNSc, or EdD. As to the nature of these programs, Grace (1978) and Murphy (1981) have described the development of doctoral programs in three phases: Phase I (inception to 1959) is characterized by focusing on education *for* nurses for functional roles; Phase II (1960–69) is characterized by a focus on education *for* nurses in a second discipline, referred to as nurse scientist training; Phase III (1970 to the present) is characterized by a focus on education *in* and *of* nursing.

A review of the content of U.S. journals suggests that many report on international issues, some have articles co-authored by nurses from overseas, and others have a regular international column. But the effect of these developments, while significant, is not major. Many libraries now subscribe to international journals; yet class assignments do not often include readings from these journals. A few journals now have international representatives on their review boards.

Qualitative Perspective

The Code for Nurses (ANA, 1985) represents embodiment of the values of American Nursing. The preamble reads, in part:

> When making clinical judgments, nurses base their decisions on consideration of consequences and of universal moral principles, both of which prescribe and justify nursing actions. The most funda-

mental of these principles is respect for persons. Other principles stemming from this basic principle are autonomy (self-determination), beneficence (doing good), nonmaleficence (avoiding harm), veracity (truth-telling), confidentiality (respecting privileged information), fidelity (keeping promises), and justice (treating people fairly)" (p. i).

The values in the code, and others emanating from them, find expression in nursing theories and conceptual frameworks developed by U.S. scholars. Indeed, they permeate the nursing literature. These values are at times explicit and at other times implicit.

Why are value assumptions important? Values have important effects on people, communities, and societies; the primary concern of nursing is people—individually or in the aggregate. An understanding of behavior and the values that underlie behavior, becomes a critical starting point for designing and implementing nursing interventions. Value assumptions underlying U.S. nursing are profoundly influenced by American culture, social mores, and the biases of the people who produce this literature. Yet, a reading of U.S. literature suggests that the ideas therein are claimed to be either acultural or universal.

Most nursing theories and nursing research are developed and implemented in the United States, and therefore, can be said to be influenced by the social and cultural context of this country. In the next section, we offer specific examples of the influence of culturally-specific values and assumptions—and present comparisons or contrasts gleaned from the literature.

Graduate and Higher Education in Nursing. In the United States, it is assumed that academic study is "good" and necessary for nursing education and that higher educa-

tion (at college and university level) is even better. However, in many countries these are not assumptions; the terms often have different meanings.

Hockey (1987) draws on her knowledge and experience in European countries, and states that in some countries "higher education" refers to academic study beyond that required for qualification for practice. In addition, she explains that typically with higher education come leadership positions, even though some nurses do not wish to assume such positions. Thus she poses the dilemma in ethical terms: Is "higher education" necessary for nursing? In another poignant example from the Austrian experience, she reveals that nurse training begins at age 15, and notes that "nursing autonomy assumes a different meaning" under these circumstances (p. 77).

Another author from the same conference describes the experience of Norway and its dilemmas which highlight value conflicts and value differences of a significant magnitude for that country. The main dilemma posed by Haugen Bunch (1987) is whether Norwegian nurses should study in the United States or in Norway. Each choice is described as having significant consequences for Norwegian nursing. She describes the choices as (a) studying social and natural sciences, (b) developing nursing science, or (c) blending the two. At the University of Bergen (Norway), where an Institute of Caring Sciences was established in 1979, many believe that caring is not subject to scientific inquiry, that nursing cannot be both holistic and scientific, that science may compromise the nursing discipline, that nursing can use relevant scientific principles from other disciplines, and that there is no need for a separate nursing science. Thus, if nurses study in Norway, with its tutorial educational model, their role models will not be nurses and they will learn the traditions of other disciplines rather than of nursing. If, on the other hand, they study in the United States, they will be socialized in nursing's scientific tradition and will have nurse role models. Haugen Bunch warns that for those educated in the U.S. there will be the danger of bringing back to Norway "undigested American knowledge that is presented as 'Norwegian truisms'—forgetting the need for value clarification so that the knowledge will fit Norwegian culture and traditions" (p. 103). Throughout her presentation she emphasizes the importance of adapting and testing theories and concepts before, "being applied and integrated to the Norwegian culture" (p. 103).

Nursing Science and Japan.   According to a Japanese nurse who did graduate work in the United States, Japanese nurses have imported nursing knowledge and literature since the end of the 19th century. The works of many American authors and theorists have been translated into Japanese by exchange nurses and by those who came to the U.S. for master's and doctoral degrees (Minami, 1987). Minami claims that many of these nurses "were not aware of the differences between the Japanese and American cultures or social context" (p. 66), and claimed that nursing was universal. She describes fundamental differences in the cultural milieu of the two countries that make concepts developed in one country inapplicable or irrelevant in the other. She also describes dilemmas faced by American-educated Japanese nurses in functioning in their home settings. Communication differences, for example, exist in eight areas: physical proximity; self disclosure; trust in words; boundary in human relationships; commitment and contract; dependency and independence; autonomy and independence; and confrontation (p. 70). She says that Americans communicate with language while Japanese communicate with empathy; and she provides examples. These differences are characterized by Boyacigiller and Adler (1991) as high-context or low-context cultures. The external environment, the situation, and non-verbal behavior determine communication in high-context cultures like the Japanese, and subtlety, facial expression, relationship, and timing are valued. In low-context cultures like the USA, meaning comes from the spoken word and legal contracts are valued.

Multicultural Knowledge Development in the United States

Rapid change in the demographic composition of the U.S. population has occurred within the past several decades. Some demographers estimate that by the twenty-first century, one-third to one-half of the population will be other than Euro-Caucasian. Thus a reversal is anticipated whereby groups that were minorities will collectively become the majority. The importance of a change of such magnitude is immense. An appreciation for diversity and for the varying needs of people who are different—with regard to any number of characteristics—is needed. Nowhere is this appreciation more compelling than in health care and nursing.

A small group of nurse investigators has been developing research and theory that is culturally sensitive. In a recent American Academy of Nursing monograph (AAN, 1995), a group of authors define culturally-competent care as that which "takes into account issues related to diversity, marginalization, and vulnerability due to culture, race, gender, and sexual orientation" (p. 4). In their assessment of the state of knowledge development in this area, the authors identify the dearth of principles to guide selection of culturally sensitive research questions and selection of culturally appropriate methodologies. Many nursing programs do not offer content relevant to this area and fewer still require doctoral students to enroll in seminars about cross-cultural nursing.

The authors of the AAN monograph (1995) identify two metatheories and studies based on them that have shown promise of generating knowledge that is culturally sensitive. One theory is Leininger's (1985), wherein she posits that care, as the essence of nursing, is universal across cultures, although its forms and expressions may vary. The authors cite a number of nursing studies in which Leininger's theory helped researchers generate knowledge related to cultural care. The other metatheory cited is the "self-care deficit theory" (Orem, 1991). This theory enables study of self-care practices used by diverse social groups. Its relevance for populations in a number of European countries—as well as Mexico and Thailand—is being studied by a network of collaborators (AAN, 1995).

In addition to the two metatheories, others are being developed that are referred to as "situation specific theories" (AAN, 1995). Examples are studies of Middle Eastern immigrants (Lipson, Reizian, & Meleis, 1987; Meleis, 1981; Meleis & Jonsen, 1983), patterns of health-seeking behaviors among Arab children (May, 1985), and post-partum transition among Arab women (El Sayed, 1986). The authors contend that, collectively, such studies can be synthesized to provide conceptualizations of patterns of responses to health-illness transitions, thus enabling development of a situation-specific theory in a particular population (AAN, 1995, p. 10).

Methodological concerns in the conduct of research with ethnically and racially diverse groups have received increasing attention as well. The U.S. Department of Health and Human Services (1990) has recently stipulated that ethnically and racially different groups be included as research subjects. Porter and Villarruel (1993) provide a cogent analysis of research issues and propose a set of guidelines to be considered for the design of research. Consideration of appropriate sensitivity is reflected in conceptualizing and conducting research, including each step of the research process and investigator activities. It is implied that unless these design considerations are present and deliberately addressed, the relevance and applicability of the outcome of the research to diverse populations would be questionable.

Other Knowledge Development Strategies. Over the years, nurses in many countries have identified their inability to describe nursing practice, client populations, or geographic areas as a serious constraint (Clark, 1994). To meet this need, and to contribute to knowledge development for nursing, various classification systems have been developed. The Nursing Minimum Data Set was developed by Werley in the late 1960s (Werley & Lang, 1988) and in turn spurred other developments.

In the early 1980s, a classification of nursing diagnoses was proposed by the North American Nursing Diagnosis Association, where the phenomenon of concern is patient status (McLane, 1987). More recently, the Nursing Interventions Classification (NIC) project was developed. The use of nursing diagnoses and NIC are becoming widespread in the United States and internationally. Such standardization has many advantages: it helps expand nursing's knowledge base, provides a common language to communicate the functions of nursing, provides shared understanding of nursing practice across national and cultural boundaries, and highlights the distinctive contribution nursing makes toward solving health problems. The International Council of Nurses currently has a project in progress with these goals in mind (Clark, 1994). Although we do not know how the different knowledge development strategies will evolve, significant developments are providing the basis on which to build continuing work by nurse scholars in doctoral programs around the world.

Next Steps

Some authors discuss the urgent need to develop nursing knowledge relevant to the health of the global community (Meleis, 1993). A Western perspective generally pervades organizing concepts and frameworks in nursing and thus is a dominating influence in knowledge development and research. Meleis expressed concern that U.S. nursing doctoral programs may be producing nurse scientists who do not challenge Western perspectives, particularly in terms of definitions and assumptions related to nursing phenomena.

In 1997 we are at a critical juncture for American nursing science. Given the global society in which we live, nursing science now faces the challenge of moving to its next phase of development, which we call "becoming globally relevant." This movement entails a variety of activities and changes in the way we do science, a responsibility that should be shared by scientists in the U.S. and internationally. We need to test nursing models, propositions, and hypotheses in several countries; include relevant content in educational programs; provide opportunities for doctoral students to develop nursing research internships abroad; involve international scholars in editorial review boards; increase the representation of international authors in U.S. journals and vice versa; encourage international students to focus their dissertations on topics pertinent to their countries; integrate collaborative international research in the ongoing work of scientists in leading nursing institutions throughout the world, and expand the criteria for promotion and tenure to include such activity.

We hope the questions raised in this essay will be viewed as opportunities by the global nursing community. If future discussions result in recognition of the challenges facing nursing knowledge development and doctoral education throughout the world, then our purpose will have been served.

REFERENCES

American Academy of Nursing. (1995). *Diversity, marginalization, and culturally-competent health care: Issues in knowledge development*. Washington, DC: Author.

American Nurses Association. (1985). *Code for nurses with interpretive statements*. Kansas City, MO: Author.

Boyacigiller, N.A., & Adler, N.J. (1991). The parochial dinosaur: Organizational science in a global context. *Academy of Management Science, 16(2)*, 262–290.

Clark, J. (1994). The international classification of nursing. In J. McCloskey, & H.K. Grace (Eds.). *Current issues in nursing* (4th ed.) (143–147). St. Louis, MO: Mosby-Year Book.

Colling, J.C., & Liu, Y.C. (1995). International nurses' experiences seeking graduate education in the United States. *Journal of Nursing Education, 34(4)*, 162–166.

El Sayed, Y.A. (1986). *The successive-unsettled transitions of migration and their impact on postpartum concerns of Arab immigrant women*. Unpublished doctoral dissertation, University of California, San Francisco.

Fenton, M.V. (1994). Development of models of international exchange to upgrade nursing education. In J. McCloskey, & H.K. Grace (Eds.). *Current issues in nursing* (4th ed.) 202–206. St. Louis, MO: Mosby-Year Book.

Grace, H. (1978). The development of doctoral education in nursing: An historical perspective. *Journal of Nursing Education, 17(4)*, 17–27.

Haugen Bunch, E. (1987). International perspectives and implications for doctoral education in nursing: Norwegian perspective. In *International perspectives and implications for doctoral education in nursing* (97–105). Portland, OR: Oregon Health Sciences University School of Nursing.

Hockey, L. (1987). Ethical issues in higher education in nursing. In *International perspectives and implications for doctoral education in nursing* (75–85). Portland, OR: Oregon Health Sciences University School of Nursing.

Ketefian, S., & Redman, R.W. (1994). The changing face of graduate education. In J. McCloskey, &

H.K. Grace (Eds.). *Current issues in nursing* (4th ed.) (188–195). St. Louis, MO: Mosby-Year Book.

Leininger, M.M. (1985). Ethnography and ethnonursing: Models and modes of qualitative data analysis. In M.M. Leininger (Ed.). *Qualitative methods in nursing*. New York: Grune & Stratton.

Lipson, J.G., Reizian, A., & Meleis, A.I. (1987). Arab-American patients: A medical record review. *Social Science and Medicine, 24(2)*, 101–107.

May, K.M. (1985). *Arab-American immigrant parents' social networks and health care of children*. Unpublished doctoral dissertation, University of California, San Francisco.

McCloskey, J.C., & Bulechek, G.M. (1994). Standardizing the language for nursing treatments: An overview of the issues. *Nursing Outlook, 42(2)*, 45–63.

McLane, A.M. (1987). *Classification of nursing diagnoses: Proceedings of the seventh conference*. St. Louis, MO: Mosby-Year Book.

Meleis, A.I. (1981). The Arab-American in the Western health care system. *American Journal of Nursing, 6*, 1180–1183.

Meleis, A.I., & Jonsen, A. (1983). Ethical crises and cultural differences. *The Western Journal of Medicine, 138(6)*, 889–893.

Meleis, A.I. (1993). A passion for substance revisited: Global transitions and international commitments. In *Proceedings of the 1993 Annual forum on doctoral nursing education* (5–22). St. Paul, MN, University of Minnesota School of Nursing.

Minami, H. (1987). Reflections of the cultural and social milieu on the development of nursing science in Japan. In *International perspectives and implications for doctoral education in nursing* (63–74). Portland, OR: Oregon Health Sciences University School of Nursing.

Murphy, J.F. (1981). Doctoral education in, of, and for nursing: An historical analysis. *Nursing Outlook, 29(11)*, 645–649.

Orem, D.E. (1991). *Nursing: Concepts of practice* (4th ed.). New York: McGraw-Hill.

Porter, C.P., & Villarruel, A.M. (1993). Nursing research with African American and Hispanic people: Guidelines for action. *Nursing Outlook, 41(2)*, 59–67.

Splane, V.H., & Splane, R.B. (1994). International nursing leaders. In J. McCloskey & H.K. Grace (Eds.). *Current issues in nursing* (4th ed.) (49–56). St. Louis, MO: Mosby-Year Book.

US Department of Health and Human Services. (1990). *Healthy people 2000: National health promotion and disease prevention objectives. Superintendent of documents*. Washington, D.C.: US Government Printing Office.

Werley, H.H., & Lang, N.M. (Eds.). (1988). *Identification of the nursing minimum data set*. New York: Springer.

Zwanger, L. (1987). International perspectives and implications for doctoral education in nursing: The Israeli case. In *International perspectives and implications for doctoral education in nursing* (17–43). Portland, Or: Oregon Health Sciences University School of Nursing.

Part III

NURSING'S METAPARADIGM: CONCEPTUALIZATIONS OF NURSING AND HEALTH

Each discipline has a specialized body of knowledge that includes its philosophy, theories, and frameworks or models. The discipline's major concepts reflect its scope of knowledge. Nursing's metaparadigm represents its scope of practice and consists of four major concepts—nursing, health, client/person, and environment. These concepts were first introduced in the 1970s by Dr. Jacqueline Fawcett, and later generally accepted as the major building blocks for nursing theories and models. Although each nurse theorist was expected to have specific definitions for all four concepts, not all theorists provided clear definitions, and each defined the concepts according to her own philosophical views and assumptions.

Nursing is usually described as both a science and an art, however, the scope and boundary of nursing practice varies according to each theorist. In recent nursing literature, there have been numerous articles discussing the specific ontological and epistemological underpinnings of different nursing theories to justify their structure. Theorists' underlying philosophy, along with their own particular ontological and epistemological beliefs, determine how each defines nursing and health. Ontology and epistemology are branch of philosophy called metaphysics. Ontology refers to specific claims by a philosophers about the nature and structure of their beliefs, and their assertions can differ radically or be contradictory to others views. Epistemology is concerned with the origin and structure of knowledge in relation to whether there are sufficient and necessary conditions for justifying or refuting the limits and possibilities of specific knowledge.

Health has also consistently been a major concept in nursing's metaparadigm, yet there is little agreement on the meaning of health among nurses and other health care professionals. Commonly accepted definitions include: the absence of disease or symptoms of illness; the ability to perform one's role satisfactorily; the ability to perform self-care activities; the ability to adapt to change and health problems; and, attaining self-actualization or exuberant well-being. Within nursing, no two theorists define health in the same way, yet each nurse's personal definition of nursing and health serve to guide the client's identified goals and ultimately determine nurses's actions, or how they practice nursing. The following chapters present several nurse theorists' and scholars' different perspectives on nursing and health.

In 1993, five nurse theorists —Imogene King, Madeleine Leininger, Rosemarie Parse, Hildegard Peplau, and Martha Rogers—participated in a panel discussion on nursing. A transcript of these theorists views was provided by Mary Huch, entitled "Nursing and the Next Millennium." The theorists discuss such topics as 1) caring as the essence of nursing; 2) the value of developing nursing theory; 3) what constitutes nursing research; and, 4) the role of advanced practice nurses. The divergent viewpoints of these renown theorists may challenge and stimulate your own thoughts and perspectives about the meaning of nursing practice, theory and research, and your future role as an advanced practice nurse.

In her article, "Nursing: The Ontology of the Discipline," Pamela Reed proposes that nursing is an inherent human process of well-being that is manifested by both complexity and integration in human systems. Dr. Reed cites the work of various theorists to support her view that human and nursing processes involving complexity and integration to achieve a client's well-being are the substantive focus of the nursing discipline. She recommends adoption of her definition of nursing for the metaparadigm, and views nursing as creative actions to facilitate the client's well-being.

Joy Johnson critically examines and analyzes relevant literature on the art of nursing, in her chapter "A Dialectical Examination of Nursing Art." She identifies five conceptualizations related to the art of nursing, which include the nurse's ability to: 1) grasp meaning in patient encounters; 2) establish a meaningful connection with patients; 3) skillfully perform nursing activities; 4) rationally determine an appropriate course of nursing action; and 5) morally conduct nursing practice. Each of these is discussed with examples from nurse theorists' and others' work to support them.

In her article on nursing ethics, Dr. Sally Gadow explains the basis for ethical decision making, how changes occurred, and how each type affects both the individual client and nurse. She begins with ethical immediacy (subjective immersion), which means ethical decisions reflect the values of family, religion, tradition, and the community. This type of ethical decision is an unreflective and uncritical certainty about what is considered "good," and allows no room for discussion. Ethical universalism (rational detachment) is based on using objective principles, theories, codes, and laws that are unconditional to make ethical decisions. This method eliminates all subjectivity, and everyone is considered equal. Ethical engagement (relational narrative) moves beyond strict objectivity and considers each individual as unique, so that different perspectives, including the client's, are considered. Engagement of care respect by health providers is obtained through dialogue and interpretation of the meaning of an experience to the client. Dr. Gadow discusses the strengths and limitations of each approach to ethical decisions. She recommends that they be considered layers, and as co-existing possibilities that are mutually complementary in making ethical decisions.

In her article, "Expressing Health Through Lifestyle Patterns," Nola Pender describes the shift in nursing science toward a unitary view of humans, concomitant with a rejection of the health-illness continuum. Dr. Pender believes that health is a primary life experience in which illness is superimposed. She compares her view with those of several other nurse scholars, then offers five dimensions of health—affect, attitude, activity, aspirations, and accomplishments. Each of these dimensions is thoroughly clarified and explained. Lastly, she recommends that health be defined in a positive, comprehensive, and humanistic manner.

Afaf Meleis provides a thought-provoking and critical analysis on the meaning of health in her article, "Being and Becoming Healthy: The Core of Nursing Knowledge." She begins with a discussion on the diverse definitions of health among nurses and health care providers, then suggests the need for a unifying, global definition. Dr. Meleis' main point is that health is more a social matter among poor people worldwide because scarce community resources, limited access to care, and inadequate knowledge and an ability to prevent disease, have a far greater impact on their health and illness. For those above poverty, health is often based on lifestyle choices and one's personal responsibility, which is not acceptable nor applicable to those constrained by societal or economic conditions. Dr. Meleis challenges nurses to consider multiple societal and environmental factors that influence health and to move beyond the traditional view that health is the "client's responsibility."

10

Nursing and the Next Millennium

MARY H. HUCH, RN, PhD

On March 19, 1993, in Toronto, Canada, at Discovery International, Inc.'s, Biennial Nurse Theorist Conference, five theorists participated in a panel discussion on: caring as an essence of nursing; the value of continuing to develop nursing theory; what constitutes nursing research; the role of advanced practice nurses. The theorists were Imogene M. King, Madeleine M. Leininger, Rosemarie Rizzo Parse, Hildegard E. Peplau, and Martha E. Rogers. Marlaine C. Smith was the moderator and presented the questions to the panel. (Keywords: Advanced practice, Caring, King, Leininger, Nursing knowledge development, Nursing research, Nursing theory development, Parse, Peplau, Rogers.)

Question 1: Is nursing the study of caring in the human health experience?

Dr. Leininger:
Well, I think you already know my answer. Caring is the essence of nursing and I think what Newman, Sime, and Corcoran-Perry did was add caring to the human health experience. So they were really saying, in terms of my theory, that caring is the health experience. But it's more than just the experience, because caring also reveals a lot more about some patterns of behavior and sometimes caring has explanatory value. If you look at the phenomenon of care itself, there's a whole world of knowledge out there to discover. I am pleased that Newman et al. are beginning to see and value caring with the human; this is long overdue. I was stunned when I found out that caring was left out of the metaparadigm in the late 1900s. We had already begun the

caring explication in the 1960s. So, as you know, I have held that caring is the overall concept, and then we have the environmental context. Health flows from care, because if you know care and caring, you then can predict health and well-being. Experience is only one aspect of all this; there's philosophy, there's expression, there are patterns—the linguistic things that you have to examine. And so I say we're moving in the right direction. In our international work we have care as a central, dominant domain of nursing. That's what we're about, and that's what we'll continue to look at until we have established it firmly as the root and the basis. I also take the position that many disciplines are studying health, and health is a unique and important dominant area within nursing. But it is care that will explain health, and that's a different pitch and a very important one.

Dr. King:
If caring is a process, I don't know how it can become a major concept in the nursing meta-

Source: Huch, M. (1995) Nursing and the Next Millennium. *Nursing Science Quarterly* 8(1) 38–44. Reprinted by permission of and copyright © 2002 Sage Publications, Inc.

paradigm, because concepts are terms such as perception and health, and they're not processes. And so I have a little problem with that. I also believe that if you use a particular process that leads to a positive outcome, and I think that's what my process and my theory are about, you automatically are caring. We've always had nursing care as part of our literature and history. And what is it? I haven't seen yet in the literature the characteristics that make up care or caring, and I think that's where we have a problem. Maybe I haven't read the right thing.

Dr. Parse:

I think caring is a ubiquitous term; it is not the central phenomenon of nursing. The human-universe-health process is the central phenomenon. The definition of caring is "to be concerned for something or someone," and I think many people in many disciplines are concerned about others. Physicians care, plumbers care, mothers care, and physical therapists care. Caring in the human health experience is not the proper way to state the phenomenon of concern to nursing. That particular phrase forces all the theories and frameworks to take up the issue of caring, and I don't believe that it is a central concept. We talk about human-universe-health process, and we look at the theories and frameworks in relation to that process, and all of the theories do address that. Most of them do not address caring as a central focus. Now, do I think that nurses care or should care? Yes, of course, I do. My disagreement is with elevating the term caring to the conceptual level where we have unitary human being or the human-universe-health process. I would suggest an alternative—that human-universe-health process is the central phenomenon of nursing. That should be our guide—that would be what the theories and frameworks should address—and then our particular practice and research would be guided by those theories and frameworks.

Dr. Peplau:

Up until now it's been pretty much Madeleine Leininger out on a limb all by herself with all the rest of us sawing it off. I don't want to come up the sharpest saw, because Madeleine is a good friend and she does good things for the profession, but I really don't believe that caring is the essence of nursing. I think that the way it's defined, it's a big scrap basket and it covers everything. It's almost a synonym for nursing practice or it's an alternate for the word nursing. I've read some of the caring literature, although I must admit I don't read much of it, but recently I've read a little more than usual. Three men nurses in Scotland have a paper which is about to be published in which they take on the whole concept of caring. They sent it to me for critique and comment and my name is on it, so when it comes out, you'll know I have the saw in hand. I don't know that there's any real benefit to defining what the essence of nursing is, but, if I'm forced to, I would say that it has to do with the nurse and patient in a relationship interacting in such a way that the patient's difficulties are remedied and the patient receives some substantial benefit as a consequence of having this interaction with a professional nurse who is knowledgeable and intellectually competent. I think the one thing that bothers me the most is that nursing has been primarily a woman's profession. We need to move as rapidly as possible to get more men into the profession. The word caring has been associated with women down through the ages and has not been particularly attuned to the behavior of men. And so, in essence, I think when you say caring is the essence of nursing, you are excluding men until the present reformation or transformation or metamorphosis occurs in which men are allowed to be caring individuals who can cry if they want to and hold babies and change diapers and wash dishes and do all of the other things that women do. By the same token, women can get into businesses and be career-oriented and make money and do all the other things that down through the ages men have done so that we have more androgyny in nursing. The percentage of men nurses in the United States has gone up a little bit. I think it's about 3 to 5% now, something like that, but it needs to go up a great deal more because we need a gender mix in order for nursing to reach its full potential. We need the benefits of both men and women. Although I applaud Madeleine's efforts and the efforts of others who have been thinking about caring and have been writing a great deal about it, I do not believe it belongs exclusively to nurses. We have carpet care for instance. We have people who care for your animals. We have all kinds of advertisements on television about how somebody cares for me, my dentist certainly cares, my dental hygienist is a caring person. I have experienced nursing care in a very limited degree in my lifetime experience because I've been phenomenally healthy. But I can't say that the nurses were more caring than the physician I had in that instance or that they were more caring than some of the teachers that I've had in my lifetime or the professional colleagues that I've had down through the years. So I don't think that we should latch onto this one concept and kind of say it belongs to us.

Dr. Rogers:

As far as caring being an effort of any field, it's sort of like the ads. You know mothers love their babies; if a mother cares, she'll give her child Castoria. And if she loves her spouse and cares about him, she'll feed him Nutri-Grain. Now you know, as I have said many, many other times, I happen to believe that everybody ought to care. But any idea that it is an identifying note for nursing is making us look right foolish. Because while we all care, unless there is knowledge that goes before, there is nothing to care with, and I think it's about time that we begin to value knowledge of

some sort. Now, I think this gets into the idea of unique knowledge in nursing. Are we, with our old dependency, going to run off to every other field and say, you tell us what to do and we'll go do it? It's time that we bury the whole idea of caring as the essence of nursing and begin to look at some substance.

Dr. Leininger:

Well, I just want to assure you, it isn't going to be buried. We are moving forward. I feel like I'm in my first seminar with new students. The students come in and say, I don't know what there is to learn about caring. And before we finish and after they get into the body of knowledge, which is really quite substantive, they change their view. As you know, we have over 175 different care constructs. Care is even more important than some of the other things. We have opened a whole body of knowledge that's going to help us in many ways. That people care and banks care is what we call the lay generic perspective. We look at what is professional care. How do we know *that* care? What is it that makes it what it is, and how do we demonstrate it? So I think that when you get into this and begin to systematically study caring, you open some interesting things transculturally and genderwise. As an anthropologist, I know that care has been a part of the male and female world. Margaret Mead proved this very early in her work from 1928 to 1948. I'm not saying care is only exclusive to nursing. I am saying that care is the essence, and I will hold to that. It is the central dominant domain and that must be explicated in this century and into the future. I know other people use care, but I'm saying care has been with us and the least understood and the most ubiquitous because we haven't attended to it. I would gladly refer to nearly 40 some books now on the phenomenon of care and over 2,000 articles. If we get care established as a substrate, this will be one of our major unique contributions to the world at large. I invite you to the International Caring Conferences to really get the substrate. It is exciting to see how it's being teased out and it's not an emotional movement. It is a full substantive knowledge based on care.

Dr. Rogers:

Madeleine, you know I respect you and I love you and I think you've made some major contributions, but I have to ask the critical question when it comes to theory and to theoretical knowledge. What we do is care, but before *we* can *do*, we have to *know*, and that's my point. What do we *know* first before we can exhibit care?

Dr. Leininger:

Caring is the action modality. What you need is to understand what is behind the body of knowledge that is related to care. What all does care mean to you as a professional nurse? What is that knowledge first? You cannot apply and do caring unless you know the phenomenon of care. That's what you have to systematically study.

Dr. Rogers:

I might start off with Patrick Henry. I disagree with everything you say, but I will defend to the death your right to say it! I think as far as research is concerned, whether it's in caring or how to teach or supervise or whatever else, we do need research. Whether one wants to label something care or caring, fine, but that's not the basic knowledge of nursing, and, I think, here again I get concerned when you make the statement about what anthropologists are doing. If nursing is nothing but anthropology, then let's go hire some anthropologists. Give them some manual skills and be done with it. But nursing is no more anthropology than anthropology is physics. Now I'll admit there might be some physical anthropologists who might want to play with physics, but I think we need to give further

thought to how we are using terms. Is there something to know in nursing? Knowledge in another field is not knowledge in nursing.

Dr. Leininger:

I'm not saying it's anthropology; you're missing the point. Knowledge is open to the world—there are no boundaries to knowledge. And just as you are interested in looking at space and energy in physics and that is not nursing, but you can abstract out; you can look at how you use knowledge within the perspective of nursing. It is how we develop the nursing knowledge. We are free to use any knowledge, but it's how we transform it, how we change it to be within nursing, and care is within nursing and has been since the beginning.

Question 2: It has been suggested that the uniqueness of nursing knowledge is not an issue for the next millennium. It may have been an issue in nursing as we struggled for identity as a young discipline, but now as a mature and respected discipline, we can abandon this struggle for identity and work together in interdisciplinary teams to build knowledge around selected phenomena related to health. Meleis offered this view in an article on theory development in the 21st century. So I would like each of you to think about that idea and give your thoughts and opinions.

Dr. Peplau:

Well, the whole notion of uniqueness in nursing has indeed been a 20th-century issue, but I thought it was broader than unique knowledge. Rather, the question is what is unique or what are the unique aspects of nursing per se? From my standpoint, what is unique about any profession are the phenomena which the professional must understand and be able to explain in some theoretical sense and the ability to provide theory-based treatment that will bring about a beneficial outcome. So to me, the issue was never nursing knowledge but rather the broader question of uniqueness. I think there's no doubt that the 21st century is quite likely to be the century of the professional nurse. I think we have come quite a distance now in developing theoretical sophistication, practical know-how, and a good deal of knowledge and information about organizations and networking and publishing and all of that, so that I think we're well on our way.

Whether or not we're going to be on an interdisciplinary team as a participating practitioner or a theory generator or a research assistant or a research participant is a longstanding issue, and I think that issue will continue. But, in terms of our getting away from the theory and moving in that direction totally, I think that would be a great mistake. One of the reasons that I think so comes out of my own experience. In the '40s and '50s I was a member of many important governmental committees which made decisions about government money and where it should go in terms of training grants and research grants and things like that. Additionally, I also was on some World Health Organization consultations in the same vein, and, inevitably, these committees or meetings were interdisciplinary. The one thing that I observed fairly early on was that as nurses we were coming pretty much empty-handed. When it came to talking about what it was that we did, we could always come up with an activity. We could say, we make beds and we pass out medicine and we take temperatures. So we could say what we *did* but not what we *knew*, or what we *understood*, or what the phenomena of nursing were. What were the kinds of phenomena patients presented to nurses about which they were supposed to be knowledgeable and about which they were supposed to provide a beneficial service? When those kinds of questions were raised, we began to stretch it and blow it up and make it up as we went along. I can tick off some of the nurse leaders who,

along with me, would get together afterward and discuss how we did that day. Had we persuaded the boys that we really had this body of knowledge which was called nursing knowledge which, of course, at this point we didn't have? Remember, in the United States we didn't even have a nursing journal until 1952, and then they had to beat the bushes to get articles for it because there was so little research being conducted. That situation has changed. We have a lot of information, a lot of research results and theory development. We have the international theory conferences on a biennial basis now, so that we have many ways to say what it is that nurses know. So when we get into an interdisciplinary meeting we don't come empty-handed. But it would be a grave mistake to say that we know all that we must know. Or that we must stop the development of finding out more in order to get in and work with other disciplines in terms of what we should do, which is the main point of interdisciplinary work in treatment centers, unless you're going to be involved doing the research for them. If you go empty-handed to the interdisciplinary team, you go gravely disadvantaged, and you are then very vulnerable to being put in the position of hand-maiden instead of colleague.

Dr. Rogers:

I think the whole business is still a great deal back at the area of nothing to know in nursing, and I think until we resolve that we're in trouble. Yesterday someone asked who thought should be head of the schools of health sciences in which nursing along with occupational therapy and physical therapy and health education were a part. What did I think of the need for a separate school for nursing? I think that unless we assume our responsibility for a body of scientific knowledge unique to nursing we will be lumped with other professionals. I think that when we get to what is unique, we're dealing with the uniqueness of any science, the phenomena of concern. One of the problems we've gotten into is we are still so oriented to *doing* that people talk about phenomena as really task-oriented. A few years ago Kellogg paid for a large study by the American Association of Colleges of Nursing. There was this large volume put out about associate degree education and baccalaureate education. They did mention in a couple of sentences the need for a liberal arts base, but the report didn't say much, and then there were pages of numbered lists of activities that all nurses should know how to do. There was not one activity that could be construed as knowledge in nursing. And I am talking about nursing knowledge and the use of nursing knowledge. Now, as long as we operate on that basis, as long as we add up parts and come up with something what we label nursing that is not more nursing than it is any other field, we will not gain the respect of any intellectual or academic group in terms of a knowledge base for nursing. It's interesting that people are very happy to say, well, yes, nursing is concerned with human beings and their environments and as long as you don't define your terms and keep it open, nobody gets into a hassle. But when you begin to define your terms, then, somehow, it looks a little hard. It isn't hard. Either we recognize nursing as a science with its own unique phenomenon of concern and an organized abstract system to underwrite it, or we agree to become a conglomeration.

Dr. Parse:

We, and others like us, have spent our lives carrying out the uniqueness of nursing. And so I think that in the 21st century the carving out of nursing as it grows and develops its theories and frameworks will continue. Nursing is a scientific discipline, just like psychology and physics and sociology. We are all independent; we are separate. And scholars from those disciplines do not give up their identities and do not

stop developing their sciences. No one says to them, well, now you have become sophisticated enough in the development of the phenomena for sociology, so you can move to interdisciplinary groups and you can study phenomena from different perspectives. Sociologists do not study the psychologist's perspective. Psychologists do not study the chemist's perspective or the physicist's. So, I think nursing should stay on the track and continue to evolve the theories and frameworks that we have through research. We need to continue in that way to further specify the discipline. We can move toward much greater specificity. Then we can go to that interdisciplinary table with something in our hands that is very significant. We can be colleagues with scholars of other disciplines and not move into a handmaiden's position. We are unique. We must continue to develop that uniqueness, and in no way would I agree with Meleis where she says that we should leave this theoretical perspective behind and just work on phenomena in general. I think that in coming to an interdisciplinary table, each one brings a different perspective, and I think that nursing's perspective is extremely important there. So, I would encourage all of us to continue to develop the specificity of nursing science.

Dr. King:

This idea just absolutely jarred all the things that I have worked on in the last 30 years. I disagree, but I haven't read Meleis' article. I believe we cannot stop this whole scientific movement called theory development.

Dr. Leininger:

We are still at the beginning of nursing knowledge development, and I think our colleagues have said that. So, we have a whole area ahead of us, and it would be really tragic to shortcut it. That's a lot of foolishness! In any discipline, scholars build, refine, debate, critique, and continue to develop.

Dr. Parse:

I would like to just make a comment that I thought about while Madeleine was speaking. I didn't go through it in the '50s as you did. But I have one major concern about the doctoral programs and the education that our doctoral students are receiving. Many of our doctoral students across the country are invited to do research that is grounded in sociology or psychology or philosophy or in some other area, and they do not utilize the nursing frameworks or theories as guides to research. That is a great concern of mine because I think if we are going to build the discipline, the only way to do it is by building the knowledge of the discipline. If one chooses a framework from outside of the discipline, for example, from a sociological perspective or a psychological perspective, then the research findings enhance that particular discipline. The knowledge, of course, can be used by nurses. We can use any knowledge, the whole world of knowledge. There are very few doctoral programs in this country that require students to utilize nursing frameworks as guides for their research, and that is tragic.

Dr. Leininger:

We ask the question, so what has this got to do with meaning? We already built a body of knowledge. And students have to start right from that base to begin to really systematically examine and study from there.

Dr. Parse:

And I know that you do require nursing theory-based research at Wayne State. But there are many PhD programs that do not. The other concern, too, is somewhat related. It is the way we do research. All of us have spoken in some way about both qualitative and quantitative research. Unfortunately, in many of the doctoral programs if the students want to do qualitative research, there is no one to guide them. Even though you have done it for years,

Madeleine, the first books in nursing on qualitative research were only published in 1985 and 1986. I would encourage doctoral students to go to programs where they can connect with faculty who are working on ideas for research that are of interest to them. When I have my editor's (*Nursing Science Quarterly*) hat on, I sometimes see manuscripts, particularly ones reporting qualitative research, that have weak methodologies. Students are disappointed when their research papers are rejected, because they had assumed their doctoral programs were providing proper guidance for conducting research. We as faculty must be willing to say to students, "Look, this is not my particular area, so I cannot guide it." We have a responsibility to the discipline to educate new scholars properly since these persons will guide and lead the knowledge development in nursing in the next century.

Dr. Peplau:

Well, I just wanted to comment that in essence what Meleis says in that article is enough already on the theory business. Let's go interdisciplinary. And that seems to be a pattern that we've had in nursing. In earlier years when nurses did a research project (and they had to do that in order to get faculty status in academia), they did one itty-bitty little research project and then they said, "Okay, I have done it now; I have done my research." You see the same thing going on in psychiatric nursing, where biomedicalization came in and the biological, biochemical explanations of mental illness got dumped in this "decade of the brain." The nurses pass pills and watch for complications and chart and act as physicians' assistants, as a matter of fact. Then, of course, as Madeleine pointed out, the federal grants office in Washington said that grants must be multidisciplinary, so nurses say, "Okay, if that's where the money is, forget nursing. Let's drop it in a ditch somewhere; after all, we already have all these theories." There's almost a lack of stick-to-it-iveness in nursing. We don't dig very deeply into something. We do it for a little while and then something more interesting comes up or something with money attached to it comes up, and we move on to that. And I find this very ominous. Certainly we don't have enough theory. I could tick off a dozen good research projects where we need theory in order to help nurses to know what to do with a patient who has certain kinds of phenomena. So, I would be absolutely horrified if the nursing population took Meleis seriously on this one.

Question 3: What makes *nursing* research *nursing* research? Must it utilize a nursing framework?

Dr. King:
I wouldn't take a conceptual framework as a basis for a study I wanted to do. I would take a theory and I would test it. To me a conceptual framework is too broad and comprehensive.

Dr. Parse:
Would you agree, Imogene, that the research should be utilizing nursing knowledge? Like in your own system, it would come from the conceptual framework and move into a theory and then be tested. Wouldn't you agree that it has to be nursing knowledge?

Dr. King:
Rosemarie, we've not been at research long enough. We don't have a history of research that tells us that we really have nursing knowledge.

Dr. Parse:
Okay, so you don't think we have nursing knowledge?

Dr. King:
No, because we haven't studied it enough.

Dr. Leininger:
I just want to say another important area that has been growing is the development of theories within the qualitative paradigm. Grounded theory is an example of how you would generate theory from the use of that method. But it is not unique. We now have nearly 20 different distinct methodologies that fall within the qualitative paradigm. Not all theories are tested within the qualitative approach. They are systematically examined to meet the goals and the objectives of the qualitative research project. So, I think there is a lot of opportunity for nurses to do some of these things.

Dr. Peplau:
Well, we have been arguing that for many years. It's nursing research if a nurse does it. It's nursing research if it's done on a nursing service. It's nursing research if it's done on a nursing problem that a patient presents to a nurse. It's nursing research if it uses nursing theory. You know, you could go on down the list. What I wanted to say was that the definition of nursing, which was accepted by the American Nurse Association, and to some extent by the International Council of Nurses, is that nursing is the diagnosis and treatment of human responses to actual and potential health problems. Now, there are a whole bunch of human responses to actual health problems, not to mention potential ones, about which we know nothing as nurses. Some of them I have experienced of late, and I wish somebody would study the exhaustion effect of vigilance. What is the human response to continual vigilance associated with aging, associated with hallucinations, associated with multiple personalities, associated with any number of conditions, strokes, for instance? Now, it seems to me that's something nurses ought to know and know intimately. We have an increasing population of aging people. They are going to have this

problem of vigilance, and they are going to have some kind of response. There's nothing in the literature that I know of on that. We have a whole large area where theory generation is the important thing and then you go and test it. Now you might use a theoretical framework or some kind of theoretical orientation to guide the observation, and I have no problem with that. But I would like to see nurses doing research in which they observe and interview and get patients to describe their own experience, and I am hoping some of that will come out of Parse's theory because she is big on the experiential end. And I am hoping that her students will go and ask people to describe their long-range, long-term experiences, of having a stroke, or whatever. I would like to see a lot of that go on, but I don't expect it will for a long time. I think when you want to go interdisciplinary instead of dealing with more research related to nursing, I think there is going to be less and less of that and we get on to bigger generalizations and bigger generalities and bigger scrap baskets and know less and less about it. But it is in a human response area that we are supposed to know something.

Dr. Rogers:

I think we are doing with research some of the same things we do in talking about nurses when people say a nurse is a nurse, and researchers are researchers are researchers. Everybody is not equipped to do research, everybody doesn't want to, and is there any reason that everybody has to? Certainly people ought to be curious, certainly they ought to read the literature, but we have lots of different kinds of research. Some of the fight over qualitative and quantitative, I think, is like a playback of Descartes and Bacon when they got into the fight over deductive and inductive reasoning. Not too far back, I am sure you all remember, the big hurrah that came up around chaos theory. And it really was a

fancy fad. Fortunately, it is sort of dying away a little bit, but I think it provides an excellent illustration of how we get caught between new realities and changing times and people. When I first got into chaos theory, I read two or three articles that appeared in *Science News* and they didn't bother to include the fine print in there and I thought, oh, boy, with chaos theory, somebody else is believing in the unpredictable besides me. Now, when the chips are down and you begin to get into the whole business, chaos is from an old worldview. There is nothing new about the idea of chaos theory; it had been proposed 30 to 40 years ago and had been worked on then. But what they were saying was, since the human being is not very knowledgeable and he can't possibly know everything, then of course he can't predict everything. Then there was a great big but; but if the human being did know everything, it would all be laid out and he could predict everything. In other words, the same old absolutist philosophy that was supposedly pushed out of the way around the turn of the century when Einstein and some of the others came along. Well, Einstein had trouble with it. At any rate, we are getting into a new reality, a new worldview. I know several of the others on the program here mentioned the idea of emerging worldviews and changing knowledge and that sort of thing. A new worldview that we are moving into now is just as big a shift as when life moved out of the waters onto dry land. Now we are moving into something very, very different. And on an everyday basis, the kinds of things that we have been studying or talking about or wanting to predict about in some distant future simply aren't going to be around to be predicted. Moreover, tools that have been developed out of our old worldviews are not valid for research in new realities. In other words, when one begins to study chaos theory or the idea of unpredictability within a new reality, then it really doesn't matter whether humans know everything or not. In an evolving, continuously changing world, things are unpredictable. There is no absolutism. Now, chaos theory is fading, and I think it will go away because it has perhaps served its purpose. I think it's an excellent example of how we have to recognize that the future cannot be measured according to the past, and that we are not living in the same world. About research, I think we need to be much more specific and recognize what it is that we are talking about and that it's all right for some people not to do research. "Publish or perish" is going to drive all of us crazy yet.

Question 4: There is a move toward the funding of programs for primary care practice or nurse practitioner-type programs. What is your opinion about the movement of primary care or nurse practitioners, and how do you see that related to nursing theory, or does it have any relationship at all?

Dr. Peplau:
Well, it's not hot on my agenda. I suppose you all know that the term now is advanced nursing practice and under that come nurse practitioners and clinical nurse specialists. By my logic, this pulls a specialist down to the level of nurse practitioner, some of whom have graduate degrees, but many of whom have only their RN diploma from a hospital school and maybe four months of training after that. So I find it's a leveling thing. Nobody in nursing can get a little further ahead than anybody else. We can't have specialists and we can't have experts of any kind. Maybe we are at the point where we can't have theorists because they are too smart or they know too much or they know something I don't know. But anyway, we always have this leveling back to a nurse is a nurse is a nurse. So, I have trouble, great trouble, with the advanced practice rubric; however, it's into the political system now and it's in the association's terminology,

so I would guess that it's here to stay. From my viewpoint, every nurse is a practitioner. I mean a nurse practitioner. The attempt to dignify it was originally a political thing. It came at the time in the United States when the American Medical Association began training physician assistants, and nurses were very unhappy at that point. I happened to be the ANA president, so I was the unhappiest of all. And we let it be well-known. As I recall, Martha Rogers called a conference to really deal with this issue, and I was one of the people who helped her deal with it on the podium. In any case, because we were so unhappy about it, our government threw us a bone, gave us money and said, okay, you have this money to train nurse practitioners. So then we had the terrible dilemma of should we take the money and let all those nurses get a little training, however limited, or should we say, keep your money—we will run our own show, which would offend all those politicians and, you know, might have long-term effects. So, anyway, the money was taken and nurse practitioners were turned out in great numbers. They organized. There are more of them than there are clinical nurse specialists. And, as a consequence, they have been running the show. It's one place where money drove the change in practice, and I am sure that has happened many, many times.

Dr. King: At one point, 20 years ago when I met some of the first nurse practitioners, they were in a 3-month training program. And when I saw the first one in a practice setting where this nurse was behaving like a physician, I said to her, "What makes you different from these master's-prepared clinical nurse specialists?" And she said, "Well, I do physical diagnosis." Now that was the behavior. And I said, "Well, I thought that was the basis for the practice of medicine." She said, "No, that's the basis for the advanced practice of nursing." I never saw this nurse ever behave like a nurse. She was like a mini-doctor who teamed up with a couple of doctors and did all of their physical assessments. I don't know why that made me feel negative toward that title. Since then, master's programs have been preparing nurse practitioners. In an attempt to differentiate nurse practitioners from clinical nurse specialists early on, we did say the nurse practitioner extended nursing into medicine and the clinical specialist had an expanded nursing role.

Dr. Rogers:
There is a clear-cut difference between a practitioner of nursing and a nurse practitioner. I think the use of the term nurse practitioner was an old con name to get nurses to accept something that to me is nothing in the world but a physician's assistant. I think Hilda mentioned, that in Washington the bill was set up so anybody who was an RN could take 2 months to 2 years or whatever was needed and be labeled a physician's assistant or a nurse practitioner and be paid for doing it. When it comes to what this means in terms of nursing, I would wonder why in the world nurses want to extend into medicine. I will repeat again, Nightingale said medicine and nursing should never be mixed up. Nurses do not need medicine in order to practice nursing. And if we practiced nursing, we would know that. Now, we certainly ought to learn to work with other groups, and it's a shame that nursing and medicine do not work with each other very well.

Dr. Leininger:
I think a lot of what we're going to see in this next period is what I call partnership care. How do we work with partners in the community? And how does nursing make its contribution in that partnership?

Dr. Parse:
There was an article in *The American Nurse* which specified that nurses who were moving to advanced nursing practice were very important because patients who met with them said they were friendlier and nicer than physicians and they were cheaper and we could probably be able to pay them better in our health care system. I am very concerned that nurses will be used in that way in the United States, that just because we are cheaper, that we will be asked to practice in ways that will help to decrease the cost of health care.

Dr. Peplau:
That concept that nurses are cheaper is demeaning for nursing, very demeaning, and nurses should be aware of what they are agreeing to be part of in the health care reform.

SUMMARY

This panel discussion among the nurse theorists on key issues related to nursing knowledge development and practice provided the audience with an opportunity to hear various views articulated by leading scholars in the discipline. The diversity of perspectives expressed in dialogues such as this reveals the richness of nursing science.

11

Nursing: The Ontology of the Discipline

PAMELA G. REED, RN, PhD, FAAN

The purpose of this article is to contribute to clarifying the ontology of the discipline by extending existing meanings of the term nursing *to propose a substantive definition. In this definition, nursing is viewed as an inherent human process of well-being, manifested by complexity and integration in human systems. The nature of this process and theoretical implications of the new nursing are presented. Nurses are invited to continue the dialogue about the meaning of the term and explore the implications of nursing, substantively defined, for their practice and science. [Keywords: Deconstruction, Knowledge development, Metaparadigm, Ontology, Postmodernism]*

Distinguishing the term *nursing* as a noun from its use as a verb was put forth most profoundly by Rogers (1970), whose vision extended the scholarship of earlier nursing theorists to thrust nursing forward to be recognized as both a scientific discipline as well as a professional practice. It is time, however, to push back the frontier once again, beyond these two important understandings of nursing, by proposing a new meaning of nursing. With this new meaning, the term itself represents the nature and substance of the discipline. In other words, *nursing* is the ontology of the discipline.

The ideas put forth here are done so in the spirit of accepting Watson's (1995) "postmodern challenge" to exploit the climate of deconstruction of nursing (see Rampragus, 1995; Reed, 1995) to extend and, by some degree, reconstruct current understandings of nursing. Smith's (1988a) article outlined the ongoing dialogue about two meanings of nursing, as a verb and a noun. This dialogue is revisited here for the purpose of further clarifying what is the ontology of the discipline, long considered a crucial question by seminal thinkers in nursing (Ellis, 1982; Rogers, 1970; Roy, 1995).

CONTINUING THE DIALOGUE: NURSING AS A PROCESS OF WELL-BEING

It is proposed here that there exists a third and perhaps most basic definition of nursing in which nursing represents the *substantive* focus of the discipline. Disciplines are characterized by their substantive focus: archaeology is the study of the archaeo, or what is ancient and primitive; astronomy is the study of the astro, astronomical phenomena such as the motion and constitution of celestial bodies; biology is a branch of knowledge about biol, or living matter; chemistry deals with the processes and

Source: Reed, P. (1997). Nursing: The ontology of the discipline. *Nursing Science Quarterly.* 10(2):76–79. Reprinted by permission of and copyright © 2002 Sage Publications, Inc.

properties of chemical substances; physics is the study of physical properties and processes; psychology is the study of the psyche, referring to mental processes and activities associated with human behavior; and nursing, the discipline, is proposed here to be the study of nursing processes of well-being, inherent among human systems.

This meaning of nursing, as an inherent process of well-being, derives in part from the root word, nurse, defined as a process of nourishing, of promoting the development or progress of something. The meaning also derives from synonyms of nurse meaning to heal, to foster, to sustain (Laird, 1971; *Webster's New Collegiate Dictionary*, 1979). These descriptions signify that nursing involves a process that is developmental, progressive, and sustaining, and by which well-being occurs.

The Inherent Nursing Process

The theme of human beings' inherent nursing processes as the substantive focus of the discipline is supported in nursing theorists' works from Nightingale in 1859, to the mid-20th century writings of Henderson, to the contemporary turn-of-the-century ideas of Schlotfeldt. Nightingale (1859/1969) wrote about the person's "innate power" and the inner "reparative process." Henderson (1964) eloquently symbolized the power of the nurse within, describing nursing as "the consciousness of the unconscious, the love of life of the suicidal, . . . the eyes of the newly blind, a means of locomotion for the infant, . . . the voice for those too weak or withdrawn to speak" (p. 63). Watson (1985) referred to "self-healing processes," and Schlotfeldt (1994) stressed human beings' "inherent ability and propensity to seek and attain health." In addition, this nursing process is not necessarily based upon a reversal of a disease process, but more upon a moving forward, to

gain a sense of well-being in the absence or presence of disease.

The discipline's understanding of how a nursing process is manifested is shifting away from the mid-20th century mechanistic conception of nursing as a process external to patients and conducted by the nurse, that is, the old nursing process. The process of nursing is viewed now more from a relational perspective, congruent with contextual and transformative conceptions of the world (see Newman, 1992; Pepper, 1942). Nursing is a participatory process that transcends the boundary between patient and nurse and derives from a valuing of what Rogers (1980, 1992) described as human systems' inherent propensity for "innovation and creative change."

"Human systems" refers to an individual or a group of human beings (Rogers, 1992, p. 30). As such, human systems, whether in the form of individuals, dyads, groups, or communities, emanate and participate in nursing processes. Nursing processes may be manifested, for example, in the grieving that an individual experiences, in the caring that occurs among people and their families and nurses, in the healing practices shared by a culture, or in many other as yet undiscovered patterns of nursing. Today, these patterns may be described as intentional or unconscious, automatic or contemplative, relational or chemical, or simply unknown. Nevertheless, with continued nursing research, education, and practice, nursing processes can be learned and knowingly deployed to facilitate well-being. Murphy's (1992) visionary book, for example, addresses some of these possibilities. He proposes a future wherein people are more aware of their innate healing potential and employ it to more purposefully enhance health.

Nightingale did not invent nursing, described here in terms of an inherent propensity for well-being. Just as earthquakes existed before geologists and photosynthesis before botanists, nursing processes existed in human beings, ultimately described by Nightingale (1859/1969) as that which nurses were to facilitate by placing the patient in the best situation possible. It follows, then, that nursing does not belong exclusively to certain groups of people, such as "well" persons or professional nurses; it belongs to human nature.

Defining the substance of the discipline of nursing in terms of a well-being process inherent among human beings does not negate the importance of knowledge of factors that interface with nursing to influence well-being and healing. Examples of these factors, often the focus of study in ancillary professions and disciplines, include the environmental, financial, cultural, surgical, and pharmacological. However, any sense of well-being involves, most basically, a nursing process. The quest for nursing is to understand the nature of and to facilitate nursing processes in diverse contexts of health experiences.

The Nature of Nursing Processes

What is the nature of nursing processes that distinguishes them from other human processes? It is proposed that the intersection of at least three characteristics—complexity, integration, well-being—distinguishes human processes as nursing; specifically, nursing processes are manifested by changes in complexity and integration that generate well-being. Importantly, other distinguishing characteristics of nursing processes may be identified as the dialogue continues beyond this article.

This new understanding of the nature of nursing processes derived from various theorists' work, such as von Bertalanffy's (1981) systems view of human beings; Rogers' (1970, 1992) science of unitary human beings; Lerner's (1986) developmental contextualism; and complexity theory (see Kauffman, 1995; Waldrop, 1992). While the translation of these theorists' ideas may not be entirely congruent

with those presented here, their ideas nonetheless can help inform development of a new nursing ontology.

Human beings are viewed as open, living systems and not as passive but intrinsically active and innovative. As an open system, human systems are capable of self-organizing, where *self* refers to the system as a whole. Self-organization is an inherent capacity for generating qualitative change out of ongoing events in the life of a system and its environment.

In his seminal work on development, Werner (1957) explained this process of qualitative change as his "orthogenetic principle," which posits that living organisms change over time from lower to higher levels of differentiation and integration. Werner (1957) called this change "development," in contrast to mechanistic processes of change, which are not developmental.

Similarly, Rogers' (1980) principles of homeodynamics describe the inherent innovative patterning of change that occurs in open systems, both environmental and human. Her three principles of helicy, resonancy, and integrality together depict the nature of qualitative change in human beings in terms of ongoing movement from lower to higher levels of diversity.

Complexity theorists (for example, Kauffman, 1995; Waldrop, 1992), and developmentalists (for example, Lerner, 1986; Werner, 1957) in particular have clarified a distinction between quantitative and qualitative change, both of which are necessary for development; contrasting terms such as complexity and order, and differentiation and organization, depict this distinction. Similarly, two distinct forms of change can be identified in Rogers' (1980, 1992) works, namely diversity and innovation (Reed, 1997).

Because of the articulation between quantitative and qualitative change, human systems are not simply complex systems (SCS) but rather are complex innovative systems

(CIS) (see Stites, 1994). In the context of nursing, then, nursing processes entail at least two forms of change, complexity and integration.

Complexity. Complexity refers to the number of different types of variables that can be identified in a given situation. A variable is simply something that varies (*Webster's*, 1979). Complexity occurs when human systems experience or express variables (for example, life events, physiologic events) as parts, separated from the whole, rather than as patterns of the whole. So, for example, complexity is evident when loss of a loved one or chronic illness introduces many new and seemingly disconnected variables into an individual's life, on various levels of awareness. Increasing complexity means change in quantity (size or number) not change in quality of the whole; this would become chaotic were it not accompanied by corresponding changes in integration.

Integration. Integration refers to a synthesizing and organizing of variables such that there is a change in form, not just change in size or number of events. A certain level of complexity is needed for integration to occur. Integration is evident, for example, when people construct meaning or identify a pattern in the variables or events experienced. Integration may also occur on levels of awareness that are not yet so readily apparent. Integration is trans*form*ative, involving qualitative change in form.

Well-Being

While changes in complexity and integration may be used to explain many facets of human development and systems' changes, this process may also be used to understand health, healing, and well-being. The rhythm between complexity and integration is proposed here to be a means by which innovative change occurs, as a manifestation of the underlying process called nursing. Thus, well-being may be explained in part by changes in complexity that are tempered by changes in integration. Complexity provides life with diversity, specialization, and depth in experiences, whereas integration provides organization, coherence, and breadth.

Examples of nursing processes are abundant. For example, groups incorporate new attachments or children into an organization called family. Persons with spinal cord injuries develop different pathways that link together shattered parts of life and bodily functions. Premature infants' behaviors become more innovative as they organize the complexity of their environment. Adults reminisce to integrate past life events and inevitable death. Healing after the loss of a loved one or the occurrence of chronic illness requires an integration of what seem like disjointed events and experiences, including memories of the past, future dreams, altered rhythms and routines, physical pain and other bodily symptoms, sadness, anguish, and self-doubt. Further, Sachs (1995) depicted what can be called nursing processes, through his stories about people with various maladies, such as a colorblind painter and a surgeon with Tourette's syndrome. These people were able to create a new organization that fit with their altered needs and world. These health events, in all their initial complexity and heartbreak, gave way to metamorphoses and innovation. Regardless of whether there is a "cure" that can reverse a particular ailment, well-being occurs when the particulars of a life experience are brought together and synthesized in a coherent way. Any less, and people risk feeling disintegrated, dis-associated, dis-organized.

While the centrality of well-being as a focus in nursing has been established, other disciplines also may be concerned with well-being and its correlates. However, promoting well-being based upon a perspective of the inherent process of complexity and integration is distinctly nursing.

CHALLENGING THE STATUS QUO: NURSING RECONSTRUCTED

The definition of nursing proposed here is that of an inherent process of well-being, characterized by manifestations of complexity and integration in human systems. The substantive focus of the discipline, then, is not how *nurses* per se facilitate well-being but, rather, how *nursing processes* function in human systems to facilitate well-being. The focus is, in a very basic sense, how nurses can facilitate nursing.

Refocusing the Lens

This new construction of nursing provides another lens of focus for nursing researchers and practitioners. Smith (1988b) wrote metaphorically about three different camera lenses used to view human wholeness. One in particular, the motion lens, focuses on process and rhythmic flow, and requires a "creative leap" to identify this process. Nurses typically encounter people in motion, in dynamic flow with their environment, whether in life-threatening experiences or perceived memory loss, chronic illness or acute pain.

The creative leap necessary for formulating the motion lens of nursing inquiry may be to address the rhythmic processes of complexity and integration that enhance well-being across these health experiences. From premature infants to dying adults and their families and communities, it is proposed that human systems have nursing processes, that is, inherent resources for well-being based on a capacity to integrate their complexities.

Debates on holism and on what represents the critical focus of nursing may be enlivened by including a new ontology of nursing—an ontology that transcends debates about part versus whole, person versus environment. Nursing processes are not necessarily bound by dimensions such as biologic, environmental, or social. Instead, the lens is focused on any human process that manifests complexity and integration related to well-being. Looking through this new lens, researchers and practitioners may identify a myriad of human manifestations of wholeness, whether they be labeled physiologic, phylogenic, or philosophic, that are integral to well-being.

NURSING AS A METAPARADIGM CONCEPT

Given this reconstructed view of nursing, as a substantive focus of the discipline, the term *nursing* should be a central concept in the nursing metaparadigm. In the past, for good reason, some have suggested the elimination of the term nursing from the metaparadigm (Conway, 1985). However, rather than remove the term nursing from the metaparadigm, this fin-de-siècle may be the time in nursing history to consider renaming the discipline to something other than a verb, to better distinguish the disciplinary label from the substantive focus of the science and practice.

To help clarify this distinction, a term such as Paterson and Zderad's (1976) "nursology," or another disciplinary label with the "nurs" prefix could be developed, while reserving the term nursing as the *process* word and verb that it is, for the metaparadigm. By identifying nursing as a substantive, metaparadigm concept, nurses can better claim their unique focus and clarify the ontology of their discipline.

APPROACHING THE FRONTIER

Rogers (1992) explained that one could not push back the frontier of knowledge until one approached it. This article has not been about maintaining the status quo, but about approaching a frontier so that others might join in a dialogue that pushes back the frontier a bit more. In this era of healthcare reform, the discipline must define nursing as nurses truly envision it and not necessarily as others would have it be defined. Nurses may decide against renaming the discipline as was suggested here. Nevertheless, within a broadened and partially reconstructed view of the discipline that embraces nursing at its most fundamental meaning, new understandings that blend with the old can emerge to present a fuller picture of the discipline.

Nursing (as practice and praxis) is a way of doing that creates good actions that facilitate well-being. Nursing (as syntax and science) is a way of knowing that creates goods in the form of knowledge. And nursing (the substance and ontology) is a way of being that creates patterns of changing complexity and integration experienced as well-being in human systems.

Nurses are invited to try on the substantive definition of nursing to see how it fits within the context of their practice and science. Ongoing philosophic dialogue about the ontology of the discipline will help ensure that nurse theorists are theorists of nursing in its fullest sense, and likewise, that nurse researchers are researchers of nursing, and nurse practitioners are practitioners of nursing.

REFERENCES

Conway, M. E. (1985). Toward greater specificity in defining nursing's metaparadigm. *Advances in Nursing Science, 7*(4), 73–81.

Ellis, R. (1982). Conceptual issues in nursing. *Nursing Outlook, 30* (7), 406–410.

Henderson, V. (1964) The nature of nursing. *American Journal of Nursing, 64* (8), 62–68.

Kauffman, S. (1995). *At home in the universe: The search for laws of self-organization and complexity.* New York: Oxford University Press.

Laird, C. (1971). *Webster's new world thesaurus* (rev. ed.). New York: Simon and Schuster.

Lerner, R. M. (1986). *Concepts and theories of human development* (2nd ed.). New York: Random House.

Murphy, M. (1992). *The future of the body: Explorations into the further evolution of human nature.* New York: J.P. Tarcher.

Newman, M. (1992). Prevailing paradigms in nursing. *Nursing Outlook, 40,* 10–13.

Nightingale, F. (1969). *Notes on nursing: What it is and what it is not.* New York: Dover (Original work published 1859)

Paterson, J. G., & Zderad, L. T. (1976). *Humanistic nursing.* New York: Wiley.

Pepper, S. P. (1942). *World hypotheses: A study in evidence.* Berkeley: University of California Press.

Rampragus, V. (1995). *The deconstruction of nursing.* Brookfield, VT: Ashgate.

Reed, P. G. (1995). A treatise on nursing knowledge development for the 21st century: Beyond postmodernism. *Advances in Nursing Science, 17* (3), 70–84.

Reed, P. G. (1997). The place of transcendence in nursing's science of unitary human beings. In M. Madrid (Ed.), *Patterns of Rogerian knowing* (pp. 187–196). New York: National League for Nursing Press.

Rogers, M. E. (1970). *Introduction to the theoretical basis of nursing.* Philadelphia: F. A. Davis.

Rogers, M. E. (1980). A science of unitary man. In J. P. Riehl & C. Roy (Eds.), *Conceptual models for nursing practice* (2nd ed., pp. 329–337). New York: Appleton-Century-Crofts.

Rogers, M. E. (1992). Nursing science and the space age. *Nursing Science Quarterly, 5,* 27–34.

Roy, C. L. (1995). Developing nursing knowledge: Practice issues raised from four philosophical perspectives. *Nursing Science Quarterly, 8,* 79–85.

Sachs, O. (1995). *An anthropologist on Mars: Seven paradoxical tales.* New York: A. Knopf.

Schlotfeldt, R. (1994). Resolving opposing viewpoints: Is it desirable? Is it practicable? In J. F. Kikuchi & H. Simmons (Eds.), *Developing a philosophy of nursing* (pp. 67–74). Thousand Oaks: Sage.

Smith, M. J. (1988a). Nursing: What's in a name? *Nursing Science Quarterly, 1,* 142–143.

Smith, M. J. (1988b). Perspectives of wholeness: The lens makes a difference. *Nursing Science Quarterly, 1,* 94–95.

Stites, J. (1994). Complexity research on complex systems and complex adaptive systems. *Omni, 16* (8), 42–50.

von Bertalanffy, L. (1981). *A systems view of man* (P.A. La Violette, Ed.). Boulder: Westview Press.

Waldrop, M. M. (1992). *Complexity: The emerging science at the edge of order and chaos.* New York: Simon and Schuster.

Watson, J. (1985). *Nursing: Human science and human care.* Norwalk, CT: Appleton-Century-Crofts.

Watson, J. (1995). Postmodernism and knowledge development in nursing. *Nursing Science Quarterly, 8,* 60–64.

Webster's new collegiate dictionary. (1979). Springfield, MA: G. & C. Merriam Co.

Werner, H. (1957). The concept of development from a comparative and organismic point of view. In D. B. Harris (Ed.), *The concept of development* (pp. 125–148). Minneapolis: University of Minnesota Press.

12

A Dialectical Examination
of Nursing Art

JOY L. JOHNSON, RN, PhD

Literature relevant to the art of nursing is immensely diverse and fragmented. This state is problematic in that progress in understanding nursing art cannot be made until the subject of nursing art is clearly delineated. In light of the need for conceptual clarity regarding nursing art, a dialectical study was undertaken to identify the distinct conceptions of nursing art that are represented in the nursing literature. The examined discourse was that contained in the works of 41 nursing scholars published between 1860 and 1992. The analysis revealed five distinct conceptualizations that can be identified as the art of (1) grasping meaning in patient encounters, (2) establishing a meaningful connection with the patient, (3) skillfully performing nursing activities, (4) rationally determining an appropriate course of nursing action, and (5) morally conducting one's nursing practice.

It is often said that nursing is an art and a science. Unfortunately, what is meant by the term *nursing art* is not well delineated or understood. In examining the theoretical issues nurses have concerned themselves with, it is clear that the majority of time and effort has been spent considering the nature of nursing science. Although numerous descriptions and definitions of nursing art have been suggested, little effort has been expended to analyze those definitions or to enter into a dialogue regarding the nature of nursing art.

Science alone will not solve all of the problems of nursing. Nursing is, after all, a practice discipline. Guidance regarding the use or application of scientific findings does not emanate from nursing science itself. As Ellis indicated, nursing is much more than the application of scientific findings. The practitioner cannot just "select from a rack of ready-to-wear theories."[1(p1434)] It is therefore essential that the manner in which knowledge, judgment, and skill are used in the clinical setting be carefully considered. These phenomena fall generally under the rubric of the art of nursing. Ultimately, an understanding of nursing art will further an understanding of how excellence can best be pursued and achieved in nursing practice.

The characterization of nursing as an art is not a recent development, and the literature relevant to the art of nursing is immensely diverse. It includes works such as Nightingale's[2] *Notes on Nursing* and Benner's[3] *From Novice to Expert*. Despite the abundance of writings on the topic of the art of nursing,

Source: Johnson, J. L. (1994). A dialectical examination of nursing art, *ANS*, *17* (1): 1-14. Reprinted with permission from and copyright © 1994 Aspen Publishers, Inc.

there have been few instances in which nursing scholars have addressed one another's positions. This failure is due in part to the fact that nursing scholars have tended to pursue their conceptions of nursing art in isolation and have not considered other conceptions. Nursing scholars have not confronted one another in light of their differences, resulting in the current situation in which a plethora of diverse views concerning the art of nursing are relatively unquestioned and unexplored.

Schlotfeldt[4] pointed out that the future of the nursing profession depends on the ability of its members to identify and resolve issues. Yet nurses will be unable to resolve issues related to the art of nursing unless the subject at issue is clearly set forth. Walker identified the need for such an analysis when she argued that the controversy regarding the art of nursing "has been difficult to resolve for the point of contention has not been clearly set forth."[5(p118)] The tremendous diversity of ideas regarding the art of nursing expressed in the nursing literature will remain a source of confusion unless the diversities are put in order and rendered intelligible. When differences of opinion remain implicit, or even concealed, as in the nursing discourse relevant to the art of nursing, they cannot serve as the basis for the collective effort required to further thought.

In light of the state of fragmentation that characterizes the nursing literature relevant to the subject of nursing art, a philosophic study was undertaken to discover the common ground that underlies the differences of opinion regarding the art of nursing and to transmute the current diversity into rational and intelligible controversy. This study sought to render the existing diversity more intelligible so that a rational debate of fundamental issues can proceed and a better understanding of nursing art can be attained.

METHOD

The approach that was taken for this study was a critical examination and systematic analysis of the nursing discourse concerning the art of nursing. The method is one developed by Adler[6] and his colleagues at the Institute for Philosophical Research in Chicago to examine the controversies that surround such philosophic ideas as freedom, love, and equality. The aim of this method, which Adler[6] referred to as a *dialectical approach*, is to outline and clarify the structure of a controversy, and it involves a process of constructive interpretation. The goal of this philosophic method is to explicitly formulate patterns of agreement and disagreement. The challenge of the dialectical method is to achieve a nonpartisan treatment of positions or views. The dialectical task, therefore, involves rendering an objective, impartial, and neutral report of a many-sided discussion. Using this approach, the dialectician examines and clarifies what is implicit in the discourse. By way of constructive interpretation, the researcher attempts to find similarities and dissimilarities among the various conceptions.

Although the works examined in this study are historical in the sense that they date to a specific time and place, the intent of this study was to examine the ideas contained in them apart from their historical context. The study was in no way historical in its aim or its method. Therefore, for the purpose of this study, it was assumed that the authors concerned with the art of nursing are engaged in a continuing dialogue, even though they belong to different historical periods.

The point of departure for this study was the manifold and often confusing diversity that exists on the subject of nursing art. The general subject of nursing art includes a broad field of discourse and covers a variety of themes. Rather than seeking to include the work of every nursing author who has written on the subject of nursing art, a sample of works was required that was representative of the existing diversity of views regarding the art of nursing. Literature that was broadly related to the topic of nursing art was included in the study. In total the works of 41 authors composed the examined discourse. The findings reported here are part of a larger study[7] that examined the issues and controversies that exist regarding nursing art.

DISTINCT CONCEPTUALIZATIONS OF NURSING ART

Based on an examination of the nursing literature related to the art of nursing, it was concluded that there are diverse answers to the question, What is the art of nursing? The use of the term *art of nursing* in no way ensures that those involved in the discourse refer to the same subject. Part of the dialectical task involved determining whether there are distinct conceptions of the subject within the examined discourse. The questions that guided this determination included, Is *art* being used in the same sense? and, Does the discussion involve one subject or several distinct subjects? To identify the distinct conceptualizations of nursing art, each work was carefully read, and relevant passages believed to be germane to the topic were noted. Ties of relevance that connected the various authors were sought, and points of agreement were established. These points of agreement served to delineate each distinct conceptualization.

In examining the discourse, it was found that there were five separate senses of "nursing art." They can be described as

1. The nurse's ability to grasp meaning in patient encounters,
2. The nurse's ability to establish a meaningful connection with the patient,
3. The nurse's ability to skillfully perform nursing activities,
4. The nurse's ability to rationally determine an appropriate course of nursing action, and
5. The nurse's ability to morally conduct his or her nursing practice.

It should be pointed out that although the authors who have written about nursing art provide evidence for the construction of these conceptions, the identification of these conceptions is not theirs per se. It should also be noted that although these subjects are mutually exclusive, most authors have conceptualized nursing art as consisting of more than one ability; therefore, these authors are viewed as addressing more than one conception of nursing art. Finally, it cannot be concluded that an author's apparent silence on a particular conceptualization of nursing art indicates a denial of that conceptualization. The descriptions that follow focus primarily on the similarities of thought regarding each conception, rather than the issues, or points of disagreement, that exist regarding these conceptions.

Ability to Grasp Meaning in Patient Encounters

The situations that confront nurses are often characterized by uncertainty, ambiguity, and indeterminacy.[8] This is due in part to the fact that nursing practice situations are complex. The complexity of a patient's situation can be further compounded when patients are unable to articulate their needs, either because they are unaware of the needs or because they are incapacitated.[9] Consequently, the nurse must grasp the meaning of each particular patient situation and determine what in the situation is relevant. For select authors,[3,8-33] nursing art involves the ability to grasp meaning in patient encounters. According to these authors, the artful nurse, as compared to the nurse who lacks art, can grasp what is significant in a particular patient situation. The term *grasping meaning* is used here to describe the process of attaching significance to those things that can be felt, observed, heard, touched, tasted, smelled, or imagined, including emotions, objects, gestures, and sounds.

Although marked variation can be found among the descriptions of the authors who have been construed to conceptualize nursing art as the grasping of meaning, several points of agreement can be found. First, nursing art is seen as based in an immediate perceptual capacity and is not affected by the intellect. This capacity to grasp meaning is often referred to as intuition. Rather than being based in reflection, or reasoning, the art of nursing according to this view is based in an immediate perceptual capacity that is more integrated than simple sensation and more concrete than intellection; it is based in a capacity that involves the external senses as well as the imagination.

Using this capacity, the artful nurse attributes meaning to things that are felt, observed, or imagined. It is the artful nurse who can *sense* the meaning or significance of a situation, such as when a patient is distraught; *perceive* patterns, such as the set of signs and symptoms that indicate when a patient is going into cardiogenic shock; have a *feel* for what he or she is doing; or *sense* what should be done, such as *knowing* when to use humor to help relieve the tension of a situation. Thus, Chinn and Kramer stated, "Esthetic knowing is what makes possible knowing what to do with the moment, instantly, without conscious deliberation."[14(p10)] Nursing art is thought to involve the direct apprehension of what is to be done, or what is the case, and is unmediated by concepts. The immediacy of the art of grasping meaning was emphasized by Benner and Wrubel, who argued that "the person does not assign meanings to the situation once it is apprehended because the very act of apprehension is based on taken-for-granted meanings embedded in skills, practices, and language."[9(p42)]

A second point of agreement is that the art of grasping meaning results in a form of understanding that defies accurate or complete description. The insights gained by this perceptual ability are thought to be tacit, nonpropositional, personal, and as such incommunicable. Carper, for example, argued that esthetic knowing is gained by "subjective acquaintance, the direct feeling of an experience"[13(p149)] and that this knowing defies discursive formulation. The meanings that the artful nurse grasps are concrete and individual, pertaining to a particular patient situation (e.g., this particular patient that I am nursing and can observe in front of me who happens to have had an appendectomy), rather than abstract, pertaining to patients in general (eg, appendectomy patients). Orlando emphasized this distinction when she stated that the nurse must distinguish between general principles and "the meanings which she must discover in the immediate nursing situation in order to help the patient."[25(p1)]

A third point of agreement to be found is that the art of grasping meaning is a perceptual ability that can be honed and developed over time. Rew,[31] for example, argued that the nurse can learn to become sensitive to the signals and feelings that he or she experiences and, over time, can learn to understand their significance. Similarly, Newman[21] argued that nurses can learn to attend to and trust their inner experiences. Benner[3] contended that perceptual abilities are formed by previous experiences and by immersion in the present perceptual environment. Consequently, the information taken in by the senses is endowed with meaning. According to Benner,[3] it is through experience that the nurse learns to immediately focus on what is relevant in a patient situation and to grasp its meaning. Using past experiences, or foreknowledge, the artful nurse has the ability to recognize patterns and can therefore make sense of ambiguous, unstructured situations. According to Benner, "Past concrete experience . . . guides the expert's perceptions and actions and allows for a rapid perceptual grasp of the situation."[3(pp8-9)]

Finally, according to those who affirm this first conception of nursing art, the art of nursing is a holistic capacity. The nurse's perceptual ability allows him or her to immediately grasp the meaning of a situation, instead of piecing together an understanding of what is happening. In contrast, the nurse who is not artful must assess every minute detail, breaking down a situation into its component parts to discover what is of significance. Benner and Wrubel described the artful capacity as " a perceptual awareness that singles out relevant information from irrelevant, grasps a situation as a whole rather than as a series of tasks, and accomplishes this rapidly and without incremental deliberative analysis of isolated facts or bits of information."[10(p13)]

Ability to Establish a Meaningful Connection with the Patient

The connection between the nurse and the patient is considered by many authors* to be of particular importance, particularly in the current era of increasing technology. Many emphasize that it is the artful nurse's interactions that can bridge the gap introduced by technology and that such interactions can promote "wholeness and integrity in the personal encounter, the achievement of engagement rather than detachment, and . . . [denial of] the manipulative impersonal orientation."[13(156)] *Connection*, as it is used here, refers to an attachment, or union, that occurs between patients and their nurses. The term *connection* is used because, unlike the term *relationship*, it

*References 13-18, 21-24, 26-30, 34-43.

encompasses short-term or fleeting encounters as well as long-term associations. According to these authors, a meaningful connection between the nurse and the patient is central to the provision of nursing care, since it is through this connection that services such as physical and emotional support are offered and accepted. Kim,[39] for example, pointed out that the core of nursing resides in human-to-human actions. Similarly, Gadow suggested that the central question in nursing is not, How can we help them [patients] to recover? but, instead, How can we recover them [and] overcome the distance between us?[16(p12)]

The second conception of nursing art is distinguished by four major points. First, it is contended that nursing art is nondiscursive; that is, it is expressed in the nurse's actions or behaviors. According to those who hold this second conception of nursing art, the art of nursing is "unmediated by conceptual categories."[13(p154)] It cannot be expressed through words; instead, it is expressed in the concrete actions and gestures of the artful nurse in response to a particular patient. Paterson and Zderad argued that "nursing is an experience lived between human beings"[28(p3)] and that nursing art is evident in the synchronicity between the nurse and the patient.

Second, it is contended that its expressive nature constitutes an essential characteristic of nursing art. Chinn and Kramer maintained that this expression takes the form of "human actions—words, behaviors, and other symbols—that give communicable form to what we know."[14(p6)] Although it is agreed that nursing art is expressive, there is little agreement regarding what exactly is expressed in nursing art. For some authors, emotions play an important role in the origin of art. For example, Watson[41] argued that through their art, nurses express emotions or feelings. The work of Peplau[29] suggested that the expression of nursing art is appropriately limited to the expression of sentiments such as concern, compassion, and caring. Paterson and Zderad,[28] on the other hand, suggested that nursing art involves the expression of the nurse's state of being.

Third, it is argued that the art of nursing occurs in relation to another human being. The ideas of philosopher Martin Buber[44] are echoed frequently in the works of authors who have conceptualized nursing art as the ability to establish a meaningful connection. Buber[44] posited that relationships are of two kinds. The first is a subject-to-subject, or "I-Thou," relationship, which is a relationship of connectedness and affirmation of another person's being. The second type of relationship is subject to object, or "I-It," which arises out of a stance of separation and detachment, in which the individual is differentiated over and against a world of objects. Authors who hold that nursing art is establishing a meaningful connection with the patient contend that nursing art can only occur when the nurse stands in a subject-to-subject relationship with the patient. For example, Paterson and Zderad stated, "If she enters into genuine relation with the patient (I-Thou) her effective power (caring, nursing skills, hope) brings forth form (well-being, more-being, comfort, growth)."[28(p92)]

Finally, the authors who support the view that nursing art is the ability to establish a meaningful connection are in agreement regarding the necessity of authenticity on the part of the nurse. Bishop and Scudder argued that "the inauthentic nurse merely plays the role of nurse rather than really *being* a nurse."[34(p102)] It is held that the artful nurse must be genuine; any attempt to mask or hide feelings will serve only to distance the nurse from the patient, thereby threatening the relationship between the nurse and the patient. Parse[26] referred to this authenticity as genuine or true presence. Similarly, Watson asserted that "the degree of transpersonal caring (in this sense of unity of feeling) is increased by the degree of genuineness and sincerity of the nurse."[41(p69)]

Ability to Skillfully Perform Nursing Activities

The conceptualization of nursing art as the skillful performance of nursing activities is one of the earliest conceptions of nursing art found in the nursing discourse.[2,3,5,9-12,45-59] It is from this view that we see in early nursing curricula the attainment of nursing skills being referred to generally as the "nursing arts." Price contended that nursing art involves the ability to "recognize the nursing needs of the patient and to develop skill, through practice, in various procedures designed to answer those needs."[54(p19)] According to the authors who hold the view that nursing art is the ability to skillfully perform nursing activities, the artful nurse is one who has a demonstrable capacity to effectively carry out nursing procedures and techniques. *Skill*, as it is used here, refers to a developed proficiency or dexterity. *Nursing activities* are all those tasks, procedures, and techniques that a nurse carries out in his or her practice.

The focus of these authors' conceptualizations of nursing art is an array of activities both manual and verbal in nature. For example, we see in the work of Nightingale[50] a list of behaviors that the good nurse must demonstrate. These behaviors include such things as moving silently through the sickroom, keeping constant watch over the sick, and airing out the sickroom on a regular basis. Nightingale[50] expected the artful nurse to do more than understand these edicts. She expected these behaviors to be instantiated in the nurse's practice; the artful nurse knows more than what is to be done, she knows "how to do it."[50(p1)] Wiedenbach[58] numbered among the skills the nurse must possess the ability to perform back rubs, to take a pulse, and to help a patient walk as well as the ability to handle necessary equipment, such as a cardiac pacemaker and the circular-electric bed: "These skills involve manipulations and techniques—

executed with finesse to achieve desired results."[58(p28)]

Those who hold this third conception of nursing art were found to be in agreement regarding three central points. First, according to the authors, the art of nursing is primarily a behavioral ability; that is, it involves observable actions and focuses on the process of doing, rather than the process of knowing. As such, it is concerned with the nurse's demonstrable ability, not his or her knowledge per se. Heidgerken made this distinction clear when she stated, "The principles, procedures, and technics, or science, of nursing are learned in the classroom. The art, or skill, of nursing is learned on the ward."[48(p9)] Although there is agreement among the authors who hold this third conception that nursing art is ultimately a behavioral ability, there is no consensus regarding the role that one's intellectual capacity plays in the art of nursing. Some theorists argue that the activities must be intelligently performed. Montag,[49] for example, contended that skill without understanding is mere imitation. Similarly, Heidgerken[48] contended that the memorization and demonstration of step-by-step procedures will not produce an artful nurse. Tracy, on the other hand, contended that "the nurse should have so mastered her procedures that the minimum of thought is needed for their use."[57(p29)] Similarly, Benner and Wrubel[9] argued that nurse's everyday actions are effective not because they think about them, or base them on theory, but because they have a sophisticated repertoire of reactions.

Second, those who conceptualize nursing art as skillful performance of nursing activities are in agreement about the claim that nursing art can be learned. Key to learning the art of nursing are persistent practice and repetition. Goodrich maintained that practical experience for student nurses should be "sufficiently long to allow of a constant repetition of procedures."[47(p42)] Heidgerken, however, warned that practice alone is not enough and that "the attitude of the learner, the will to improve, and eradication of mistakes are all equally as important as practice."[48(p54)]

Finally, there is also evidence of agreement regarding the fact that certain criteria can be used to judge the art of nursing. When discussing the art of nursing, these theorists inevitably use descriptors such as fluidity of movement, adroitness, coordination, and efficiency. Stewart indicated that nursing art involves "manual dexterity, lightness, steadiness, quickness of movement, strength, endurance, and that complete coordination of head and muscle which cannot be acquired except by long, directed training."[55(pp324-325)] Similarly, Heidgerken[48] argued that the artful nurse's activities must have the appropriate form; elimination of excess movements, appropriate timing, force, and coordination are among the qualities that characterize the activities of the artful nurse.

Ability to Rationally Determine an Appropriate Course of Nursing Action

For those* who support the fourth conception of nursing art, intellectual activity is essential to the performance of nursing care. According to this fourth conception, nursing art refers to the nurse's ability to rationally determine an appropriate course of nursing action. The term *rational ability*, as it is used here, refers to the intellectual ability to effectively draw valid conclusions from existing knowledge.

This fourth conception of nursing art is characterized by five points of agreement. First, it is argued that nursing art is practical in nature. According to these authors, the aim of this ability is the determination of an appropriate course of action. Nursing art, it is argued, is action oriented and not simply aimed at understanding. Beckstrand,[60] for example, contended

*References 2, 4, 5, 25, 39, 40, 45, 46, 48-53, 55, 56, 58-78.

that the aim of nursing art is the control of practice. Dickoff and James[62] concluded that nursing art is concerned ultimately with producing nursing situations. Similarly, Orlando contended that nursing art is a rational capacity that is aimed at "helping the patient."[25(p70)]

Second, it is contended that there is an underlying discipline on which nursing art rests. All of the authors who contend that nursing art is a rational ability emphasize the importance of knowledge, specifically scientific knowledge, to nursing art. Orem stated, "The art of nursing is the nurse's quality or habit of reasoning and judging correctly about the design and production of the kind and amount of nursing needed according to the principles or laws of nursing itself. Science and technique are 'the first necessary conditions for honest art.' The point of view of nursing as art therefore encompasses the point of view of *nursing as knowledge.*"[52(p24)]

Arguments about the importance of knowledge for nursing art are often tied to the claim that nursing is a profession. Abdellah and her colleagues, for example, argued, "Professionalization of nursing requires that nurses identify those nursing problems that depend for their solution upon the nurse's use of her capacities to conceptualize events and make judgments about them. Nurses need to become skilled in recognizing both overt and covert nursing problems, in analyzing them in terms of relevant principles and in working out courses of action by applying nursing principles."[45(p11)] It was assumed by Abdellah et al.,[45] as it was by all of the authors who support this fourth conceptualization of nursing art, that the nursing profession possesses a distinct body of knowledge and that this body of knowledge provides the foundation for nursing practice.

Leininger[73] also contended that nursing art is based on scientific knowledge. She believed that nurses must, if they are to be effective, "scientifically care" for their patients. *Scientific caring*, according to Leininger, "refers to those

judgments and acts of helping others based upon tested or verified knowledge."[73(p46)] The importance of knowledge to artful practice is echoed by all of the authors. Kim stated, "Knowledge is antecedent to action."[39(p146)] And Diers contended that "nursing practice is done consciously, if not always with a formal plan, that it is not done mindlessly."[65(p31)] Finally, Rogers claimed that "the art of nursing develops only as it incorporates more and more of science unto itself. The nature of its art lies in the core of scientific knowledge it embodies."[75(p32)]

The third point of agreement regarding the art of rationally determining an appropriate course of nursing action is that it presupposes that nurses possess a thorough understanding of what is before them and the actions they should take. According to this perspective, the artful nurse solves problems by selecting the intervention that is best suited to the intended end. This process of instrumental problem solving involves a thorough consideration of the facts of a situation and is made rigorous by the application of scientific theory. For example, Johnson[70] argued that an artful nurse thinks "logically, soundly, and searchingly" about the causes and effects in a given nursing situation. The key point is that the artful nurse's actions are not "automatic" or "blind" but instead are grounded in an intellectual activity, in which knowledge or information of certain kinds is considered to determine which actions will result in the best possible patient outcome.

Fourth, it is contended that the art of rationally determining an appropriate course of nursing action involves a process of logical reasoning in which scientific principles and theories are applied to problems identified in practice. According to this view, the artful nurse uses evidence to reason through the best course of action to be followed. Beckstrand described this process in the following manner:

Once the conditions requiring changes in the client's situation are determined, a practitioner examines the situation to identify the possibility of making the changes desired. First, a practitioner uses scientific knowledge of necessary and sufficient conditions to determine if desired changes are realizable. Next, a practitioner examines the situation to determine whether conditions for achieving the desired changes exist. . . . As a result, the set of realizable outcomes in practice is determined by what is scientifically possible within the exigencies of the practice situation.[61(p177)]

The steps of the nursing process (assessment, planning, implementation, and evaluation) are seen as the steps that an artful nurse takes to ensure quality patient care. The emphasis of this approach is on deliberate, systematic, and scientifically based care.

Finally, it is contended by those who hold the fourth conception of nursing art that the art of nursing can be judged according to certain standards. They agree that the appropriateness of a nursing action can be judged on the basis of whether the identified course of action enabled the practitioner to attain his or her identified goals or standards. For example, Henderson[37] contended that a nurse's art can be evaluated according to the degree to which the patient has reestablished independence. Some authors have suggested additional criteria for evaluation. Dickoff, James, and Wiedenbach,[63] for example, suggested that nursing art can be evaluated using the criteria of coherency, palatability, and feasibility.

Ability to Morally Conduct One's Nursing Practice

For a final group of authors,* nursing art involves the ability of the nurse to practice

_____
*References 2, 3, 9, 11, 15-18, 34-38, 47, 48, 50-53, 60, 61, 67, 68, 79-81.

morally: The nurse is obligated to practice in such a way that seeks to avoid harm and to benefit the patient. The term *moral*, as it is used here, refers to that which is good, or desirable, for human beings. These authors are in agreement regarding four central points. First, it is held that good or excellent nursing practice is, by necessity, moral in that it is directed toward the good of the patient. As Goodrich stated, "So much is nursing of the essence of ethics that it is consistent to assert that the terms good and ethical as applied to nursing practice are synonymous."[47(p5)] Conversely, the view that nursing art can under any circumstances be amoral or immoral is antithetical to this position. Indeed, for these authors, the moral aspect of nursing cannot be separated from the notion of excellence in nursing, either existentially or analytically. This is the case, it is argued, because unlike the fine arts, nursing is an art that deals directly with human beings. Artful nursing, Curtin[79] asserted, is inextricably entwined with human life and the achievement of particular human ends.

According to those who hold that nursing is a moral art, a nurse may be technically competent and knowledgeable, yet if he or she does not make moral choices in the performance of patient care, he or she is not artful. Lanara[81] argued that values and ideals must guide the nurse's care. In a similar fashion, Gadow[17] posited that good nursing is more than a cluster of techniques in that it involves a commitment to a moral end and is directed and judged by that end. This position is also supported by Bishop and Scudder, who argued that the artful nurse's ability consists in more than the ability to efficiently complete tasks: "[The] technician uses techniques which are evaluated by efficiency; whereas, the professional makes decisions which are evaluated by the good."[34(p69)]

Second, it is held that the possession of skill and knowledge are necessary, but not sufficient, conditions for the moral conduct of nursing practice. Indeed, it is presupposed by many of these authors that the artful nurse must be competent in his or her practice. As Curtin[80] pointed out, the license to practice nursing does not include permission to practice poorly. In stating that one is a professional, one is claiming a certain level of competence.

Third, it is argued by those who hold that nursing art is the ability to morally conduct one's practice that nursing art involves a commitment to care competently for patients. Curtin stated that "although knowledge and skill are integral to the practice of a profession, the foundation consists of the performative declarations professed by its practitioners and the fidelity of the practitioner to these promises."[80(pp101-102)] The moral responsibility to nurse well involves a commitment not only to nurse a patient competently, but to "sustain excellent practice in the face of unreasonable demands and lack of appreciation on the part of patients."[35(p37)] The artful nurse not only must be competent, but must also consistently demonstrate competence in his or her practice, no matter how arduous the circumstances.

Finally, the notion that the artful nurse must possess moral virtues is reiterated in various forms by all of the authors who ascribe to the notion that the art of nursing is of a moral nature. Expressed in all of their works is the belief that the artful nurse must be properly motivated in his or her action. Rather than being motivated by self-aggrandizement or expediency, the artful nurse is motivated by care and concern for others. Benner and Wrubel suggested that the same act done in a caring and uncaring way may have different effects and that only a nurse who cares about his or her patients will notice small differences in their behaviors and create unique solutions to patient problems: "Caring makes the nurse notice which interventions help, and this concern guides subsequent caregiving. Caring causes the nurse to notice subtle signs of improvement or deterioration in the patient. In fact, caring . . . is required for expert human practice."[9(p4)]

Accordingly, the nurse who does not care about his or her patient cannot nurse well. Lanara[81] argued that the ability to care about patients rests on the nurse's capacity to love others and that nurses, inspired by the ideal of love, will care not only for, but about, their patients. It is love, according to Lanara,[81] that allows the nurse to transcend obstacles and become heroic in his or her nursing practice.

CONCLUSION

Through the identification of these five conceptions of nursing art, nurses can begin to understand the structure of the discourse regarding nursing art. Once one goes beyond the description of the five conceptions identified, differences of opinion can be found among the authors who affirm a particular conception of nursing art. Indeed, each of the five conceptions is a subject of controversy in that each comprises numerous conceptual, existential, and normative issues.

It is evident that although nursing scholars have written about the subject of nursing art, few have acknowledged one another's conceptions. Indeed, to date there has been little recognition that different conceptions of nursing art exist. When one examines the discourse regarding the art of nursing, it is clear that not all of the authors agree about the nature of nursing art. This state of affairs is consistent with the state of the nursing discourse in general. Kikuchi and Simmons accurately characterized this state of affairs when they stated,

> Although nursing scholars are prone to speak or write on the same topic, use the same words, or express a common interest in knowledge development, there is very little in their productions to indicate that they share to any great degree a common understanding, a coming-to-

terms, that would allow for the minimal topical agreement required before questions can be commonly interpreted, controversies identified, issues debated, and answers commonly agreed upon.[82(p3)]

It is hoped that the identification of distinct conceptions of nursing art will facilitate productive debate and analysis among nursing's scholars.

The method employed in this research is limited in that it does not answer the question, What is nursing art? The next step must be taken: to examine each of these conceptualizations in detail to determine which conceptualization or group of conceptualizations is sound. The findings of this study provide the groundwork for future philosophic analyses, thereby bringing nursing one step closer toward a sound conception of nursing art. It is only when a sound conception of nursing art is developed that nursing will be able to answer questions regarding how nursing art should be pursued and developed. It is hoped that nursing scholars in the future will dispute the nature of nursing art more explicitly and extensively.

REFERENCES

1. Ellis R. The practitioner as theorist. *Am J Nurs.* 1969;69:1434-1438.
2. Nightingale F. *Notes on Nursing: What It Is, and What It Is Not.* New York, NY: Dover; 1969.
3. Benner P. *From Novice to Expert: Excellence and Power in Clinical Nursing Practice.* Menlo Park, Calif: Addison-Wesley; 1984.
4. Schlotfeldt RM. Resolution of issues: An imperative for creating nursing's future. *J Prof Nurs.* 1987;3:136-142.
5. Walker LO. *Nursing as a Discipline.* Bloomington, Ind: Indiana University; 1971. Dissertation.
6. Adler MJ. *The Idea of Freedom, I: A Dialectical Examination of the Conceptions of Freedom.* Garden City, NY: Doubleday; 1958.
7. Johnson JL. *Toward a Clearer Understanding of the Art of Nursing.* Edmonton, Alberta, Canada: University of Alberta; 1993. Dissertation.
8. Tanner C. Curriculum revolution: the practice mandate. In: *Curriculum Revolution: Mandate for Change.* New York, NY: National League for Nursing; 1988:201-216.
9. Benner P, Wrubel J. *The Primacy of Caring: Stress and Coping in Health and Illness.* Menlo Park, Calif: Addison-Wesley; 1989.
10. ———. Skilled clinical knowledge: The value of perceptual awareness. *Nurs Educ.* 1982; 7(3): 11-17.
11. Benner P. The role of experience, narrative, and community in skilled ethical comportment. *ANS.* 1991;14(2):1-21.
12. Benner P, Tanner C, Chesla C. From beginner to expert: Gaining a differentiated clinical world in critical care nursing. *ANS.* 1992;14(3):13-28.
13. Carper BA. *Fundamental Patterns of Knowing in Nursing.* New York, NY: Teachers College, Columbia University; 1975.
14. Chinn PL, Kramer MK. *Theory and Nursing: A Systematic Approach.* 3rd ed. St. Louis, Mo: Mosby–Yearbook; 1991.
15. Gadow S. Clinical subjectivity: Advocacy with silent patients. *Nurs Clin North Am.* 1989; 24:535-541.
16. ———. Beyond dualism: The dialectic of caring and knowing. Presented at the conference "The Care-Justice Puzzle: Education for Ethical Nursing Practice" at the University of Minnesota; October 13, 1990; Minneapolis, Minn.
17. ———. Nurse and patient: The caring relationship. In: Bishop AH, Scudder JR, eds. *Caring, Curing, Coping: Nurse, Physician, Patient Relationships.* Tuscaloosa, Ala: University of Alabama Press; 1985:31-43.
18. ———. Body and self: A dialectic. *J Med Philos.* 1980;5:172-185.
19. Moccia PA. A critique of compromise: Beyond the methods debate. *ANS.* 1988;10(4):1-9.
20. ———. *A Study of the Theory-Practice Dialectic: Towards a Critique of the Science of Man.* New York, NY: New York University; 1980. Dissertation.
21. Newman MA. The spirit of nursing. *Holistic Nurs Pract.* 1989;3(3):1-6.
22. ———. *Health as Expanding Consciousness.* St. Louis, Mo: Mosby; 1986.
23. ———. Newman's theory of health as praxis. *Nurs Sci Q.* 1990;3:37-41.
24. ———. Sime AM, Corcoran-Perry SA. The focus of the discipline of nursing. *ANS.* 1991; 14(1):1-6.
25. Orlando IJ. *The Dynamic Nurse-Patient Relationship: Function, Process and Principles.* New York: G.P. Putnam's Sons; 1961.

26. Parse RR. Human becoming: Parse's theory of nursing. *Nurs Sci Q.* 1992;5:35-42.

27. ———. *Man-Living-Health: A Theory of Nursing.* New York, NY: Wiley; 1981.

28. Paterson JG, Zderad LT. *Humanistic Nursing.* New York, NY: National League for Nursing; 1988.

29. Peplau HE. The art and science of nursing: Similarities, differences, and relations. *Nurs Sci Q.* 1988;1:8-15.

30. ———. *Interpersonal Relations in Nursing: A Conceptual Frame of Reference for Psychodynamic Nursing.* New York, NY: G.P. Putnam's Sons; 1952.

31. Rew L. Nurses' intuition. *Appl Nurs Res.* 1988;1:27-31.

32. ———. Intuition in decision-making. *Image J Nurs Schol.* 1988;20:150-153.

33. Tanner CA. The nursing care plan as an instructional method: Ritual or reason? *Nurs Educ.* 1968;11(4):8-10.

34. Bishop AH, Scudder JR. *The Practical, Moral, and Personal Sense of Nursing: A Phenomenological Philosophy of Practice.* Albany, NY: State University of New York Press; 1990.

35. ———. Nursing ethics in an age of controversy. *ANS.* 1987;9(3):34-43.

36. ———. *Nursing: The Practice of Caring.* New York, NY: National League for Nursing Press; 1991.

37. Henderson V. The nature of nursing. *Am J Nurs.* 1964;64(8):62-28.

38. ———. Excellence in nursing. *Am J Nurs.* 1969;69:2133-2137.

39. Kim HS. *The Nature of Theoretical Thinking in Nursing.* Norwalk, Conn: Appleton-Century-Crofts; 1983.

40. ———. Structuring the nursing knowledge system: A typology of four domains. *Schol Inq Nurs Pract.* 1987;1:99-114.

41. Watson J. *Nursing: Human Science and Human Care: A Theory of Nursing.* New York, NY: National League for Nursing; 1988.

42. ———. The lost art of nursing. *Nurs Forum.* 1981;20:244-249.

43. ———. Caring knowledge and informed moral passion. *ANS.* 1990;13(1):15-24.

44. Buber M; Smith RG, trans. *I and Thou.* 2nd ed. New York, NY: Charles Scribner's Sons; 1958.

45. Abdellah FG, Martin A, Beland IL, Matheney RV. *Patient-Centered Approaches to Nursing.* New York, NY: Macmillan, 1960.

46. Abdellah FG, Levine E. *Better Patient Care Through Nursing Research.* New York, NY: Macmillan; 1965.

47. Goodrich AW. *The Social and Ethical Significance of Nursing: A Series of Addresses.* New York, NY: Macmillan; 1932.

48. Heidgerken LE. *Teaching in Schools of Nursing: Principles and Methods.* Philadelphia: Pa: Lippincott; 1946.

49. Montag MI. *The Education of Nursing Technicians.* New York, NY: G.P. Putnam's Sons; 1951.

50. Nightingale F. *Training of Nurses and Nursing the Sick* [Microfiche, Adelaide Nutting Historical Nursing Collection]. London, England: Spottiswoode; 1899.

51. ———. *Suggestions for Thought to the Searchers After Truth Among the Artizans of England* [Microfiche, Adelaide Nutting Historical Nursing Collection]. London, England: George E. Eyre & William Spottiswoode; 1860.

52. Orem DE. *Nursing: Concepts of Practice.* 4th ed. St. Louis, Mo: Mosby-Yearbook; 1991.

53. ———. The form of nursing science. *Nurs Sci Q.* 1988;1:75-79.

54. Price AL. *The Art, Science and Spirit of Nursing.* 2nd ed. Philadelphia, Pa: W.B. Saunders; 1960.

55. Stewart IM. The aims of the training school for nurses. *Am J Nurs.* 1916;16:319-327.

56. ———. Practical objectives in nursing education. *Am J Nurs.* 1924;24:557-564.

57. Tracy MA. *Nursing: An Art and a Science.* St. Louis, Mo: Mosby; 1938.

58. Wiedenbach E. *Clinical Nursing: A Helping Art.* New York, NY: Springer; 1964.

59. ———. The helping art of nursing. *Am J Nurs.* 1963;63:54-57.

60. Beckstrand J. The notion of a practice theory and the relationship of scientific and ethical knowledge to practice. *Res Nurs Health.* 1978;1:131-136.

61. ———. The need for a practice theory as indicated by the knowledge used in the conduct of practice. *Res Nurs Health.* 1978;1:175-179.

62. Dickoff J, James P. A theory of theories: A position paper. *Nurs Res.* 1968;17:197-203.

63. Dickoff J, James P, Wiedenbach E. Theory in a practice discipline: Part II. Practice oriented research. *Nurs Res.* 1968;17:545-554.

64. Dickoff J, James P. Taking concepts as guides to action: Exploring kinds of know-how. In: Nicoll LH, ed. *Perspectives on Nursing Theory.* 2nd ed. Philadelphia, Pa: Lippincott; 1992:576-580.

65. Diers D. *Research in Nursing Practice.* Philadelphia, Pa: Lippincott; 1979.

66. ———. Learning the art and craft of nursing. *Am J Nurs.* 1990;90:65-66.

67. Dock LL. *Short Papers on Nursing Subjects*. New York, NY: M. Louise Longeway; 1900.

68. Dock LL, Steward IM. *A Short History of Nursing: From the Earliest Times to the Present Day*. 3rd ed., rev. New York, NY: G.P. Putnam's Sons; 1937.

69. Donaldson SK, Crowley DM. The discipline of nursing. *Nurs Outlook*. 1978;26:113-120.

70. Johnson DE. A philosophy of nursing. *Nurs Outlook*. 1959;7:198-200.

71. ———. The nature of a science of nursing. *Nurs Outlook*. 1959;7:291-294.

72. ———. Theory in nursing: Borrowed and unique. *Nurs Res*. 1968;17:206-209.

73. Leininger M. Caring: A central focus of nursing and health care services. In: Leininger MM, ed. *Care: The Essence of Nursing and Health*. Thorofare, NJ: Slack; 1984:45-59.

74. ———. *Care, Discovery and Uses in Clinical and Community Nursing*. Detroit, Mich: Wayne State University Press; 1988.

75. Rogers ME. *Reveille in Nursing*. Philadelphia, Pa: F.A. Davis; 1964.

76. ———. *An Introduction to the Theoretical Basis of Nursing*. Philadelphia, Pa: F.A. Davis; 1970.

77. ———. Nursing science and art: A prospective. *Nurs Sci Q*. 1988;1:99-102.

78. Schlotfeldt RM. Structuring nursing knowledge: A priority for creating nursing's future. *Nurs Sci Q*. 1988;1:35-38.

79. Curtin LL. The nurse as advocate: A philosophical foundation for nursing. *ANS*. 1979;1(3):1-10.

80. Curtin L. The commitment of nursing. In: Curtin LL, Flaherty MJ, eds. *Nursing Ethics: Theories and Pragmatics*. Bowie, Md: Robert J. Brady; 1982:97-102.

81. Lanara, VA. *Heroism as a Nursing Value: A Philosophical Perspective*. Athens, Greece: Sisterhood Evniki; 1981.

82. Kikuchi JF, Simmons H. Prologue: An invitation to philosophize. In Kikuchi JF, Simmons H, eds. *Philosophic Inquiry in Nursing*. Newbury Park, Calif: Sage; 1992:1-4.

13

Relational Narrative:
The Postmodern Turn in Nursing Ethics

SALLY GADOW, RN, PHD

A philosophy of nursing requires an ethical cornerstone. I describe three dialectical layers of an ethical cornerstone: subjective immersion, objective detachment, and relational narrative. Dialectically, the move from immersion to detachment is the turn from communitarian to rational ethics, replacing traditions with universal principles. The move from universalism to engagement is the turn from rational to relational ethics, replacing detached reason with engagement between particular selves. Conceptually, the three layers correspond to premodern, modern, and postmodern ethics. I propose that the layers be viewed not as stages, but as elements that coexist in an ethically vital profession, and I conclude with an illustration of their coexistence in a clinical situation.

A philosophy of nursing requires an ethical cornerstone, because a profession is informed by moral ends. Discussions of ethics in nursing usually are framed in the categories of philosophical ethics, such as deontology, virtue, and consequentialism. While useful for locating nursing ethics within the disciplinary context of philosophy, the categories are not helpful because they manifest no internal relationship to each other, no connection within an encompassing framework. Without a coherent framework, ethics cannot provide the cornerstone for a philosophy of nursing.

In the hope that establishing philosophical connections among different ethical approaches will lead to the construction of an ethical cornerstone, I offer a method for understanding different ethical views within a dialectical framework. The framework I describe is a triad of ethical layers: subjective immersion (ethical immediacy), objective detachment (ethical universalism), and intersubjective engagement (relational narrative)—corresponding, respectively, to premodern, modern, and postmodern ethics (see Figure 13.1). After a brief discussion of dialectic, I describe each of the three layers and conclude with an illustration of their coexistence in a clinical situation.

DIALECTIC

The method of developing a philosophical dialectic is adapted here from the work of Hegel (1807/1977). A brief elaboration of method is important to the thesis of this discussion, namely, that premodern, modern, and post-

Source: Gadow, S. (1999). Relational narrative: the postmodern turn in nursing ethics. *Scholarly Inquiry for Nursing Practice*. 57 – 69. Used by permission of Springer Publishing Company, Inc.

modern ethics represent a dialectical relationship among different ethical approaches in which none of the three can stand alone and only their coexistence constitutes a sound basis for practice.

The nature of dialectic can be expressed as mediation. Mediation is the negation of simplicity, resulting in increasing complexity as each new level of differentiation is in turn negated, producing further distinctions. At the same time, the opposition among distinctions is itself mediated. Negativity, in other words, becomes increasingly positive as the original opposition is qualified by a new relationship in which once antithetical elements are no longer mutually exclusive but become mutually enhancing.

A clinical example of dialectic is the experience of injury and rehabilitation (Bloom, 1992; Gadow, 1982).[1] Before injury, the body is experienced as a taken-for-granted immediacy that accomplishes the aims of a person, such as climbing stairs, without reflection or even awareness.[2] An injury negates that immediacy in two ways: the body opposes the aims of the self by its inability to climb, and the inability is itself the antithesis of the lost immediacy.[3] Rehabilitation negotiates a new relationship between body and self. While the body remains an other for the self (an otherness the injury produced), harmony between them is cultivated through attentiveness to the injured part. That cultivated unity based on care entails the possibility for climbing stairs as a cooperative, rather than an unconscious, activity of body and self.

A characteristic rhythm is associated with dialectic because of the three phases of simplicity, opposition, and reconciliation. The formulaic description of dialectic as thesis-antithesis-synthesis, however, can be deceptive; it masks the principle of ongoing self-negation at the heart of dialectic. No phase is exclusively thesis, antithesis, or synthesis. Each phase serves as antithesis of the one before,

and each synthesis becomes a new thesis as its own unity is further differentiated. The rehabilitated body, for example, can train for a marathon, involving further cycles of immediacy, opposition, and reconciliation.

If an inherent telos is assumed, a dialectic will move inexorably toward culmination. Hegel insisted on a telos, but I do not. Without a telos, the movement of mediation can proceed indefinitely. Without closure, a dialectic of ethical levels such as I propose can give rise to further cycles of differentiation. Ethics, in other words, need not culminate in the postmodern. Indeed, the most interesting question evoked by a dialectic of premodern-modern-postmodern ethics may be, "What now?" Given the nihilism sometimes associated (mistakenly, I believe) with postmodern ethics, treating it as the thesis for a new set of negations might be a fruitful sequel to the discussion that follows.

PREMODERN IMMERSION: ETHICAL IMMEDIACY

In a dialectical framework the first level is immediacy. In ethical terms, immediacy is an unreflective and uncritical certainty about the good. A certainty powerful enough to resist reflection originates outside an individual in order to avoid being undermined by particularity. Certainty about the good, if it is to be more than personal conviction, must derive from a source that transcends the individual, such as religion, family, customs, or the ethos of a profession.

Ethical immediacy is an experience of certainty that needs and allows no explication; it is nondiscursive. That, in fact, is its power. A discursive description of a morally good nurse can be argued and revised, requires consideration, and has to be consciously accepted in order to have power. In contrast, a nondiscur-

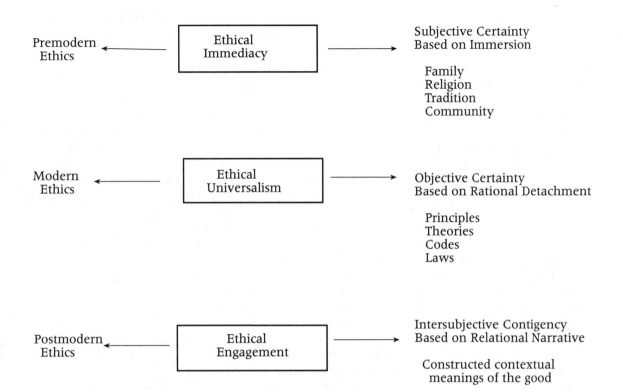

Figure 13.1. Triad of Ethical Layers.

sive portrayal—an image rendered in film, a virtue modeled by a mentor—bypasses deliberation to gain acceptance. With a cultural, professional, or religious basis for certainty, a nurse intuits the good directly, without recourse to reflection. That immediacy is the phenomenon I call immersion: a nurse is immersed in a tradition that provides an ethical appraisal of the situation, as well as immersed in the situation itself. Depending on the tradition, that appraisal may dictate, for example, that nurse-assisted suicide is wrong (or that it is right). Whatever the tradition, immersion offers a degree of certainty unavailable to the other ethical layers because it is nonreflective. It needs no defense.

The strength of immersion as an ethical approach is the solidarity it achieves. Nurses and patients sharing an unquestioned view of the good are united in their attempt to realize that good. Differences in interpretation may arise between individuals, but the foundational unity that grounds their values prevents differences from becoming divisive. Similarly, within an individual, ethical immediacy prevents fragmentation of the self that can result from self-questioning and critique. Immediacy serves to maintain the self—and the group—as a coherent, harmonious whole. Immersion and immediacy, in other words, describe community. "In community persons cease to be other, opaque, not understood, and instead become mutually sympathetic, understanding one another . . ., fused" (Young, 1990, p. 231). Immediacy, like a spell, would be broken by the detachment needed to explain or defend it. Defense is unnecessary in a community characterized by a common tradition, but few nurses practice in such a community. One of the hallmarks of contemporary nursing is the decline of moral immediacy (Benjamin & Curtis, 1992). In place of actual groups united by a single worldview, there are diffuse disciplines (Foucault, 1975/1979) and discourses (Bordo, 1993). They invite a form of immersion, but they unite individuals through abstract ideology rather than community identity (Gouldner, 1978).

Community-based certainty is not obsolete, however. Its contemporary form is communitarian ethics. Communitarians regard individuals as situated within a natural community such as the family, neighborhood, or nation, a community of origin that anchors personal identity and guarantees moral certainty (MacIntyre, 1981). For communitarians, immersion is the ideal form of moral knowledge and the only basis for ethical certainty.

Because the likelihood of a shared community is low for contemporary nurses, ethical immediacy will be challenged in most settings. Merely identifying an ethical issue (Should we allow this person to die?) undermines immediacy, since ethical issues do not arise in a premodern approach. Once a question is posed, there are two choices. One is to reinforce certainty using force, such as shame or exclusion, against the questioner, thereby ending inquiry and reinstating immediacy. The other option is to answer the challenge by articulating the basis for certainty. That response, however, entails translating subjective certainty into objective forms (language and reasons) that another could understand, and, in so doing, immediacy is shattered. When a person surfaces from ethical immersion to defend a view of the good, certainty is compromised and immediacy is lost.

MODERN DETACHMENT: ETHICAL UNIVERSALISM

Dialectically, the move away from immediacy produces its opposite, rational objectivity. Historically, the rational turn is symbolized by the Enlightenment celebration of reason as liberator from the Dark Ages of superstition, parochialism, and feudalism (Poole, 1991). In health care, too, an ethics based on rational principles has been heralded as a moral enlightenment following an era of professional feudalism known as paternalism (Beauchamp & Childress, 1994).

Because immersion in unquestioned certainty is an extreme form of ethical knowing, its antithesis too is uncompromising. Rationality counters subjectivity with principles that are categorical and unconditional. Detachment provides the distance needed for objectivity, for viewing from a vantage point outside, instead of inside, a situation. Freed from the limiting perspective of particularity, reason equals universality. The modern turn in ethics aims at overcoming the relativity of competing parochial certainties by producing one incontestable system of universal principles.

The strength of ethical universalism is epitomized by the principle of respecting individuals equally. Respect for individuals is based on the rational autonomy that each person possesses, the ability to transcend personal feelings in making universalistic choices. Formulated another way, ethical choices respect others as ends in themselves, affirming them as rationally autonomous and capable of transcendence; individuals are equivalent units of universality (Friedman, 1993). The principle is blind to actual identities of both the agent and the other, not unlike the double-blind design that assures objectivity in science. In nursing, the principle restrains us from discriminating against patients; prevents us from coercing, oppressing, or lying to them; and prevents our treating them as mere objects, material, or means to others' ends. In short, it commits us to a contract of reciprocity in which we respect the value that they and we share as universal, free persons.

Despite the appeal of rational principles, especially in health care, they provide less certainty than they promise. Three limitations of rational ethics can be identified. First, interpretations of a principle can conflict in clinical situations. A requirement to protect life can be interpreted as maintaining physiologic functioning or as alleviating suffering. One way to reconcile the conflict involves redefining terms so that life means quality of life, but for some nurses a life is more than its quality, while for others, suffering enhances the quality of a life. For still others, a nurse's view of life is irrelevant, because only the patient's view matters. Application of a principle, in other words, compromises its universality because interpretation is required, and interpretations differ according to the perspectives of the people involved.

A second limitation is the contradiction that universalism, alleged alternative to force, governs by force when it insists on the suppression of particularity, stripping from persons and situations their lived reality. Universal principles provide ethical knowledge in a situation only if all cases are alike but actual issues and the people involved are not identical. The only way a principle could provide solutions would be by force, that is, by requiring a nurse to suppress particular knowledge about a situation and blindly apply the principle; but that reduces a professional from an ethical agent to an automaton.

A feminist critique of universalism identifies a third limitation of rational ethics. That critique exposes the cultural hegemony of reason, specifically the oppressive authority of those whose status affords them the luxury of transcendence as long as others remain bound by conditions of hunger, exhaustion, or pain (Benhabib, 1992). Ethical universalism is founded on a dualist metaphysics in which reason is the essence of humanness, and other aspects (especially emotions and the body) are inessential, unruly, and, ideally, transcended. Because universalism values persons as transcendent, it devalues those experiences, already marginalized by dualism, that are not fully controllable, such as illness and suffering. The moral high ground of rationality becomes synonymous with privilege and power instead of the equality it promised.

The question raised by a critique of rationalism is whether nondualist respect is possible, valuing persons as irreducibly ambiguous: particular and universal, embodied and intellectual, emotional and rational. Dialectically, nondualist respect represents an ethical level beyond both immersion and detachment as sources of certainty, a third level characterized by uncertainty and engagement.

POSTMODERN ENGAGEMENT: RELATIONAL NARRATIVE

The move beyond rational objectivity in ethics can be considered an existential or postmodern turn. In existentialist ethics, the uniqueness of individuals is their essential feature. A self has a particular perspective as a situated subject. Transcendence is only the ability to imagine and appreciate different perspectives, not to assume a universal view from nowhere. The situated self encompasses not only rationality but emotion, imagination, memory, language, the body, and even other selves. Individuals are intrinsically relational; existential subjectivity is intersubjectivity.

Respect for persons as existential selves involves more than detached regard for abstract autonomy; it entails attentive discernment and valuing of an individual as unique. Dillon (1992) describes this discernment as care respect, because its valuing of particularity parallels that of care ethics. The valuing of persons requires perception of each one's uniqueness, and perception involves engagement. In contrast to rational ethics, which demands detachment in order not to perceive people concretely or respond to them personally, care respect conveys "cherishing, treasuring, profoundness of feeling" (p. 120).

The engagement of care respect is the opposite of ethical objectivity; it is personal responsiveness to the particular other, a relation between individuals that is grounded in the ambiguity of their being at once encumbered and free, situated and transcendent. Engagement cannot be regulated by principles; they would remove the relation from its grounding in actual persons and orient it toward external authority. Codes have no authority to command engagement. The only form that moral authority takes is authorization, the call from the other commanding concern simply by being the other. "The moral call is thoroughly personal, . . . the command is not universalizable" (Bauman, 1993, p. 51).

The move from rational principles to existential engagement is a postmodern turn. Postmodern ethics can be characterized as embracing contingency, refusing certainties, and resisting the modern drive for unity, order, and foundations (Bauman, 1995; Tester, 1993). Postmodernism expresses its resistance by dismantling the fixed meanings rationalism has constructed. Every form of order becomes a target for deconstruction, from the social, sexual, and political to the epistemological and metaphysical, but none is as inimical to postmodern ethics as the hermeneutic order, the modern hierarchy of meanings. In that hierarchy, rational meanings are authoritatively assigned, fixed rather than fluid, and ranked by their degree of objectivity. A diagnosis of HIV, for example, is assigned its correct meaning by clinical experts, the meaning remains constant among experts, and the assigned meaning

ranks higher on the hermeneutic scale than an emotional or imaginative interpretation by a person with the diagnosis. Significantly, experiences that pose the greatest threat to rational control—dying, illness, pain, dementia—become objects of the strictest hermeneutic control, often with disabling consequences. A social construction of aging, for example, as decline and deterioration can be more disabling than physical changes accompanying aging. From a postmodern perspective, the modern oppression through meanings represents hermeneutic terrorism in which experience is held hostage to authority.

Postmodernism destabilizes the hierarchy of meanings by displaying them as contingent, demonstrating that any interpretation of an experience can be revised because other meanings are always available. Moreover, no uninterpreted basis exists from which to decide objectively among meanings, "no neutral ground on which to stand and argue that either torture or kindness is preferable" (Rorty, 1989, p. 173). Our most trusted ethical certainties are our own creation. We may choose kindness rather than torture, but there is no authorization for our choice. Without a higher authority than ourselves, we have no certainty that our meanings are better than those of others. Ethically, we are on our own, without a metaphysical warrant from either religion or reason.

Meanings are contingent because they are human creations, but the most radical contingency is that of meaningfulness itself. The very enterprise of making meaning is conditional, never assured. It depends on our continuing acts of interpretation, always subject to the possibility that we may be overwhelmed into silence and incapable of interpretation. Scarry (1985) describes intense pain as world-destroying. Grief, fear, and despair also can unmake the meanings that comprise a person's world, including the central meaning of the person as meaning-maker. If disintegration of both world and self are possible, then meaningfulness itself, not just one or another meaning, is radically uncertain.

Radical contingency is not captured by the nihilist certainty that life is meaningless. That certainty in fact reassures us that there is no possibility of meaninglessness. Radical contingency is more serious. It lacks the comfortable universality of nihilism. It is the concrete possibility in each situation that meaning might not be created, a human interpretation might not be voiced in time to keep the world from ending. If I can say, at least, "this pain is meaningless," I am safe from meaninglessness. If I can say nothing because language is powerless or my voice is silenced, then my world ends.

Dismissing end-of-the-world talk is hubris, the modern certainty that there can be no gap in the plenum of meanings, no abyss into which one could fall. Nurses rarely indulge in that hubris. Most have glimpsed the abyss through a patient's eyes. At the edge of the abyss ethical certainties fail, and nothing remains except possible engagement between nurse and patient; but engagement is enough (without it a patient is alone, no matter how many nurses are present). The ethical narrative a nurse and patient compose through their engagement interprets the situation, saving it, for the moment, from meaninglessness.

Narrative meaning is communicative, the saying of something another can understand; it represents a "moral party of two" (Bauman, 1993, p. 82). Beyond that, it requires that at least one of the two is not silenced by their situation, remaining able to imagine and voice an interpretation: one of the two serves as their poet. "In times of strangeness, . . . by being strangers together, people and poet reconstitute an internal homeland" (Cixous, 1993, p. 26). That homeland for nurse and patient is the narrative they compose together, the words of their engagement.

Engagement includes the danger that the poet too will fall silent. By joining another in vulnerability, I myself become vulnerable, and the other's pain may silence me. Wordless, I can only turn to the other for meanings, as did the poet Akhmatova (1983), waiting with the other mothers outside Leningrad prisons, writing her poems with their words. In engagement, even authorship is contingent; "if Akhmatova, mother among mothers, writes with the mothers' meager words, then the mothers are also poets among poets" (Cixous, 1993, p. 27). In composing a narrative between nurse and patient, it does not matter who is author, because each is poet; it matters only that there are enough words between them to make a story.

The attempt to compose meanings, given their contingency, is flawed from a modern standpoint. The ethical knowledge created through a relational narrative is particular, contextual, and nongeneralizable; even its authorship is ambiguous when one person speaks with the other's words. An ethical narrative fails all criteria for objective knowledge, and terms like poem or story only further demean it in the rationalist view.

Dialectically, however, rationalism is flawed by its suppression of engagement as avenue to ethical knowledge. From a postmodern standpoint, modern ethics fails to grasp a significant feature of human experience, its narrative nature (Carr, 1986). To claim that "we lead storied lives" (Connelly & Clandinin, 1990, p. 2) is not only to point out that crafting stories is an important human activity, but, more fundamentally, to assert that an experience, in order to be my experience, has narrative form; it has to be fitted into the rest of my experience with a connecting meaning, a thread of sense, even if sensible only for me. To make sense of experience is to make the narrative connection, to relate otherwise inchoate events to my story, the life I am living as mine (LeGuin, 1989).

Nursing has (re)discovered narrative as a form of coherence in the absence of encompassing certainties. Through narrative intervention patients can be helped to create emancipatory narratives, that is, to revise disabling into enabling views that allow movement toward a self with possibilities (Sandelowski, 1994). Ethical narratives are emancipatory in their portrayal of a good toward which a person can move. Because individuals are particular, situated, and self-interpreting, the most faithful way to know the good they seek is through their own accounts, their personal ethical narratives. At times of vulnerability, however, personal narratives can fail, just as ethical certainties fail in the face of radical contingency. In those moments a new narrative is needed, and help may be needed to compose it. Ethical narratives created by patient and nurse from the homeland of their engagement are thus more than individual accounts: they are relational narratives.

Because a relational narrative expresses engagement, it extends beyond the particularity of either person alone but does not extend beyond their relationship; it is more than personal but not universal (Gadow, 1994, 1995). It embodies intersubjectivity, an alternative to both the subjectivity of immersion and the objectivity of detachment. The paradox of a relational narrative is that it narrates uncertainty, but in so doing can offer a safer home, existentially, than would be found in subjective or objective certainty. Either of those would cost the nurse and patient their relationship. Their lived reality together would be displaced. The aim of relational narrative is to provide a place of shared, and therefore safer, contingency. By combining contingencies through engagement, persons are able to coauthor an interpretation that may be more inhabitable than either of their individual narratives as they seek a new form of the good.

A DIALECTICAL FRAMEWORK IN PRACTICE

I have proposed that the philosophical cornerstone of nursing is dialectically layered rather than unitary. The question now emerges: What would the dialectic among different ethical layers look like in practice?

A dialectic can be reduced to ideology by theorizing a telos that draws the movement toward a final level. To avoid that reduction and its coerciveness, I suggest that the three ethical approaches be regarded not as successive stages in the profession's advance, but as possibilities coexisting in an ethically vital practice. Dialectic offers a way of envisioning contradictory approaches as intrinsically related. None of the three is fully intelligible without its connection to the others. Each complements the limitations of the other two. Dialectic as a philosophical framework is more than a heuristic device for conceptualizing nursing. It is a also a framework for the continuing development of the discipline. If otherwise opposing approaches can be appreciated as inseparable, they may then be acknowledged in practice as being mutually enhancing instead of oppositional. Nursing becomes more than a moral high ground from which difference is excluded. It becomes, instead, a region of existence large enough to accommodate, even encourage, diversity among those who live there.

Just as a geographic region cannot be conveyed in its totality by a map, an existential region cannot be captured in a theory, but something of its vitality can be rendered by images. In a beginning attempt to answer the question of how a dialectical framework might look in practice, I offer instead of theory a metaphor and a clinical example that may serve as an impetus to further exploration.

The flourishing of premodern, modern, and postmodern ethics in nursing can be imagined metaphorically as the biodiversity of a coral reef where different life forms integrate and where organisms even after their death provide a structure that supports life. At the level of immediacy, we are immersed in ethical currents that carry us safely through situations where reflection would be impossible. When crosscurrents require us to reflect and to hold a position, an edifice of ethical principles offers a structure for steadying ourselves. Finally, there are situations where no edifice can alleviate our vulnerability, and in those cases we can only turn to each other and together compose a fragile new form of the good.

To illustrate, I consider the reef-like situation described by Schroeder (1998) in which Carole (mother) and Morgan (daughter) found themselves while Morgan spent the first 3 months of life undergoing surgical heart repairs, inept and relentless technical procedures, and near-fatal nursing and medical errors. Schroeder's description does not indict professionals for being unethical, but displays instead the inevitable collisions when a mother's immersion in her daughter's danger meets the detachment of ethical objectivity.

> "How can she be in congestive heart failure if I'm rooming-in?"

> He looked impatiently at me. "You're a nurse. Call the intensive care nursery if her respirations go over 60".

Instead of calling, Carole brought her baby into bed with her, pulled the blanket over them, and unplugged the phone, mutely sinking into the quicksand of isolation that immersion becomes when no hand is offered.

Hands eventually were offered from each of the three ethical layers. All of them were essential to the survival of both mother and child.

1. From the urgency of another mother's immersion in her own child's situation:

> "Get her out of here no matter what," she whispered, . . . "Get her out of here if she is getting better at all"

And from the same mother, the offer of community in an informal group where mothers' stories to each other kept them from drowning in the immediacy of their children's pain.

2. From the honesty of a nurse who countered institutional hierarchy with her own ethical autonomy:

> One day, Lea told me that the physicians at this hospital were unable to do anything further for Morgan. . . . Although she merely confirmed what I had already been thinking, I was unable to summon the strength to act upon my thoughts without her support. I now know that Morgan would have died in that hospital cubicle if Lea had not risked angering the physicians and telling me the truth.

3. From a nurse whose overtures opened the door to a different story, to engagement instead of isolation:

> Carolyn would ignore my hostile looks and sit with me at Morgan's bedside on work breaks . . . Her words and presence began to fill some of the emptiness inside me. Although I would never admit it to her, I began to look forward to her visits, and eventually we began to communicate on a level very foreign to our previous working relationship

And from a nurse who transcended moral duties:

> Cathy came out of the ICU and said that they were trying to get her off the heart-lung machine now; "I'll be right back to let you know," she said, and walked back into the ICU. I stared at the door, awestruck at her bravery. She'll have to let me know, I marveled, now she can't just stay behind those doors and let someone else tell me the news. I felt ready to handle anything, almost exhilarated that someone would risk so much when it wasn't even required

The coral reef that I believe Schroeder describes is ethically layered. Modern, premodern, and postmodern elements alternately prevailed. The situation would have been ethically diminished by an absence of any of the elements. Philosophically, the dialectical nature of nursing entails the presence of all of them. Without a telos to drive the dialectic, there is no basis on which to insist that nursing limit itself to one. The postmodern turn only makes explicit an element that has been implicit; it does not establish a superior ground from which to dismiss the others. In the case of Carole and Morgan, no single element was decisive in determining the ethical course to pursue. They did escape, as the first mother urged, but not before a nurse had urged moving to a better hospital where surgery was successful, and not until other nurses had offered engagement as alternative to immersion.

A dialectical ethical narrative such as Schroeder provides is the equivalent of a relational narrative that a nurse and patient together create. Both narratives are layered with voices from immediacy and objectivity in a continuing tension that cannot be resolved in favor of either without destruction of the narrative's relational nature, its contingency and vitality. The postmodern turn is not an advance that dismisses immersion and detachment as ethical approaches. It is instead a turn toward the absurd, as Camus (1955) would call it, the cultivation of a life "without appeal" (p. 39) in which the longing for certainty and the impossibility of certainty are both embraced passionately. From a modern or premodern perspective, that contradiction is absurd in the sense of being hopeless. From the postmodern perspective, an absurd life is filled with "a wild kind of hope" (Schroeder, 1998, p. 20).

The practice of an absurd life, an absurd ethics, is dialectical because it grants at once the validity of subjective and objective ethics. In nursing the story of that practice can only be intersubjective, a relational narrative. The narrative is layered with voices of immersion and detachment like a medieval motet in which several voices simultaneously sing parts of the text that counter and complement one another (Gadow, 1999). Perhaps the fact that a philosophical cornerstone can be compared metaphorically to a phenomenon as ephemeral as a song is one more indication of the postmodern turn in nursing ethics.

REFERENCES

Akhmatova, A. (1983). *Poems*. New York: Norton.

Bauman, Z. (1993). *Postmodern ethics*. Oxford, England: Blackwell Publishers.

Bauman, Z. (1995). *Life in fragments: Essays in postmodern morality*. Oxford, England: Blackwell Publishers.

Beauchamp, T., & Childress, J. (1994). *Principles of biomedical ethics* (4th ed.). Oxford, England: Oxford University Press.

Benhabib, S. (1992). *Situating the self: Gender, community and postmodernism in contemporary ethics*. London: Routledge.

Benjamin, M., & Curtis, J. (1992). *Ethics in nursing* (3rd ed.). Oxford, England: Oxford University Press.

Bloom, L. R. (1992). How can we know the dancer from the dance?: Discourses of the self-body. *Human Studies, 15*, 313–334.

Bordo, S. (1993). *Unbearable weight: Feminism, western culture, and the body*. Los Angeles: University of California Press.

Camus, A. (1955). *The myth of Sisyphus and other essays*. New York: Vintage Books.

Carr, D. (1986). *Time, narrative, and history*. Bloomington, IN: Indiana University Press.

Cixous, H. (1993). We who are free, are we free? In B. Johnson (Ed.), *Freedom and interpretation: The Oxford Amnesty Lectures, 1992* (pp. 14–44). New York: HarperCollins.

Connelly, F., & Clandinin, D. (1990). Stories of experience and narrative inquiry. *Educational Researcher, 19*(5), 2–14.

Dillon, R. (1992). Respect and care: Toward moral integration. *Canadian Journal of Philosophy, 22*, 105–131.

Foucault, M. (1979). *Discipline and punish: The birth of the prison* (A. Sheridan, Trans.). New York: Vintage Books. (Original work published 1975)

Friedman, M. (1993). *What are friends for? Feminist perspectives on personal relationships and moral theory*. Ithaca, NY: Cornell University Press.

Gadow, S. (1982). Body and self: A dialectic. In V. Kestenbaum (Ed.), *The humanity of the ill: Phenom-*

enological perspectives (pp. 86–100). Knoxville, TN: University of Tennessee Press.

Gadow, S. (1994). Whose body? Whose story? The question about narrative in women's health care. *Soundings, 77,* 295–307.

Gadow, S. (1995). Clinical epistemology: A dialectic of nursing assessment. *Canadian Journal of Nursing Research, 27,* 25–34.

Gadow, S. (1999). *I felt an island rising: Interpretive inquiry as motet.* Manuscript submitted for publication.

Gouldner, A. (1978). *The dialectic of ideology and technology: The origins, grammar, and future of ideology.* Oxford, England: Oxford University Press.

Hegel, G. W. F. (1977). *The phenomenology of spirit* (A. V. Miller, Trans.). Oxford, England: Clarendon. (Original work published in 1807)

LeGuin, U. (1989). Some thoughts on narrative. In U. LeGuin (Ed.), *Dancing at the edge of the world: Thoughts on words, women, places* (pp. 37–45). New York: Harper & Row.

MacIntyre, A. (1981). *After virtue.* Notre Dame, IN: University of Notre Dame Press.

Poole, R. (1991). *Morality and modernity.* London: Routledge.

Rorty, R. (1989). *Contingency, irony, and solidarity.* Cambridge, England: Cambridge University Press.

Sandelowski, M. (1994). We are the stories we tell: Narrative knowing in nursing practice. *Journal of Holistic Nursing, 12,* 23–33.

Scarry, E. (1985). *The body in pain: The making and unmaking of the world.* Oxford, England: Oxford University Press.

Schroeder, C. (1998). So this is what it's like: Struggling to survive in pediatric intensive care. *Advances in Nursing Science, 20,* 13–22.

Tester, K. (1993). *The life and times of post-modernity.* London: Routledge.

Young, I. (1990). *Justice and the politics of difference.* Princeton, NJ: Princeton University Press.

14

Expressing Health through Lifestyle Patterns

NOLA J. PENDER, RN, PhD, FAAN

Few concepts have received more attention from health professionals and the public during the last decade than health. This is largely due to the emergence of disease prevention and health promotion as global priorities. Unfortunately, the nature of health as a positive life process is poorly understood. Theoretical formulations of health often lack specificity and existing measures almost without exception reflect a narrow clinical perspective of health as the absence of disease. The purpose of this chapter is to propose a system for classifying expressions of health of persons in their entirety and to suggest related indicators of high-level health.

During the last decade nursing, as well as other health disciplines, has recognized the limitations of medical and technological approaches for improving the quality of life and health of the world's population. Major changes in social, political, and environmental conditions of living and the life ways of large segments of society are necessary, if significant improvements in health are to occur during the next century. Thus, disease prevention and health promotion have become global agendas with the potential for achieving health goals unattainable previously through curative interventions. The escalating commitment to health promotion among nations raises important questions concerning the nature of health. What is the *critical essence* of that which is to be promoted? A review of relevant scientific literature confirms that health as a human life span process is poorly understood.

Historically, illness, not health, has been the primary concern of the health professions and mortality and morbidity the indicators of "health" used most frequently (Smith, 1981). Therefore, it is not surprising that in reviewing studies of health, Terris (1975) identified the following illness-related approaches to health assessment: measurement of impairment, assessment of physiological systems in relation to established norms, and measurement of performance in the context of potential decrements. The concept of health has not fared much better in nursing. Although health along with person, environment, and nursing constitute the commonly accepted metaparadigm of the discipline (Fawcett, 1984), the concept of health seems to elude clear theoretical descriptions and, to an even greater extent, useful empirical specifications. Reynolds (1988), in reviewing the measures of health used in reports of nursing research, found that, despite articulation of a holistic concept of health in dominant theoretical views within

Source: Pender, N. J. (1990). Expressing health through lifestyle patterns. *Nurse Science Quarterly, 3* (3): 115-122. Reprinted by permission of and copyright © 2002 Sage Publications, Inc.

the discipline, nurse scientists tended to use indicators derived from a clinical model as the absence of disease.

Is health such a complex human process that it cannot be studied qualitatively or quantitatively? Is high-level health a utopian state, a mirage to be fantasized but never achieved (Dubos, 1965)? On the other hand, if health can be the object of systematic investigation, can it *only* be defined by negation, that is as the absence of disease? Unwilling to settle for such a narrow definition, various health disciplines have attempted to define health from fragmented perspectives placing primary emphasis on psychological, sociological, cultural, or spiritual dimensions. Some attempts have been made to synthesize these perspectives to achieve a complete view of health. Parse (1987) refers to this approach as the totality paradigm, in which persons are considered as biopsychosocial spiritual beings responding and adapting to their environment. A major question about this additive approach is whether the whole is equal to or greater than the sum of the parts.

PERSON AND HEALTH: NEW VIEWS OF OLD CONCEPTS

Within the past two decades in nursing, there has been a significant conceptual shift toward viewing persons as unified wholes possessing integrity and manifesting characteristics that are more than and different from the sum of the parts. According to Rogers (1970),

> The unity of man is a reality. Man interacts with his environment in his totality. Only as man's wholeness is perceived does the study of man begin to yield meaningful concepts and theories. Only as man's oneness is apprehended is it possible to identify man's distinctive attributes. (p. 44)

This shift in nursing toward a unitary view of human beings has resulted in increasing reliance on the tenets of human science in addition to the reductionistic paradigm of traditional science for understanding health. How do individuals *experience* health and what *meanings* do they give these experiences have emerged as central questions within the discipline. Tripp-Reimer (1984) suggested that within nursing, health be reconceptualized to incorporate both etic and emic perspectives. In the etic perspective, objective observations without input from those observed are used to determine health. In the emic perspective, the meaning of health to individuals within their particular culture is ascertained. Concerns relevant in the latter perspective include, How is health expressed? Is the expression of health universal or culture specific? Are expressions of health qualitatively different at various developmental phases throughout the life span?

In contrast to the totality paradigm based primarily on the etic perspective, the simultaneity paradigm (Parse, Coyne, & Smith, 1985) captures the emic perspective. Within the latter paradigm each person is viewed as a synergistic being in open, mutual, and simultaneous interchange with the environment. In this context health is a wholistic unfolding of humans in interaction with the environment in which all the elements or dimensions of health are experienced as a unitary phenomenon. Based on Rogers's theory of unitary human beings, Newman (1979) defined health as the totality of the life process evolving toward expanded consciousness. Parse (Parse et al., 1985), also in the Rogerian tradition, described health as a "process of becoming uniquely lived by each individual . . . a nonlinear entity that cannot be qualified by terms such as *good, bad, more,* or *less.* Unitary man's health is a synthesis of values, a way of living . . . a continuously changing process that man cocreates" (pp. 9-10). Definitions with similar themes have been offered by Pender (1982), who described health as the actualization of inherent and acquired human potential and Watson (1988) who defined health as harmony with self and environment. A new approach for combining objective (etic) and subjective (emic) health perspectives is needed to avoid a conception of health in which observable physical and behavioral aspects are viewed as separate or in oppositional relationship to experiential aspects. It is the author's belief that both perspectives are valuable and can coexist within the discipline of nursing.

Along with acceptance of a unitary view of health, there is an increasing tendency in nursing to reject the health-illness continuum which Newman (1979) criticized on the grounds that it maintains a false dichotomy by polarizing health at one end of the continuum and illness at the other end. If nursing is to facilitate a client's movement toward health on the health-illness continuum, this must *always* be away from illness. An "either-or" dichotomy precludes the existence of high levels of health in the presence of a disability or chronic illness. This belief, if carried to its logical conclusion, would imply that health promotion efforts are futile for millions of Americans young and old who have a chronic disease incurable by existing medical means. Health promotion would only be considered appropriate for the favored few without any evidence of disease, thus disenfranchising the poor, the old, and the disabled of services directed toward optimizing their health. To address this dilemma, Newman (1979) suggested a synthesis of the concepts of diseases and nondisease into an integrative concept of health.

Taking another theoretical approach to the problem posed by the health-illness continuum, Pender (1987) described health as the primary life experience with illness superimposed on health. Health can exist without illness, but illness never exists without health as its context. When illness occurs, it is synthesized as part of the ongoing health experience modifying it in varying ways—changing the quality of the experience, and *decreasing* or *increasing* overall feelings and perceptions of health. Unlike Parse (1981), who rejects the idea of health as existing to varying degrees, Smith (1981) views health as a comparative term. It has long been recognized that all persons free of disease are not equally healthy. It is the degree to which health is present from both objective and subjective points of view that should be mutually assessed by nurse and client. It is only on the basis of both perspectives that effective efforts can be directed toward appropriate health enhancement activities.

The dominant definition of health espoused by a society has profound political and economic implications because the dimensions of that definition and their associated measures often become major social concerns. Frequently, programs of national and international scope are established to bring about positive changes in the identified indicators of health (McDowell & Newell, 1987). Thus, the discipline of nursing faces one of its biggest challenges in decades—how to best articulate the dimensions of health of persons in their entirety and develop valid and reliable indicators of health as a unitary phenomenon. Such indicators must be articulated with a level of conceptual clarity that permits communication of this perspective to other health disciplines and the public. The clinical view of health as the absence of disease has been the dominant definition in the United States for decades. It is time for a paradigmatic shift to a unitary conception of health that will enable society to deal capably with the multiplicity of factors now known to have an impact on health status.

As nursing moves forward in developing a unitary concept of health, strongly influenced by the tenets of human science, the discipline should not lose sight of empiricism as a viable approach to health-related research. Some questions asked about health are best addressed within a traditional science paradigm. For example, health processes outside of conscious awareness may be observable using highly sophisticated methods and techniques (Norbeck, 1987). Nursing can provide leadership to the health disciplines in blending the approaches of traditional and human sciences. Differences between the two paradigms should not be interpreted as conflict but as integrative tension that promotes creativity in scientific endeavors (Kritek, 1989).

HEALTH AS PATTERN

Rogers (1970) identified the energy field as the fundamental unit of the universe for the science of nursing. The human and environmental fields are coextensive and in an intimate relationship. Pattern is the distinguishing characteristic of an energy field, which becomes more complex throughout the life span. Persons shape their own health experiences to a considerable extent as they make choices from the options available to them (Parse, 1981). Innate to energy fields are generative powers that can facilitate positive patterning and repatterning, resulting in progressively healthier conditions of being, as objectively measured and subjectively reported.

There is no single, universal health pattern that all human beings share. Health when viewed as a lived experience, that is, within the emic perspective, represents many alternative realities. Only individuals can reveal the hidden meanings that they create for health. Although health has many different shades of meaning, there are recurring themes or commonalities that persons report as expressions of health when queried as to what health means to them. The critical question is, What are the varying human patterns most indicative of health?

DIMENSIONS OF THE HEALTH EXPERIENCE

In 1981, Smith proposed a model of health with four dimensions reflective of existing lit-

erature: the clinical dimension defining health as the absence of disease, the role performance dimension describing health as competent performance of socially defined roles, the adaptive dimension characterizing health as flexible adjustment to changing life situations, and the eudaimonistic dimension viewing health as exuberant well-being. Laffrey (1986) operationalized Smith's model in a scale intended to determine the extent to which individuals viewed health along each of these dimensions. In further research Woods and colleagues (1988) supported the health conception model of Smith in a study of 528 women who were asked, "What do you mean when you say you are in good health?" Their work contributed to the further elaboration of the eudaimonistic view of health identifying nine images consistent with this dimension: actualizing self, practicing healthy life ways, positive self-concept, positive body image, social involvement, fitness, effective cognitive function, positive mood, and harmony.

Parse (Parse et al., 1985) conducted a phenomenological study of 400 men and women who were asked to write descriptions of a personal situation in which a feeling of health was experienced. Recurring themes were identified for persons of differing ages. As an example, the recurring themes for persons between 20 and 45 years of age as expressed within the theoretical framework of man-living-health were: spirited intensity, fulfilling inventiveness, and symphonic integrity.

CLASSIFYING EXPRESSIONS OF HEALTH

In this section, a system for classifying human expressions of health is proposed. Five dimensions of human health expression are organized further into 15 subcategories as shown in Table 18.1. This framework for studying health has emerged as a result of discussions with colleagues, review of the literature, and

TABLE 18.1.   Classification System for Expressions of Health

Affect			
Serenity	*Harmony*	*Vitality*	*Sensitivity*
Calm	Close to God	Energetic	Aware
Relaxed	Contemplative	Vigorous	Connected
Peaceful	At one with the universe	Zestful	Intimate
Content		Alert	Loving
Comfortable		Fit	
Glowing		Buoyant	
Happy		Exhilarated	
Joyous		Powerful	
Pleasant		Courageous	
Satisfied			

Attitudes		
Optimism	*Relevancy*	*Competency*
Hopeful	Useful	Purposive
Enthusiastic	Contributing	Initiating
Open	Valued	Self-motivating
Reverent	Caring	Self-affirming
Trustful	Committed	Innovative
	Involved	Masterful
		Challenged

Activity		
Positive Life Patterns	*Meaningful Work*	*Invigorating Play*
Eating a healthy diet	Setting realistic goals	Having meaningful hobbies
Exercising regularly	Varying activities	Engaging in satisfying leisure
Managing stress	Undertaking challenging tasks	activities
Obtaining adequate rest	Assuming responsibility for self	Planning energizing diversions
Avoiding harmful substances	Collaborating with coworkers	
Building positive relationships	Receiving intrinsic or extrinsic	
Seeking and using health information	rewards	
Monitoring health		
Coping constructively		
Maintaining a health-strengthening environment		

Aspirations	
Self-Actualization	*Social Contribution*
Growth or emergence	Enhancement of global harmony and interdependence
Personal effectiveness	Preservation of the environment
Organismic efficiency	

Accomplishments		
Enjoyment	*Creativity*	*Transcendence*
Pleasure from daily living	Maximum use of capacities	Freedom
Sense of achievement	Innovative contribution	Expansion of consciousness
		Optimized harmony between man and environment

reflection on 5 years of quantitative and qualitative research conducted by a health promotion research team (S. N. Walker, K. R. Sechrist, M. F. Stromborg, & N. J. Pender.) in which the health and health practices of approximately 2,000 adults were studied. The following assumptions undergird the proposed classification:

1. Integration of the views of clients as well as health professionals is essential to derive a useful definition of health.
2. Health is a manifestation of person/environment interactional patterns that become increasingly complex throughout the life span.
3. Some human health patterns can be directly observed, others must be self-reported.

The five dimensions within the classification are expressed in common language and the alliteration, although originally unintended, may be useful. Each of the five dimensions of health expression—affect, attitudes, activity, aspirations, and accomplishments—should be assessed in terms of daily fluctuations as well as evolving patterns over time. The five dimensions are proposed as culture-free whereas some of the 15 subcategories and potential indicators may be culture-specific. Tools already exist to measure some of the suggested indicators; for others, approaches to description and/or measurement remain undeveloped. Consistent with a unitary view of human beings, a comprehensive assessment tool could be constructed to assess all of the dimensions simultaneously.

AFFECT

Sensation and emotion are fundamental attributes of humanness that are expressions of wholeness or unity (Rogers, 1970). *Affect* as used here is intended to denote emotions and feelings as subjectively experienced. Affect can be assessed best through personal report, but facial expressions, body positions, or gestures, as well as an increasing array of technologic measures (biofeedback, electromagnetic resonance imaging), can provide some indication of internal emotional states. The link between emotions and illness has been suspected for centuries, but little has been known about feelings as an expression of health. Recent research in psychoneuroimmunology indicates that person/environment interactions and accompanying emotional responses may moderate immune function (Kiecolt-Glaser & Glaser, 1987). Certain emotional patterns such as serenity and harmony may enhance immune competence; their polar opposites may impair immune capabilities. There is also considerable evidence that physiological changes related to activity have an impact on emotions. For example, production of endogenous opiates or internal tranquilizers can contribute to emotional experiences of comfort and calm (Watkins & Mayer, 1982).

Feelings and emotions have a direct effect on the quality of the lived experience of health. The emotions identified in Table 18.1 are those frequently reported as expressions of high-level health. *Serenity* is a sense of tranquility, a peaceful inner state, amid life's ebb and flow. *Harmony* emanates from feelings of relatedness to God and/or the universe and is sometimes described as a feeling of being at peace with nature and fellow humans. *Vitality* is a sense of energy and power. *Sensitivity* is intense knowing of self and others. Feelings of serenity, harmony, vitality, and sensitivity at any moment reflect much more than the current life situation. Human beings have the unique ability to evoke emotions in response to remembered events from the past or anticipated events in the future. This capacity provides persons with the power to transcend current situations; to be unbound by time and space. Persons may be calm, content, or even joyous in the face of difficult situations because of their vision of a greater good to be attained in the future.

Exploration of emotions as important expressions of health presents many exciting challenges to the research community. Current research on the connections between emotions and illness need to be recast in a positive perspective. Research questions from this viewpoint might be, What person/environment interaction patterns encourage positive emotions? Which emotional patterns or fluctuations in patterns are healthful, which are unhealthful, and are these effects general or person-specific? Are different emotional profiles expressive of health at different points in the life span? What interventions on the part of health professionals assist clients in achieving positive emotional patterns? What self-care strategies can increase the frequency of positive emotions? Do emotions perceived as negative detract from or at times promote health?

Emotions can be a positive integrative force (Rogers, 1970). It is the richness of emotional experience that is uniquely human. Research approaches must be used that capture this richness as well as rhythms and fluctuations in emotional patterns. Recent scientific breakthroughs in understanding emotions will fuel increased interest and expanded research efforts in this area in the next decades.

ATTITUDES

Language, thought, and the ability to form attitudes and beliefs characterize unitary human beings and result from innate capacities to abstract and image features or person/environment interaction. Humans not only think in concepts and relationships but give meanings to such abstractions. According to Rogers (1970) persons seek to organize the world of experience and make sense of it and can do so because of the capacity for rational thought. Attitudes structure the way persons see their world and, like emotions, express persons' values and priorities.

Attitudes can be developed in relation to specific situations, events, or actions. Life in its entirety can be viewed as an event. As such, persons develop attitudes or beliefs about their own personal lived situation as well as the life process as a shared experience with others. It is these general attitudes or beliefs that are proposed to profoundly influence health.

Attitudes expressive of high-level health are presented in Table 18.1. These are recurring cognitive themes in the literature and in more than 75 in-depth interviews conducted by the author and her colleagues with persons considered to have stellar health behaviors. Three subcategories of attitudes have been proposed: optimism, relevancy, and competency.

Attitudes toward life, its value, meaning, and ultimate worth are reflected in the subcategory of *optimism*. Beliefs that all will end well despite life's changing circumstances and that there are possibilities for personal growth even in difficult situations is expressed through an optimistic outlook. Optimism is enhanced by reverence for life and trust in God or the orderliness of the universe. Optimism expands openness to creative possibilities in life patterns.

Relevancy is grasping one's place in the world with an appreciation for unique, personal contributions. Relevancy is expressed through self-respect and a feeling of acceptance by others as a useful and contributing member of society. Persons experiencing a sense of relevance are caring, committed, and involved in life. Relevancy also has an eternal time frame by which persons come to appreciate the importance of their personal existence within infinite time and space.

Competency is expressed in personal clarity about actual and potential capabilities and belief in the power to channel capabilities into meaningful patterns of work and play. Competent persons actively initiate challenging life situations. They are interactive rather than passive, challenged rather than threatened, and self-affirming rather than self-debasing. Perceptions of personal competency are transferred to fellow humans with resultant appreciation of their unique patterns and emergent potential.

Positive attitudes and beliefs express high-level wellness. They are an integral part of health as a lived experience.

ACTIVITY

Movement is an alternative to language for communicating thought (Engle, 1984). Activity reflects patterns of energy distribution as well as person/environment rhythmicity. Movement is a means whereby space and time become experienced reality (Newman, 1979). Movement augments awareness of human and environmental fields. According to Newman, the total pattern of movement reflects the organization or disorganization of the thought and feeling processes of the individual. Activity expressive of health facilitates the fuller emergence of personal potential. Three dimensions of activity considered expressive of health are positive life patterns, meaningful work, and invigorating play (see Table 18.1).

Positive life patterns go beyond isolated health practices to action patterns that are an integral part of life ways. Thoughtful patterning and repatterning of daily routines and rhythms through informed decision making based on an awareness of options enhance human capacity for optimal well-being. Clusters of behaviors with empirical support for their health-enhancing properties are the backbone of positive life patterns. Eating well,

exercising regularly, obtaining adequate rest, and managing stress represent behavioral clusters comprising positive life patterns. Such patterns must be sustained over time to optimize health. Exercise as one behavioral cluster expressive of health is a good example of unitary characteristics. If exercise is to be maintained, it must be of appropriate rhythmicity, periodicity, complexity, and intensity for a given human field. Human and environmental fields must have compatible activity rhythms and patterns to optimize health.

Health is also expressed through *meaningful work*. More energy is expended on work than on any other human activity. Work that is health-promoting has been characterized as challenging, varied, well-directed, interpersonally satisfying, and both intrinsically and extrinsically rewarding. In recent years attempts have been made to achieve greater harmony between human fields and work patterns. Child care, flexible time, job sharing, and use of home as a satellite work site are only a few of the examples of greater awareness of the need for compatibility between person/environment patterning and work.

The rhythm between work and *invigorating play* changes throughout life. For most children, play constitutes the major activity in which they engage. In fact, meaningful work as an expression of health may not be relevant until the preschool or school years when confronted by the "tasks" of learning. The harmonious integration of work and play often becomes disrupted in young, middle-aged, and older adult years. Young and middle-aged adults, in striving to be successful, to achieve adequate pay, and to contribute meaningfully to society, may neglect play. Some compensate for this imbalance by focusing on enjoyable aspects of work and reinterpreting work as play. Older adults often have considerable discretionary time for play but lament lack of resources for recreational pursuits or the absence of meaningful work. It is predicted that leisure time will expand for many persons in the United States in the future as efforts are made to maximize the employment rate in a large and diverse population (Bezold, Carlson, & Peck, 1986). For both younger adults on shortened work weeks and the aging population in part-time employment, meaningful hobbies, satisfying leisure activities, and energizing diversions will be increasingly important as expressions of personal health.

ASPIRATIONS

Human beings are inherently purposeful. Life is not a random series of events, but an organized unfolding of each individual in light of personal aspirations and choices. Persons choose the directions in which they evolve in light of the range of options within awareness. Unfortunately, for persons in disadvantaged groups such as the poor and some ethnic/racial minorities, the range of choices is often constricted, limiting options for self-realization. Unnecessary limitations on self-expression is dehumanizing as well as detrimental to the continuing viability and vitality of a society.

The capacity of human beings to bring about changes in human and environmental fields is important for achievement of aspirations and goals. By modifying the nature of person/environment interactions, individuals can maximize available choices. Although persons usually have considerable freedom of choice concerning the goals they will pursue, the goals selected must be compatible with those of society. Social and cultural values as well as the needs of significant others provide a context for setting goals. Inherent in humanness is the moral responsibility for the ethical selection of goals and the means used to accomplish them.

Aspirations within a society often reflect normative patterns—the usual rather than

the unusual, the average rather than the exception. Fitting in to societal norms rather than exceeding them is often condoned and encouraged to the detriment of creative change. Individuals possess unique capabilities for self-transcendence (Sarter, 1988). It is only as society encourages people to achieve their uniqueness unconstrained by normative expectations that we will have instances of maximized human health potential for systematic study.

Self-actualization and social contribution are proposed as two subcategories of aspirations needing further clarification and study in relation to human health patterns. Self-actualization is not a new term. Maslow (1970) popularized the concept in his writings as a high-level need for human organisms. *Self-actualization* is predicated on fulfilling a more basic need for self-preservation. Suggested empirical indicators for self-actualization are growth or self-emergence, personal effectiveness, and organismic efficiency. Self-actualization is an orientation toward being all one can be and fulfilling one's personal potential.

Social contribution enhances global harmony, creates health interdependence, and promotes an ecologically balanced environment for present and future generations. The community in which we live is a world community in which annihilation is an ever present threat. Social contribution as an expression of health is a sensitivity to the needs and potentials of all people, which results in responsible social actions within a particular life situation. It is through shared aspirations of aggregates that social changes supportive of health are realized.

ACCOMPLISHMENTS

Accomplishments as expressions of health can be identified as the payoffs for a life well lived. They are unencumbered by time and space and may be viewed as daily achievements, life attainments, or states to be experienced only after death. Regardless of the time frame, persons need bench marks to measure their progress, their emergence as unique human beings. Accomplishments confirm a person's selfhood as well as his or her oneness with the evolving universe.

In modern society, accomplishments are often viewed as measures of worth rather than as expressions of health. Too frequently, being and becoming are sacrificed to doing, thus destroying the balance among affect, attitudes, activity, aspirations, and accomplishments. When kept in proper perspective, accomplishments contribute to the richness of human experience. Creative achievements of human beings throughout history have markedly enhanced the quality of life for others.

Enjoyment, creativity, and transcendence are accomplishments proposed as expressive of health (see Table 18.1). *Enjoyment* is a condition in which there is heightened aesthetic awareness of the multiple dimensions of human and environmental fields. Positive emotions and thoughts predominate. Daily experiences are sources of joy. Human unfolding, its challenges and exigencies as well as successive stages of development provide continuing sources of pleasure.

The capacity for *creativity* is inherent in all human beings. It is expressed through envisioning new configurations within human and environmental fields and restructuring reality or abstractions consistent with these envisioned patterns. Creativity is experienced as performing at one's optimum, maximizing human capabilities, and accelerating diversity and complexity.

Transcendence is stretching beyond the realm of human experience toward new options and possibilities (Parse, 1981). It is experienced as freedom from constraint and expansion of human consciousness to encompass infinite time and space. It is the experience of optimum mutuality and harmony between person and environment.

Accomplishments are the expression of life purpose and thus the expression of health. Their pursuit directs human patterning and evolutionary emergence.

CONCLUDING COMMENTS

Health is a life span process, a largely subjective and private experience, only partially observable by traditional scientific methods. Although defining health only in terms of negation, that is, as the absence of disease, has been common practice for more than a century, this approach will no longer suffice in an era of increasing concern about the promotion of health and the quality of life for human populations. Health as an experience is not fragmented, it only becomes fragmented in the minds of health professionals with differing perspectives. A new view of health is needed that is positive, comprehensive, unifying, and humanistic. This article represents one attempt to move toward that goal. It is imperative that an increasing number of nurse scientists direct their efforts toward expanding our understanding of human health processes and the personal, social, political, and environmental factors affecting the health of differing populations if significant progress is to be made in optimizing health for a larger segment of the world population in the years ahead.

REFERENCES

Bezold, C., Carlson, R., & Peck, J. (1986). *The future of work and health*. Dover, MA: Auburn House.

Dubos, R. (1965). *Man adapting*. New Haven, CT: Yale University Press.

Engle, V. F. (1984). Newman's conceptual framework and the measurement of older adults' health. *Advances in Nursing Science, 7*(1), 24-36.

Fawcett, J. (1984). *Analysis and evaluation of conceptual models of nursing.* Philadelphia: Davis.

Kiecolt-Glaser, J., & Glaser, R. (1987). Psychosocial moderators of immune function. *Annals of Behavioral Medicine, 9,* 16-20.

Kritek, P. (1989, April). *Nursing research enterprise in clinical practice: An agenda for the future.* Paper presented at Northern Illinois University Annual Research Conference, DeKalb, IL.

Laffrey, S. C. (1986). Development of a health conception scale. *Research in Nursing and Health, 9,* 107-113.

McDowell, I., & Newell, C. (1987). *Measuring health: A guide to rating scales and questionnaires.* New York: Oxford.

Maslow, A. H. (1970). *Motivation and personality* (2d ed.). New York: Harper & Row.

Newman, M. (1979). *Theory development in nursing.* Philadelphia: Davis.

Norbeck, J. S. (1987). Empiricism and health promotion research. In M. E. Duffy & N. J. Pender (Eds.), *Conceptual Issues in Health Promotion: Report of Proceedings of a Wingspread Conference* (pp. 110-120). Indianapolis, IN: Sigma Theta Tau International.

Parse, R. R. (1981). *Man-living-health: A theory of nursing.* New York: Wiley.

———. (1987). *Nursing science: Major paradigms, theories, and critiques.* Philadelphia: Saunders.

Parse, R. R., Coyne, A. B., & Smith, M. J. (1985). *Nursing research: Qualitative methods.* Bowie, MD: Brady.

Pender, N. J. (1982). *Health promotion in nursing practice.* Norwalk, CT: Appleton-Century-Crofts.

Pender, N. J. (1987). *Health promotion in nursing practice* (2nd ed.). Norwalk, CT: Appleton & Lange.

Reynolds, C. L. (1988). The measurement of health in nursing research. *Advances in Nursing Science, 10*(4), 23-31.

Rogers, M. E. (1970). *An introduction to the theoretical basis of nursing.* Philadelphia: Davis.

Sarter, B. (1988). *The stream of becoming: A study of Martha Roger's theory.* New York: National League for Nursing.

Smith, J. A. (1981). The idea of health: A philosophic inquiry. *Advances in Nursing Science, 3*(3), 43-50.

Terris, M. (1975). Approaches to an epidemiology of health. *American Journal of Public Health, 65,* 1037-1045.

Tripp-Reimer, R. (1984). Reconceptualizing the construct of health: Integrating emic and etic perspectives. *Research in Nursing and Health, 7,* 101-109.

Watkins, L. R., & Mayer, D. J. (1982). Organization of endogenous opiate and monopiate pain control systems. *Science, 216,* 1185-1192.

Watson, J. (1988). *Nursing, human science, and human care.* New York: National League for Nursing.

Woods, N. F., Laffrey, S., Duffy, M., Lentz, N. J., Mitchell, E. S., Taylor, D., & Cowan, K. A. (1988). Being healthy: Women's images. *Advances in Nursing Science, 11*(1), 36-46.

15

Being and Becoming Healthy: The Core of Nursing Knowledge

AFAF IBRAHIM MELEIS, RN, PhD, FAAN

Health has been described as a central concept and the goal of nursing. The incongruence between that centrality in nursing and in other disciplines and the public's view is discussed. Other issues and views of health also are considered, including diversity and unity in conceptualizing health, the social nature and societal obligations toward the health of the individual, the lack of congruency between conceptual and empirical views of health, and health as viewed in nursing and in the international arena. Several conditions to be included in nurses' attempts in the theoretical development of health are articulated. The need for focusing on an understanding of the health-care needs of underserved populations, the potential advantage in using a feminist framework, and the integration between a static conception of being healthy and a process/dynamic/becoming conception of health are some of the strategies that can be used to develop a contextual conception of health.

Becoming healthier is a popular goal in the United States, and in the media, health has been dramatized, glamorized, fictionalized, and popularized. If one can only lose weight, exercise regularly, eat oat bran, refrain from high-fat diets and decrease cholesterol, caffeine, and alcohol intake, one will be healthy. If one can just be more beautiful, more autonomous, take a bit more control over one's life, one can be healthy. Indeed, this nation has become preoccupied with ways by which health is maintained and promoted.

Two general observations can be made about this avalanche of information on health. First, the preoccupation and focus on healthy lifestyles appear to be more a popular media endeavor than an actual reflection of social and health policies. The second interesting point is that nursing, itself, is demonstrating an equally persistent fascination with health, both as a cause and a consequence. Health phenomena figure dominantly in the writings of nurse theorists and in the research that is done by nurses. Such a focus on health is not new to nursing. In the nineteenth century, Florence Nightingale conceptualized nursing in terms of a healthy environment and focused on the nurse's ability to assist the personal healing potential of clients. This interest in health has evolved to current conceptualization and inquiry.

The purpose of this chapter is to challenge the reader to think critically about the current state of knowledge surrounding health in nursing. To facilitate this critical analysis, some

Source: Meleis, A (1990). Being and becoming healthy: The core of nursing knowledge. *Nursing Science Quarterly, 3* (3): 107-114. Reprinted by permission of and copyright © 2002 Sage Publications, Inc.

issues, questions, and challenges that need to be considered and confronted by nurses as professionals and as citizens of the world are delineated. The *first* is that, when health is considered in the United States, it is rarely associated with nurses. The public tends not to think of nurses or nursing when it considers health and well-being. In other countries, including Egypt, Saudi Arabia, Brazil, Colombia, India, and People's Republic of China, health is associated with medicine, physicians, or local healers, or more recently, with community and primary health-care workers—but not necessarily with nurses. Why is it that nurses claim health to be the focus and goal of nursing? Why do they fail to receive the recognition and acknowledgment that nursing makes a difference in the health of a nation? The *second* aspect of health that should be questioned is the ethnocentric framework for health that has emerged and is gaining support in the scientific and popular literature in the United States.

HEALTH IN NURSING

There are several ideas about health that represent the status of the concept of health in nursing today: Each of these is shared here with related questions.

Centrality of Health in Nursing

That health is central to nursing is demonstrated in discussions by theorists, curriculum developers, and metatheorists. Indeed, some metatheorists suggest that theories in nursing must be inclusive of a definition of health as both a process and an outcome (Payne, 1983). A number of disciplines may be interested in the same phenomenon, for example, how women juggle their multiple roles of mother, worker, and spouse, while maintaining an in-

tegrative self-identity. A nursing perspective necessitates the consideration of ways by which this integration is manifested in healthful patterns of living and how these patterns can be developed, maintained, or promoted.

Health also is central to medicine, public health, and the lay person who comes from a certain background, namely the lay person who has the luxury of thinking of health as a central point of life. In what way is this centrality similar to or different from the centrality of health that is claimed by nursing? What does it mean when health is said to be a basic or central concept in nursing? Does it mean that any time a research project about a significant question in nursing is developed, health must be included as an outcome? Is a theory in nursing differentiated from theories in other disciplines by its focus on health? Does health have to be defined in all works or analyses of any other concept in nursing? *The question of centrality needs to be carefully considered, particularly in view of the fact that such centrality of health in nursing is not recognized by the public or by other disciplines.*

Diversity and Unity

Another comment about health is the diversity of definitions of health in nursing. Health has been conceptualized as a state, a process of development, an actualization, an outcome, and a style of life. A number of researchers and theorists have raised questions about this diversity and the need for agreement.

The way the question is raised presupposes that there is the potential for unity of thought in the way nurses view health and that there is value in that unity. The question of diversity versus unity of thought is important and is reflected in the many debates in nursing about one theory, one philosophy, one conceptual framework. The question is not whether there should be unity or diversity of definition but what aspects of health can be agreed upon and what aspects demand diversity. Understanding of the whole experience of health would be much better served if the tension and the syntheses between unity and diversity were considered.

Recently, diversity in conceptualization has been more supported in nursing and the medical literature. There are several reasons for this support. Nursing is predominantly a female profession. Therefore, ways of knowing in nursing may be different than in other disciplines and the knowers in nursing may follow a different approach to knowledge development (Belenky, Clinchy, Goldberger, & Tarule, 1986; Schultz & Meleis, 1988).

The second point in favor of diversity of conceptualization is that types of knowledge may be different because of the nature of nursing and the diversity of nursing clients. Nursing is practiced in so many different clinical areas in so many parts of the world that a multitude of definitions for health are requisite. A definition of health that fits in a modern coronary care unit where patients recover from acute myocardial infarctions is quite different from a definition of health for patients recovering from kwashiorkor in a rural area of Zimbabwe. Recovery in the United States may involve health in terms of mobility and sleep, whereas recovery in Zimbabwe may require the ability to find food, water, and adequate nutrition.

Likewise, there are multiple levels of meaning of the wellness/illness experience in the medical literature. In presenting these meanings, Pietroni (1987) has supported the idea that clinicians should be able to understand and speak clearly about each one and apply the appropriate level of meaning to a particular practice situation. Among these levels of meaning is the *classical scientific view* of health, that is, the medical, material, and molecular indications of the presence or absence of illness. In this view the task is to repress symptoms, remove the cause, or replace the diseased part or function of the part. There also

is the *psychological/psychosomatic/psychoanalytical* view in which health and illness are considered an expression of deeper meanings. In this mode, personality structures are related to health and illness; and behavioral approaches of stress reduction, relaxation, biofeedback, and other direct interventions are used. The *preventive/promotional or anticipatory view* of health speaks the language of health risk assessment, seeking meaning through individual choices, self-care, yoga classes, fitness clubs, and control of health by clients. The *cultural/social/political view*, on the other hand, addresses the role of environment in both the disease and health processes. It dictates interventions within the context of societies, cultures, and political systems. A fifth view, or level, is the *archetypal, metaphorical,* and *symbolic.* Meanings of health are found in intuition and symbolism. Interventions within this mode are relaxation, exercise, visual imagery, psychodrama, group care, and connecting with the universe.

A final level within which health and illness can be understood is *space/time/energy and the "rhythm of spheres."* This view represents some of the writers who are well known to nurse metatheorists, such as Dossey (1982), Capra (1983), and Bohm (1980). In this mode the person is conceptualized as a "bioenergetic organism" who is governed by energy, bound by the illustration of time, but universally connected to all others. Healing is, therefore, a universal and collective concern; and health is defined in terms of the meaning given to it, to time, to space, and to the balance in the collective field forces. All of these meanings of health are interactive, and a holistic approach involves all of them.

Pietroni's (1987) view supports the need to accept diversity in definitions of health. There are appropriate times for the use of each of these modes. Health-care providers tend to have one prominent way of thinking about health; yet, the health-care needs of the client preclude the possibility of focusing only on one level of meaning. Pietroni's conceptualization also is an example of academic discussions about health in which no reference is made to nursing scholarship or practice related to health. One must ask whether nursing has no interdisciplinary influence, and if not, how can that be changed?

The quest for a single definition of health is not appropriate, possible, or useful. Keller (1981) is correct when she wrote, "Has it now become a game to create a definition of health? Or is it safer and easier to continually talk and write about health than to do something about it?" (pp. 43-44).

Although diversity should be accepted and reinforced, there is a need for unity in perspective that represents the territory of investigation, the territory for theoretical development. Human responses to health and illness situations, self-care behaviors in health and illness, client-nurse interactions, client-environment interactions, the subjective world of ill or healthy clients, coping styles, therapeutic actions that enhance recovery, and a sense of well-being are all part of that perspective, part of what provides nursing its territory. In addition, there are conditions that are essential to understanding this territory, such as patterns, trends, context, responses, and perceptions. It is not possible to study, analyze, or conceptualize health from a nursing perspective without considering these conditions.

If health is so considered and it is discovered that there are different definitions that emerge, then there is no rationale to continue the search for one definition and one approach to health. It is more useful to dialogue about the nature and degree of unity, as well as the nature of and degrees of diversity. As long as certain basic conditions that emanate from a nursing perspective are met, it is important to understand health from different philosophical approaches.

In reviewing nursing theories, research reports that focus on health, analyses of research on health, and clinical narratives, seven current models of health emerge that are being used in nursing practice, research, and theory. One way nurses have traditionally conceptualized health is as an absence of disease, a model that relies on medical knowledge (Smith, 1982). A second involves internal homeostasis, as represented by Johnson (1980). Another is the adaptation model of health, which takes Johnson's ideas one step further from internal regulatory mechanisms to adaptation with external regulatory mechanisms (Roy, 1984; Smith, 1982). A fourth is the role functioning/self-care model, which is predicated on being able to perform those role functions that society expects from a person (Orem, 1980; Smith, 1982). A fifth is the existential meanings model, which focuses on symbolism and the place of the self in an intricate web of relations among objects, subjects, nature, and in the relations that include objects, subjects, nature, and the supernatural (Patterson & Zderad, 1976; Travelbee, 1971). Another model is that which relies on space/time/energy and consciousness expansion; health is viewed in terms of awareness, personal control, personal empowerment, and mastery over body (Newman, 1986; Rogers, 1970). A final model that guides an understanding of health is the crucial/social/political model, which has been discussed by cross-cultural and critical theorists (Allen, 1986; Tripp-Reimer, 1984). An effective approach to the theoretical development of health is to address the nature of unity and diversity in these models.

Health as a Social Matter

One predominant unifying theme in these models is the role of the individual in maintaining and enhancing health. What most of these models demonstrate is that health is increasingly defined as a personal matter, one in which the individual has an obligation. The underlying assumption is that individuals are responsible for their health; families, communities, and societies are not as accountable. This perception of health is reflected in such definitions as "reaching one's optimum," "ability to take care of self," "exercising," "watching one's diet," "feeling in control," "ability to adjust to the environment," "eating a diet to prevent cancer and heart diseases," "avoiding stress," "modifying type 'A' personality." But is health really a personal matter? Can one feel and become healthy in isolation from structural constraints in the environment? Is it possible that individuals can achieve total control over their environment? Are there some groups of individuals who cannot master and control their bodies' well-being because their environments are oppressive or because they have no choices, or because they have never had the opportunity to think of their optimum capacity? Could nursing not be conceptualized in terms of the environment and interactions with the environment and, at the same time, health be considered a personal matter?

Health may be a personal matter for those individuals who are privileged and come from a white, middle-class background. For others in the United States and the rest of the world, health is a social matter. Certainly, for poor people, health is social. Pill and Scott (1982) interviewed a sample of 41 working-class women in the United Kingdom and found that half of them held fatalistic views about health and illness. This view, the authors maintain, is bound to have influenced readiness for health education, consultation behaviors, and expectations about what they want from the health-care system. What are the structural conditions that have created these fatalistic views of health? When health is viewed as a personal matter, those people in the world who are constrained by societal conditions and who represent the majority of nursing clients are assessed as abnormal. They do not fit the mold of personal perseverance and personal control over one's health. A framework of individualizing strategies for health curtails any plan of action to develop societal mechanisms for enhancement of health.

In addition to the danger of conceptualizing health as a personal matter, there is a tendency to reduce the conceptualization of health to one's bodily function or system. Health for women or women's health, for instance, has become synonymous with reproductive and maternal capacities.

> In a society that values a woman primarily for her capacity to perpetuate the species, "women's health" exists as a euphemism for obstetrics and gynecology. This view of women has existed historically in most Western cultures and helps to explain the myth that all women's problems can be attributed to wandering wombs or raging hormones. (Webster & Lipetz, 1986, p. 87)

Although this view has been changing within the last two decades, as evidenced by the increasing research in nursing about other aspects of women's health, such as violence against women, women's work, and women's aging, there still is a predominant view of women's health as reproductive health.

Broadening the conception of health of women beyond one system is not enough to capture the totality of their health. A conceptualization of health that does not encompass the views of women reduces a discussion of health to a cliche. In some current research that the author is doing in collaboration with a number of international colleagues, women have said that one of the most stressful aspects of their multiple roles is worry. They spend a great deal of their energy worrying. They worry about the economic situation, about whether they are going to be paid on time, whether their children are going to take drugs, whether their landlord is going to evict them, and whether they will have a job the next day. Well-being for these women is in relief from their worrying. Worrying for them is not a personal matter; it is a public and social matter. Health for them incorporates family, community, work, and society. It is not mastery of their body; it is strategizing with the constraints and resources of their environment to achieve a sense of well-being. Nursing can understand the health of individuals if the perspective of group, family, community, and society orientation is considered. For many individuals health cannot be separated from that of their parents, children, extended family, neighbors, and friends. Individualism is not the norm for these people and, consequently, their isolated experiences are not meaningful nor are they representative of the core of health for them.

Access to health care is another aspect of health that needs consideration. Health professionals cannot afford to address health as a concept without also addressing access to it. Definitions of health are bound by access to health care and how options for health care are perceived, and a conceptualization of health that does not include access is limited at best and erroneous at worst.

When health is seen as a community and as a social and societal obligation rather than only a personal objective, it increases the potential for structural changes. Health is relief from worry. Health is relief from fear of rape, of violations to one's self, to one's body, and to one's integrity. Health is not being robbed of defenses. Health is access and options for health care. To include innovative definitions of health is to take an activist role in helping people realize health from the perspective of social obligation. Nurses need to consider whether they have taken a proactive role theoretically, empirically, clinically, and politically in issues related to the social obligations of health.

Conceptual and Empirical Views

The incongruity between a conceptual view of health and an empirical approach to studying health in nursing has been delineated and discussed by Reynolds (1988), who views health conceptually as encompassing the whole person and incorporating the relationship between the person and the environment. Reynolds' informative review of nursing research has shown that there are very few operationalizations of health that encompass these conceptual ideas. Research about health depends on the clinical manifestations of health, that is, the number of physical and psychological symptoms. When health is considered as an outcome variable, there is a tendency to separate clinical manifestations from the experience of being healthy. Nurse scientists have not yet demonstrated a way to measure or to understand the total experience of health in a way that goes beyond the mere absence of symptoms and individual perceptions of wellness, to incorporate more than role performance or functioning. The questions to be asked here are, What do nursing's operational definitions represent? and How is health conceptualized?

In the absence of more comprehensive measures of health that are congruent with a nursing perspective, Meleis, Norbeck, and Laffrey (1989) have employed two measures of health in their research about roles of women and health. One is an objective measure that focuses on clinical manifestations of illness, and the other is a subjective measure that encompasses subjective aspects of health as perceived by the person. The Cantril ladder was used for a rating of self-health. The importance of the self-rating measure has been demonstrated by Mossey and Shapiro (1982), who found that the way people view their health is highly correlated with subsequent health outcomes. As others have repeatedly indicated, there are no measures that encompass a holistic view of health (Pender, 1987; Reynolds, 1988). Should health measures be developed to correspond with each of the different conceptualizations of health in nursing? Or should a set of conditions be developed that can be incorporated into whatever measure is used? Should the development of one holistic measure of health be abandoned in exchange for a more realistic approach that measures several dimensions of health?

Webster and Lipetz (1986), among others, have claimed that the clients' experiences of wellness and illness only can be understood in the context of their everyday lives and with information about their usual health practices and health beliefs. Clients' descriptions of their health concerns in their own words are essential in assessment, planning health care, implementing interventions, and evaluating their effectiveness. Given these criteria, what are the most effective methodologies for describing health empirically, and what are the most appropriate strategies for theory development?

Health and Primary Health Care

International colleagues are considering health from the perspective of the Alma Ata Declaration of 1978 (World Health Organization, 1978). If the potential of maintaining, regaining, or developing health and well-being are discussed without careful consideration of primary health care as a strategy to attain it, then nursing in the United States will be increasingly isolated from international nursing. Concepts that are central to primary health care are community participation, consciousness raising, appropriate local resources, access, options, and empowerment. Primary health care provides a strong community orientation. Questions to be considered include, Are any of these primary health care concepts manifestations of health? Are conceptualiza-

tions of health in nursing congruent with this view of health? Should they be?

CONDITIONS FOR THE DEVELOPMENT OF THEORY

Conceptual development must take into consideration the diversity of nursing philosophies, as well as the diverse populations served by nurses. One approach to the diversification of philosophies would be to use feminist epistemological principles as an approach to theoretical formulations related to health. Feminist researchers have identified several important epistemological principles that are congruent with the goals of nursing and that have been used as guidelines in nursing practice, although not so readily in nursing theory-building and research. These principles, as outlined by Cook and Fonow (1986), suggest that nursing (a) attend to the significance of gender and lack of gender sensitivity as a basic feature of all social life, (b) consider consciousness raising as a central and specific methodological tool in research and clinical practice, and (c) include advocacy in defining the role of the theorist, the researcher, and the clinician. Feminist theory also challenges the norms of objectivity, which assume that the subject and object of research could or should be separated, and that lack of subjective involvement is the basis for human science. One should be sensitive to the potential for exploitation of research participants, the biased participation of particular groups over others, and to ethical issues inherent in research.

Nursing could empower clients and research participants by providing them information from research and clinical expertise that assists them in changing the structural constraints that impede their well-being. These feminist principles are congruent with the nursing mission, a predominantly female constituency, the caring work of nursing, and its humanitarian values.

To consider gender as a focal theoretical category is as important as considering class and ethnicity. Careful attention to all of these concepts should sensitize nursing to the extent to which it may have built knowledge related to health based on white, male, middle-class values.

Yet, to define and describe health in ways that are not culturally, ethnically, and socially biased is a difficult task. In discussing the relationship between health and environment Allen (1981) has said,

> We may look at nursing for healthy living as providing an environment in which individuals, families, or groups can learn. This means that nursing shapes the structure for learning (through) access to knowledge and information; situations in which to discuss, share, and work with others engaged in similar pursuits; opportunity to examine, analyze, plan, and test out aspects of health behaviors with health professionals; opportunities for the community to participate in educational programs for health and to evaluate its own health status and that of its families. (p. 153)

To discuss health as a personal matter constrains the potential of understanding health as a social/environmental/societal/political one.

Conceptually, there is a need to articulate conditions that are essential to understanding health, regardless of what theory is used. These conditions, such as pattern, human rights, societal obligation, and development, can form a framework for theory development and research. Health as development implies

> progressive improvements in the living conditions and quality of life enjoyed by

society and shared by its members. It is a continuing process that takes place in all societies; few would claim that their development is complete. (WHO, 1978, p. 44)

Finally, there is a need to develop and implement nursing therapeutics that create, maintain, and promote healthy social/environmental/political contexts that emanate from lack of access and options. There is also the need for the development of frameworks to enhance health in hospitals, at home, or in administration, schools, or families.

Strategies for the Development of a Contextual Conception of Health

Several strategies could be used for the development and refinement of a conceptualization of health that is more congruent with societal needs and the mission of nursing. The *first* is to focus on investigations and theories about populations who have not been particularly central to the discipline of nursing before but are in need of nursing services; these are the underserved, the stigmatized, and the disenfranchised.

It is easier to recruit white middle-class subjects in our research studies. However, if predominantly white, middle-class heterosexual women are being selected for research, one must ask whether health is being conceptualized as having the same values as them. If we disagree, then one must ask whether there are strategies to improve the participation of other groups in research. A discipline that purports to care for the homeless and the ethnically and socially diverse should not engage in scholarship that tends to exclude women of color, working-class women, immigrants, lesbians, or any other disenfranchised group. Nursing can discuss their views only if they are included in nursing studies and theoretical work.

One of the *most important agenda items for the development of a meaningful conceptualization of health and well-being is to develop some means by which representative research participants can be recruited.* Theorizing about and investigating populations who are disenfranchised or stigmatized takes a tremendous amount of time, effort, and energy. Utilizing these populations is not cost effective. From an economic perspective, many are not likely to understand the pencil-and-paper instruments nor to respond meaningfully to structured interview questions.

There are approaches to increase participation of diverse groups in research. Cannon, Higginbotham, and Leung (1988) have demonstrated that white women who were raised in middle-class families and whose occupations were male dominated tended to volunteer and respond to request letters and media solicitations for research subjects more than other women who represented other ethnic, class, and occupational backgrounds. To get underrepresented women to participate in research, researchers have had to use what Cannon et al. (1988) termed *labor-intensive recruitment strategies*, including verbal contact, face-to-face approaches, more extensive interviews, and the conviction that the research was worthwhile. Sixty percent of the black working-class women in their sample, for instance, were recruited through such interview strategies versus 30 percent of the white working-class women. Reasons for difficulty in recruiting nonwhites included less leisure time, more skepticism about research and its motives, a fear of stereotyping, and less control over time. These constraints have to be carefully addressed and removed to enhance recruitment of diverse populations.

There are other approaches to increase diversity in research participants. Lipson and Meleis (1989) found that developing trust, modifying interviewing styles and consent procedures, providing structure for reciprocity with subjects, and nontermination of relationships were important strategies in getting first-generation immigrant subjects to participate. In another research project the provision of a modest reimbursement for time to complete the interview may have increased the diversity of the sample to more than 50 percent nonwhite participants (Meleis et al., 1989). Such an increase in participants enhances the theoretical development of health and, in turn, allows further diversity in the definition of health. International work also could help in the development of conceptualizations that represent diverse populations.

It is not enough to work in disciplinary isolation in developing a contextual conceptualization of health. It is imperative to receive recognition from members of other disciplines, as well as the public, for the roles of nurses in the health and well-being of societies. Such acknowledgment can enhance that role in influencing policies related to health. Focusing on significant questions related to health also will enhance nurses' potential in being involved in health policies.

Although there is a body of literature that either defines health, or claims it to be a central concept, or uses health as a correlate variable (eg, Shaver, 1985; Smith, 1981), it has not adequately informed clinical practice or the public. The questions to be asked are, Is the information disseminated to the public? Is the message compelling and valuable? What would be more compelling? Some questions are those that address the processes of becoming healthy and nurses' activities in bringing health to people. The "being healthy" focus in definitions of health and the "becoming healthy" questions in the face of illness, lack of access, lack of resources and within such constraints as stigma, bias, and handicap are those to which the public needs answers. These are significant questions and are more urgent and germane in terms of potential impact on social and health policy. Nurses cannot afford to spend time only on definitions. The need to develop more definitions can be supplemented with engagement in creating substantial changes for people whose health is compromised in some form or another. Some of the philosophical, theoretical, and definitional questions need to be grounded in socially significant health issues.

One can do so by asking such questions as, Is the public or legislators aware that the central focus of nursing is health? What platform is congruent with the mission of nursing as it has been defined? What platform is significant for the public, for legislators? What will make nursing visible so that it can make a statement that will be heard? One way to do so is to challenge each other to come up with questions that are not only significant but are at the cutting edge of the discipline and profession of nursing.

Instead of defining health from different perspectives, maybe it should be described and explained in terms of how people are kept healthy in spite of positive HIV or a diagnosis of AIDS, or by the strategies by which Alzheimer's patients and their caregivers become more healthy than they were before confronting the disease. How can nursing make them more healthy than they were before? How can nursing make a difference in helping overburdened single working mothers maintain their own and their children's health, or the health of the single homebound elderly? Questions such as these should be the business of nursing. Health should be considered in terms of the consumer who needs specific answers and demands specific actions.

If the view of health is broadened beyond a personal focus to include social, political, and cultural contexts, other significant questions will emerge. The development of measures that focus on clinical manifestations, subjective and objective perceptions of health, meanings associated with health, priorities, relations with the environment, and individual health as part of group health are all essential strategies in developing health as a central focus in nursing. Answers to significant questions through the development of measures that represent a nursing perspective will help provide the necessary substance for the development of middle-range theories to describe, explain, and predict health.

Being healthy, as viewed empirically, provides a static view of health that can be measured by existing measures, such as the general well-being scale, omnibus personality inventory, Cornell medical index, or the Cantril ladder. These measures represent a limited view of health that may not address what the public may consider significant. Being healthy can be reconceptualized in ways that nursing constituents and clients can relate to and understand.

Being healthy need not provide a static view of health. When considered from the perspective of clients, it is a way of life, an attitude, an outlook, a history, a context with sociocultural norms, a belief, and a tradition. Being healthy is managing, negotiating, achieving, growing, becoming, and helping others grow and become. Being and becoming healthy may be parts of a whole perception of health. Becoming healthy is hopefulness, transcending worries, realizing options, advocating, and accessing resources. Being and becoming healthy incorporate awareness, resources, opportunity, development, access, enabling, empowerment, and advocacy.

REFERENCES

Allen, D. G. (1986). Using philosophical and historical methodologies to understand the concept of health. In P. L. Chinn (Ed.), *Nursing research methodology: Issues and implementation* (pp. 157-168). Rockville, MD: Aspen.

Allen, M. (1981). The health dimension in nursing practice: Notes on nursing in primary health care. *Journal of Advanced Nursing, 6,* 153-154.

Belenky, M. F., Clinchy, B. M., Goldberger, N. R., & Tarule, J. M. (1986). *Women's ways of knowing: The development of self, voice, and mind.* New York: Basic Books.

Bohm, D. (1980). *Wholeness and the implicate order.* Boston: Routledge.

Cannon, L. W., Higginbotham, E., & Leung, M. L. A. (1988). Race and class bias in qualitative research on women. *Gender and Society, 2,* 449-454.

Capra, F. (1983). *The turning point: Science, society, and the rising culture.* New York: Bantam.

Cook, J. A., & Fonow, M. M. (1986). Knowledge and women's interests: Issues of epistemology and methodology in feminist sociological research. *Sociological Inquiry, 56*(1), 1-19.

Dossey, L. (1982). Space, time, and medicine. New York: Random House.

Johnson, D. E. (1980). The behavioral system model for nursing. In J. P. Riehl & C. Roy (Eds.), *Conceptual modes for nursing practice* (2nd ed.). New York: Appleton-Century-Crofts.

Keller, M. J. (1981). Toward a definition of health. *Advances in Nursing Science, 4*(1), 43-52.

Lipson, J. G., & Meleis, A. I. (1989). Methodological issues in research with immigrants. *Medical Anthropology, 12*(1), 103-115.

Meleis, A. I., Norbeck, J. S., & Laffrey, S. C. (1989). Role integration and health among female clerical workers. *Research in Nursing and Health, 12.*

Mossey, J. M., & Shapiro, E. (1982). Self-rated health: A predictor of mortality among the elderly. *American Journal of Public Health, 72,* 800-808.

Newman, M. A. (1986). *Health as expanding consciousness.* St. Louis: Mosby.

Orem, D. E. (1980). *Nursing: Concepts of practice* (2nd ed.). New York: McGraw-Hill.

Patterson, J. G., & Zderad, L. T. (1976). *Humanistic nursing.* New York: Wiley.

Payne, L. (1983). Health: A basic concept in nursing theory. *Journal of Advanced Nursing, 8,* 393-395.

Pender, N. J. (1987). *Promotion in nursing practice* (2nd ed.). Norwalk, CT: Appleton-Century-Crofts.

Pietroni, P. C. (1987). The meaning of illness-holism dissected: Discussion paper. *Journal of the Royal Society of Medicine, 80,* 357-360.

Pill, R., & Stott, N. C. H. (1982). Concepts of illness causation and responsibility: Some preliminary data from a sample of working class mothers. *Social Sciences & Medicine, 16,* 43-52.

Reynolds, C. (1988). The measurement of health in nursing research. *Advances in Nursing Science, 10*(4), 23-31.

Rogers, M. (1970). An introduction to the theoretical basis of nursing. Philadelphia: Davis.

Roy, C. (1984). *Introduction to nursing: An adaptation model* (2nd ed.). Englewood Cliffs, NJ: Prentice-Hall.

Schultz, P., & Meleis, A. I. (1988). Nursing epistemology: Traditions, insights, questions. *Image: Journal of Nursing Scholarship, 20,* 217-221.

Shaver, J. F. (1985). A biopsychological view of human health. *Nursing Outlook, 33,* 186-191.

Smith, J. (1981). The idea of health: A philosophical inquiry. *Advances in Nursing Science, 3*(3), 43-50.

———. (1982). Letters to the editor. *Advances in Nursing Science, 4*(3), xi.

Travelbee, J. (1971). *Interpersonal aspects of nursing* (2nd ed.). Philadelphia: Davis.

Tripp-Reimer, T. (1984). Reconceptualizing the construct of health: Integrating emic and etic perspectives. *Research in Nursing and Health, 7,* 101-109.

Webster, D., & Lipetz, M. (1986). Changing definitions: Changing times. *Nursing Clinics of North America, 21*(1), 87-97.

World Health Organization. (1978). *Primary health care: Report of the International Conference on Primary Health Care,* Alma Ata, USSR. 6-12, September 1978, Geneva.

Part IV

NURSING'S METAPARADIGM: CONCEPTUALIZATIONS OF CLIENT AND ENVIRONMENT

The nurse theorists have each defined the client, or patient, in different ways based on their philosophy, experience, and assumptions about humans. Early theorists viewed the client as a bio-psycho-social being, a person capable of adapting to illnesses, a rational, sentient being interacting within a system, or a person able to perform various levels of self-care. Later theorists defined the client as a human interacting with his environment, a human becoming through use of various senses, and a person who determines the meaning of their experiences. Each of these definitions of client fosters unique ways of viewing, assessing, and treating the client, which can range from a specific part of the body to how the client interprets the meaning of illness based on his past, present, and future life. Unfortunately, there is a paucity of articles by nurse scholars regarding a more generalized definition.

In her article on conceptualizing the concept 'client,' Dr. Hesook Kim, a renown nurse scholar and writer, recognized the need for a unified definition of client. She begins by highlighting six major categories of humans and health of nurse theorists. Then she explains how nursing's focus on a client's 'state' and the emphasis on diagnoses and treatment of clients' needs and health problems is a very narrow view based on a specific time in a client's life. Dr. Kim proposes that human living be used as the unifying perspective for conceptualizing client, based on three dimensions. The first dimension is 'body and personhood,' which includes biological make-up and existential experience as to what has been and is experienced in time and space. The second dimension consists of 'living with others,' which involves communicating and interacting in relation to one's instrumental, symbolic and affective needs. 'Living in situations' is the third dimension and refers to the context and modes of living as they are adjusted to meet contextual requirements. Dr. Kim believes that her conceptualization of client is not specific to any theory or model, but could be applied to any one, and would serve to unify nursing theory, practice, and research.

Environment as a metaparadigm concept in nursing theories and models has also been defined in various ways. Some nurse theorists describe environment as internal and external factors that influence the individual, and others view the client-environment as inseparable and in constant exchange during reciprocal interactions. And some theorists have never really defined what they mean by environment. Recently, a few nurse scholars have greatly expanded the definition to include the effects of social, political, and economic factors that influence the client's health. Patricia Butterfield encourages nurses to consider how these broad contextual factors contribute to both individual and community health problems, in her article, "Thinking Upstream: Nurturing a Conceptual Understanding of the Societal Context of Health Behavior." She admonishes nurses to become more politically active in their communities if they truly want to promote health rather than merely treating clients with common health problems.

In the 1990s, Dorothy Kleffel began exploring various perspectives for defining the meaning of environment. In her article, "Environmental Paradigms: Moving Toward an Ecocentric Perspective," she examines the traditional view of the client's immediate surroundings, then mentions the effects of regional disasters, and finally explores how broad global effects of worldwide hunger, ozone depletion, human overpopulation, and other relevant factors affect health. Dr. Kleffel analyzes the effects of three environmental paradigms — egocentric, homocentric, and ecocentric — on human's health worldwide, and encourages nurses to consider an ecocentric perspective that would encompass global environmental health for all people.

16

An Integrative Framework for Conceptualizing Clients: A Proposal for a Nursing Perspective in the New Century

HESOOK SUZIE KIM, RN; PHD

It is exciting to view the year 2000 as the beginning for a new century and a new millennium that can be based on a new resolve and a refreshing insight. In thinking and reflecting about what aspects of nursing and nursing knowledge development that should be the focus for formulating such a new resolve or a refreshing insight, pluralism comes to mind as one of the critical issues that is both important and trouble-some. Nursing has pursued multiple paths to develop knowledge with different commitments to philosophies and epistemological orientations during the past three decades. The resulting pluralism is evident not only in philosophical orientations regarding human nature and nursing, but also in theories, scientific explanations, and methods of inquiry adopted in nursing science.

During the past three decades we have put a great deal of our scientific effort into developing nursing knowledge in terms of (a) conceptualizing the key and essential phenomena of concern, (b) identifying the nature of nursing problems and different ways of solving such problems, (c) understanding fundamental human processes associated with health and illness through development of multiple

theories, (d) identifying the impact of environment on human functioning and health, and (e) advancing technical supports that enhance human health. These efforts have resulted in truly pluralistic knowledge development in nursing in terms of theories, empirical findings, and practical approaches, along with differences in philosophical and value orientations. A rich array of scientific results has provided the foundation to move nursing practice to be grounded in scientific knowledge. On the other hand, multiple theories, conflicting findings, and competing approaches to patient care have created confusion as well as a heightened sense of separation and schism between science and practice in nursing.

One of the most critical aspects of such pluralism is in regard to theories and conceptualizations about phenomena in the client domain. Client domain, identified as one of the four domains of nursing's subject matter (Kim, 1987), refers to the key area of nursing's concern for knowledge development. There has been a long-standing presumption that through the understanding and explanation about client phenomena, nursing could develop its approaches, that is, therapeutics and strategies of care regarding clients' problems. The conceptual works of early nurse scholars helped to shift nursing's orientation from

Source: Kim, H.S. (2000). An integrative framework for conceptualizing clients: a proposal for a nursing perspective in the new century. *Nursing Science Quarterly* 13 (1): 37 – 44. Reprinted by permission of and copyright © 2002 Sage Publications, Inc.

medicine and pathologies to human needs. In the ensuing decades, the relevance of these frameworks as a basis for the practice of nursing became apparent, and a series of grand theories concerned with the knowledge domain of the client were proposed and studied.

Rogers's (1970, 1992) science of unitary human beings, Roy's (Roy & Andrews, 1997) adaptation model, Orem's (1995) self-care model, Neuman's (1995) systems model, and Parse's (1998) theory of human becoming are the major grand frameworks in nursing that try to formulate and explain client domain phenomena from generalized conceptualizations of humanity and health. These and related nursing models can be categorized into six major types according to their views on humanity and health: (a) holistic processes as the modes through which humans coexist within their environment, (b) balance as the essential human characteristic that expresses human condition, (c) configuration of structural and functional aspects as an integrative basis for human functioning, (d) aggregation of parts as revealing states of the human condition, (e) experiencing as the basic form of human existence, and (f) meaning-making as the essential feature of human life.

This categorization suggests that in nursing there is diversity in the way clients and client phenomena are conceptualized and that there is no generally endorsed unified perspective regarding humans. It would be quite premature to state that nursing has firmly established specific paradigms or schools of thought based on these differing conceptualizations of humans and grand theories. However, these grand theories persist as the bases for empirical work and research, middle-range theory development, nursing curricula, and nursing practice models. In addition, knowledge development in nursing regarding client phenomena, particularly during the past decade, has also been rich and active not only in association with nursing's grand theories

but in relation to general theoretical orientations such as biobehavioral, cognitive, psychosocial, and phenomenological frameworks. Multiple paradigmatic orientations are certainly in place in nursing and are viewed to be viable and necessary aspects of nursing knowledge development and practice (Gortner, 1993; Nagle & Mitchell, 1991).

Nevertheless, there are differing philosophical positions regarding this apparent pluralism in nursing. Many scholars seem to adhere to the notion that it is both acceptable and to some degree necessary to have multiple conceptualizations of persons and different grand theories in nursing. Others argue that for multiple paradigms and grand theories to be viable as the basis for scientific knowledge development, it is necessary to have a unifying perspective that provides the focus of the nursing discipline. It is from this second position that I propose a revisioning for the knowledge domain of client as necessary to establish firmly the unique focus of nursing in the larger context of healthcare. The conceptualization of the client domain as human living is presented as both a unifying perspective and a unique focus for nursing in the new century.

HUMAN LIVING AS A METAPARADIGM CONCEPT

From the 1960s and throughout the ensuing decades, nursing's focus has been to meet patients' needs related to maintaining health or to assist individuals in their responses to health and illness. As stated in the American Nurses' Association's (1980) first social policy statements, nursing is defined as "the diagnosis and treatment of human responses to actual or potential health problems" (p. 9). This view places an emphasis on clients' problems that are specified as reactions and concerns attendant with health problems. These widely accepted orientations have firmly grounded nursing to focus on states of clients, rather than on clients as humans. These client states are not only specified in the languages of the grand theories but also in the works of nursing diagnoses classifications and other concept developments such as deficiencies, deficits, adaptation/maladaptation, balance/imbalance, homeostasis, or disturbances. Such seemingly unwitting focus on states of clients also has led nursing to view time as a discrete entity tied to states of responses and occurrences, rather than as a continuum in terms of history and trajectories, and in so doing has imposed an artificial interruption in connected human experience.

Furthermore, I believe this orientation and its subsequent developments have resulted in overemphasis on technical treatment of patients' problems, thereby shadowing the essential nursing philosophy of client care. Consequently, either by design or under pressure, professional nursing began handing over the care of certain states of clients traditionally associated with nursing to other healthcare workers and assistive healthcare personnel, while taking on tasks and responsibilities of other client states that were formerly within the professional domain of physicians. Often this reshaping of nursing's realm of responsibilities, which is usually considered unsatisfactory to us, has been attributed to political and economic pressures within the dynamics of the healthcare system. However, as Kitson (1997) states, it may also have resulted from nursing's "ineptitude and lack of appreciating what matters to us" (p. 114).

Hence, the heart of the matter is in articulating clearly what the essential and central focus of nursing is, so that it becomes the guiding post not only for knowledge development but also for nursing practice. It is not satisfactory just to say that nursing contributes to patient outcomes differently from medicine and other healthcare professionals, or to say that nursing is oriented to the promotion of health and to the care of people in illness. It is this ambiguity that needs to be addressed to avoid continued diffusion of nursing's unique contribution to healthcare. Therefore, I propose human living as the revisioning orientation of the knowledge domain of client for nursing in the new century. By orienting its mission to clients' living rather than limiting its focus to clients' states, nursing can clarify its distinctive role within the community of healthcare providers, formulate client-centered outcomes that are uniquely related to its knowledge-based practice, and ensure public recognition of its distinctive professional contribution in healthcare.

DIMENSIONS OF THE HUMAN LIVING CONCEPT

Although I believe that as a profession nursing has been always concerned with clients' living, I do not believe that it has been articulated clearly as the central focus of the discipline. The following discussion is aimed at achieving this necessary articulation. Human beings are biological and symbolic entities entrusted with bodies, selves, and histories, intertwined to carry on living by continuing, responding to happenings, appropriating and accommodating, and controlling. The concept of human living is based on ontological assumptions that accept humanness in terms of its biology, personhood, and sociality. And living as it is embedded in situations cannot be clearly viewed or fully understood out of context. Given these assumptions of biology, personhood, sociality, and context, human living constitutes three dimensions—living of oneself, living with others, and living in situations—which are coalesced through integration and intersection. These three dimensions are not partitioned sectors of living or even different aspects of living, but are integrative orientations that make human living what it is.

The essential features of humanness that frame human living are body and personhood as aspects of human selves. A human body entrusted with its appearance, makeup, concreteness, and boundedness is, to begin with, biological. But this human entity is also existential, because it exists only through what is experienced in time and space. Furthermore, a human body can be considered as a vehicle through which humans are social beings, capable of symbolizing and interacting. Thus, a human body or entity is both biological/materialistic and symbolic/cultural. On the other hand, personhood is a specification of symbolic self constructed through reflexivity, consciousness, and meaning-making, which are uniquely human qualities. Hence, human living of oneself refers to body and personhood intricately connected and mediated to project the nature of living that is uniquely human. For example, eating as one particular form of human living is not simply an act of getting food but is an act having specific personal meanings and modes of operation established through personal, social, and cultural habits and desires. Living of oneself, then, is oriented to aspects of one's life related to rhythms, intactness and appearance, capacities and limitations, body feelings and sensations, history and genealogy, desires and wants, dreams and hopes, ideas and opinions, choices, habits, and knowing. For a nursing perspective, living of oneself has a specific meaning in terms of how clients' living needs to be supported and/or guided when it is constrained by various sorts of health-related threats to the integrity of body and personhood or to the modes of living itself.

The second dimension, human living with others, is based on the sociality of humans and refers to communality of human existence. Living with others (i.e., with family, friends, colleagues, neighbors, countrymen, and citizens of the world—both intimates and strangers) involves coexisting, communicating, coordinating, exchanging, and interacting as human selves, sometimes by choice and design and other times through accidents or force, both natural and instrumental. Living with others pertains to relating one's instrumental, symbolic, and affective needs with those of others, and to making connections with others for sharing humanness. Living with others is intrinsically tied to living of oneself, in that for one to live of oneself, it is necessary instrumentally to live with others in specific ways. From the nursing perspective, living with others may be viewed to have potential for being constrained or needing to be arranged differently because of clients' health status or healthcare experiences.

Living in situations refers to the idea that living takes place in contexts and that modes of living are adjusted and modified to address contextual requirements of human existence. Situations of living may vary from ordinary life situations such as family, work, and community settings to more specialized situations such as hospitals or prisons. Situations also can be considered to be stable and continuous over time, or to be transient and changing. Living in situations involves responding to, accommodating and adapting to, managing of, engaging in, and choosing and creating contexts of one's existence. From the nursing perspective, living in situations raises questions regarding clients' relationships with their environment and accommodations or variations necessary in clients' living that are necessary, inescapable, or desirable because of situational contingencies accompanying health problems or healthcare.

RELEVANCE FOR THEORY AND PRACTICE

Focusing on human living as nursing's orientation gives a possibility to articulate nursing's unique contribution in healthcare. I believe nursing's orientation to human responses and conditions arising from actual or potential health problems, and resulting formulations in many of nursing's grand theories that emphasize clients' states, have limited the scope of that contribution. Revisioning nursing's focus emerges from shifting an attention on states to an attention on living, especially in response to the outcomes-based culture of healthcare practice. Nursing's concern with client outcomes, then, can focus on, for example, how well the client is living in this situation of healthcare, how the client is progressing with his or her living throughout this episode of care, how well the client is managing his or her living in the context of given health-related threats or problems, or with what sorts of continuity or alignment the client is carrying on his or her living. Nursing is primarily concerned with helping people to live as well as they can, whether they are experiencing acute episodes of illness or trauma, chronic disease trajectories, transient or persisting disabilities, or terminal illness. Nursing is also concerned with helping people to live as well as they can as they engage in anticipated developmental human living experiences such as giving birth, aging, and dying. Diagnosing and treating conditions, difficulties, and disturbances must not be an end in themselves but must be oriented to supporting and helping clients to find ways of living through these experiences—ways of living more creatively, more wisely, more meaningfully, and with more personal control.

The human living concept, elaborated in this way as a unifying focus for the discipline, is metaparadigmatic and hence is not tied to any specific theoretical formulation. Extant nursing theories and conceptualizations regarding clients and client phenomena, therefore, need to be reframed in relation to human living as an essential metaparadigm concept and knowledge domain in nursing. For many decades, nurse scholars have considered health, person, environment, and nursing as the essential metaparadigm concepts for nursing (Fawcett, 1984; Yura & Torres, 1975). However, as concepts these are so nonspecific that they have not been used to identify a distinctive nursing focus as a discipline and an area of study. Human living as an explication of the metaparadigm concept concerned with client and client phenomena can stipulate nursing to be concerned primarily not with health problems such as diseases, illness, or disability but with living in the context of health problems and healthcare. As shown in Figure 16.1, human living as a metaparadigm concept can embrace many theoretical concepts and phenomena of clients, which can be elaborated in terms of specific theoretical orientations.

Explanations and understanding about human responses, behaviors, processes, functioning, and subjectivity can thus be formulated, developed, and empirically examined from various theoretical orientations, such as from different grand theories of nursing as well as other theoretical frameworks. When such theoretical frameworks are interpreted within nursing practice, it would be necessary to frame nursing therapeutics in terms of the three dimensions of human living, considering it as an essential metaparadigm concept of nursing. For example, the phenomenon of being diagnosed with a chronic disease such as diabetes can be examined from various theoretical perspectives (adaptation, cognitive, or phenomenological). Ultimately, any theoretical explanation about this phenomenon must address possible ways of helping individuals who are diagnosed with chronic disease. At this point, the question of what nursing can

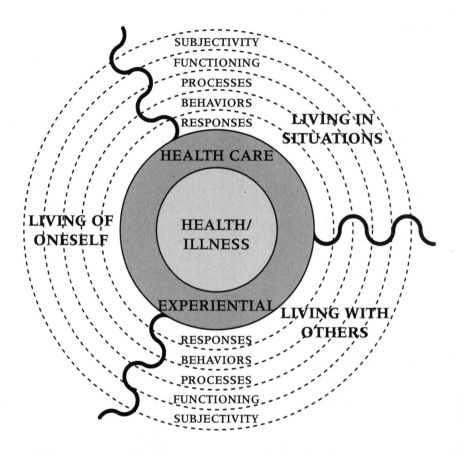

Figure 16.1. Three Dimensions of Human Living as a Metaparadigm Concept in Nursing.

do and needs to do for such clients must be framed in regard to human living in terms of living of oneself, living with others, and living in situations. This orientation means that nursing will focus on client outcomes of its practice in terms of promoting quality in human living that is understood as it is experienced—continuous, transitional, and trajectorial.

CONCLUSIONS

In this exposition, I have suggested that it is necessary to reposition nursing's focus within healthcare and uphold human living as its primary orientation. I have argued from the perspective of a pluralistic approach that allows for multiple paradigms and theories in nursing that is grounded in a unifying focus in the metaparadigm domain of client. Human living has been explained as a three-dimensional integrative dynamic of biology, personhood, and sociality. This unifying focus on human living provides a new, fresh image of nursing that can redefine and direct our role within healthcare in the emerging century. The vision it gives us is a vitalized sense of mission for nursing, through which nursing can uniquely contribute to the lives of its clients. During the past decades, nursing has established a firm alliance with the culture of science and technology, which is primarily oriented to controlling health problems. Without diminishing our involvement in the scientific problem-solving traditions, we can renew our commitment to a human-practice perspective through a unifying disciplinary focus that orients our practice to helping clients in their living within the context of health and healthcare in the new century.

REFERENCES

American Nurses' Association. (1980). *Nursing: A social policy statement.* Kansas City, MO: Author.

Fawcett, J. (1984). The metaparadigm of nursing: Present status and future refinements. *Image: Journal of Nursing Scholarship,* 16, 84–87.

Gortner, S. R. (1993). Nursing's syntax revisited: A critique of philosophies said to influence nursing theories. *International Journal of Nursing Studies,* 30, 477–488.

Kim, H. S. (1987). Structuring the nursing knowledge system: A typology of four domains. *Scholarly Inquiry for Nursing Practice: An International Journal,* 1, 111–114.

Kitson, A. L. (1997). Johns Hopkins Address: Does nursing have a future? *Image: Journal of Nursing Scholarship,* 29, 111–115.

Nagle, L. M. & Mitchell, G. J. (1991). Theoretic diversity: Evolving paradigmatic issues in research and practice. *Advances in Nursing Science,* 14, 17–25.

Neuman, B. (1995). *The Neuman systems model* (3rd ed.). Norwalk, CT: Appleton & Lange.

Orem, D. (1995). *Nursing: Concepts of practice* (5th ed.). St. Louis, MO: Mosby.

Parse, R. R. (1998). *The human becoming school of thought: A perspective for nurses and other health professionals.* Thousand Oaks, CA: Sage.

Rogers, M. E. (1970). *An introduction to the theoretical basis of nursing.* Philadelphia: F. A. Davis.

Rogers, M. E. (1992). Nursing and the space age. *Nursing Science Quarterly,* 5, 27–33.

Roy, C., & Andrews, H. A. (1997). *The Roy adaptation model: The definitive statement.* Norwalk, CT: Appleton & Lange.

Yura, H., & Torres, G. (1975). *Today's conceptual frameworks with the baccalaureate nursing programs* (NLN Pub. No. 15–1558, pp. 17–75). New York: National League for Nursing.

17

Thinking Upstream: Nurturing a Conceptual Understanding of the Societal Context of Health Behavior

PATRICIA G. BUTTERFIELD, RN, MS

This chapter addresses the issue of overreliance on theories that define nursing in terms of a one-to-one relationship at the expense of theoretical perspectives that emphasize the societal context of health. When individuals are perceived as the focus of nursing action, the nurse is likely to propose intervention strategies aimed at either changing the behaviors of the individual or modifying the individual's perceptions of the world. When nurses understand the social, political, economic influences that shape the health of a society, they are more likely to recognize social action as a nursing role and work on behalf of populations.

Despite acknowledgment that an understanding of population health is essential in professional nursing, descriptions of one-to-one relationships predominate in the literature read by most nurses. Such portrayals often emphasize the evolution of the relationship between nurse and client with minimal attention to forces outside the relationship that have been paramount in shaping the client's health behaviors. Yet for most people their cultural heritage, social roles, and economic situations have a far more profound influence on health behaviors than do interactions with any health-care professional. Examination of nursing problems from a "think small" perspective[1(p504)] fosters

inadequate consideration of these social, environmental, and political determinants of health. This perspective results not only in a restricted range of intervention possibilities for the nurse, but also in a distorted impression of clients' behaviors. An understanding of the complex social, political, and economic forces that shape people's lives is necessary for nurses to promote health in individuals and groups. If nurses are not given an opportunity to appreciate the gestalt of populations and societies, they will be unable to develop a basis for analyzing problems.

This chapter addresses the issue of overreliance on theories that define nursing primarily in terms of a one-to-one relationship and the inherent conflict between these theories and the goal of enabling nurses to promote health through population-based interventions.

Source: Butterfield, P. G. (1990). Thinking upstream: Nurturing a conceptual understanding of the societal context of health behavior. *ANS, 12* (2): 1-8. Reprinted with permission from and copyright © 1990 Aspen Publishers, Inc.

NURSING'S ROLE IN PUSHING UPSTREAM

In his description of the frustrations of medical practice, McKinlay[2] uses the image of a swiftly flowing river to represent illness. In this analogy, physicians are so caught up in rescuing victims from the river that they have no time to look upstream to see who is pushing their patients into the perilous waters. The author uses this example to demonstrate the ultimate futility of "downstream endeavors,"[2(p9)] which are characterized by short-term, individual-based interventions, and he challenges health-care providers to focus more of their energies "upstream, where the real problems lie."[2(p9)] Upstream endeavors focus on modifying economic, political, and environmental factors that have been shown to be the precursors of poor health throughout the world. Although the analogy cites medical practice, it also aptly describes the dilemmas of a considerable portion of nursing practice. And while nursing has a rich historical record of providing preventive and population-based care, the current American health system, which emphasizes episodic and individual-based care, has done woefully little to stem the tide of chronic illness, to which 70 percent of the American population succumbs.

What is the cost of a continued emphasis on a microscopic perspective? How does a theoretical focus on the individual preclude understanding of a larger perspective? Dreher[1] maintains that a conservative scope of practice often uses psychologic theories to explain patterns of health and health care. In this mode of practice, low compliance, broken appointments, and reluctance to participate in care are all attributed to motivation or attitude problems on the part of the client. Nurses are charged with the responsibility of altering client attitudes toward health, rather than altering the system itself, "even though such negative attitudes may well be a realistic appraisal of

health care."[1(p505)] Greater emphasis is paid to the psychologic symptoms of poor health than to socioeconomic causes; "indeed the symptoms are being taken as its causes."[1(p505)] The nurse who views the world from such a perspective does not entertain the possibility of working to alter the system itself or empowering clients to do so.

Involvement in social reform is considered to be within the realm of nursing practice.[3] Dreher[1] acknowledges the historical role of public health nurses in facilitating social change and notes that social involvement and activism are expected of nurses in this area of practice. The American Nurses' Association (ANA) Social Policy Statement delineates, among other social concerns, the "provision for the public health through use of preventive and environmental measures and increased assumption of responsibility by individuals, families, and other groups"[3(p4)] and addresses nursing's role in response to those concerns. However, in her review of the document, White[4] notes an incongruence between nursing's social concerns, which clearly transcend individual-based practice, and the description of nursing as "a practice in which interpersonal closeness of the professional kind develops and aids the investigation and discussion of problems, as nurse and patient (or family or group) seek jointly to resolve those concerns."[3(p19)] White[4] also notes the document's neglect of the population focus and possibilities for modifying the environment. Clearly, nursing has yet to reconcile many of the differences between operationalization of a population-centered practice and policies that define nursing primarily in terms of individual-focused care.

Three theoretic approaches will be contrasted below to demonstrate how they may lead the nurse to draw different conclusions not only about the reasons for client behavior, but also about the range of interventions available to the nurse.

THE DOWNSTREAM VIEW: THE INDIVIDUAL AS THE LOCUS OF CHANGE

The health belief model evolved from the premise that the world of the perceiver determines what he or she will do. The social psychologists[5,6] who outlined this model were strongly influenced by Lewin and the view that a person's daily activities are guided by processes of attraction to positive valences and avoidance of negative valences. From these inceptions evolved a model that purports to explain why people do or do not engage in a preventive health action in response to a specific disease threat. The model places the burden of action exclusively on the client; only those clients who have distorted or negative perceptions of the specified disease or recommended health action will fail to act. In practice, this model focuses the nurse's energies on interventions designed to modify the client's distorted perceptions. Although the process of promoting behavior change may be masked under the premise of mutually defined goals, passive acceptance of the nurse's advice is the desired outcome of the relationship.

Although the health belief model was not designed to specify intervention strategies, it can lead the nurse to deduce that client problems can be solved merely by altering the client's belief system. The model addresses the concept of "perceived benefits versus perceived barriers/costs associated with taking a health action."[6(p563)] Nurses may easily interpret this situation as a need to modify the client's perceptions of benefits and barriers. For example, clients with problems accessing adequate health care might receive counseling aimed at helping them see these barriers in a new light; the model does not include the possibility that the nurse may become involved in activities that promote equal access to all in need.

True to its historical roots, the model offers an explanation of health behaviors that, in many ways, is similar to a mechanical system. From the health belief model, one easily concludes that compliance can be induced by using model variables as catalysts to stimulate action. For example, an intervention study based on health belief model precepts sought to increase follow-up in hypertensive clients by increasing the clients' awareness of their susceptibility to hypertension and of its danger.[7] Clients received education, over the telephone or in the emergency department, that was designed to increase their perception of the benefits of follow-up. According to these authors, the interventions resulted in a dramatic increase in compliance. However, they noted several client groups that failed to respond to the intervention, most notably a small group of clients who had no available child care. Although this study demonstrates the predictive power of health belief model concepts, it also exemplifies the limitations of the model. The health belief model may be effective in promoting behavioral change through the alteration of clients' perspectives, but it does not acknowledge responsibility for the health-care professional to reduce or ameliorate client barriers.

In fact, some of the proponents of the health belief model readily acknowledge the limitations of the model and caution users against generalizing it beyond the domain of the individual psyche. In their review of 10 years of research with the model, Janz and Becker[8] remind researchers that the model can only account for the variance in health behaviors that is explained by the attitudes and beliefs of an individual. Melnyk's[9] recent review of the concept of barriers reinforces the notion that, because the health belief model is based on subjective perceptions, research that adopts this theoretic basis must take care to include the subjects', rather than the researchers', perceptions of barriers. Janz and Becker[8] address the influence of other factors such as habituation and nonhealth reasons on making positive changes in health behavior, and they acknowledge the influence of environmental and economic factors that prohibit individuals from undertaking a more healthy way of life.

The health belief model is but a prototype for the type of theoretic perspective that has dominated nursing education and thus nursing practice. The model's strength—its narrow scope—is also its limitation: One is not drawn outside it to those forces that shape the characteristics that the model describes.

THE UPSTREAM VIEW: SOCIETY AS THE LOCUS OF CHANGE

Milio's Framework for Prevention

Milio's framework for prevention[10] provides a thought-provoking complement to the health belief model and a mechanism for directing attention upstream and examining opportunities for nursing intervention at the population level. Milio moves the focus of attention upstream by pointing out that it is the range of available health choices, rather than the choices made at any one time, that is paramount in shaping the overall health status of a society. She maintains that the range of choices widely available to individuals is shaped, to a large degree, by policy decisions in both governmental and private organizations. Rather than concentrate efforts on imparting information to change patterns of individual behavior, she advocates national-level policy making as the most effective means of favorably affecting the health of most Americans.

Milio[10] proposes that health deficits often result from an imbalance between a population's health needs and its health-sustaining resources, with affluent societies afflicted by the diseases associated with excess (obesity, alcoholism) and the poor afflicted by diseases that result from inadequate or unsafe food, shelter, and water. In this context, the poor in affluent societies may experience the least desirable combination of factors. Milio notes that although socioeconomic realities deprive many Americans of a health-sustaining environment, "cigarettes, sucrose, pollutants, and tensions are readily available to the poor."[10(p436)]

The range of health-promoting or health-damaging choices available to individuals is affected by their personal resources and their societal resources. Personal resources include one's awareness, knowledge, and beliefs, including those of one's family and friends, as well as money, time, and the urgency of other priorities. Societal resources are strongly influenced by community and national locale and include the availability and cost of health services, environmental protection, safe shelter, and the penalties or rewards given for failure to select the given options.

Milio notes the fallacy of the commonly held assumption in health education that knowing health-generating behaviors implies acting in accordance with that knowledge, and she cites the lifestyles of health professionals in support of her argument. She proposes that "most human beings, professional or nonprofessional, provider or consumer, make the easiest choices available to them most of the time."[10(p435)] Therefore, health-promoting choices must be more readily available and less costly than health-damaging options if individuals are to be healthy and a society is to improve its health status.

The opportunities for a society to make healthy choices have been a central theme throughout Milio's work. In a recent book she elaborated on this theme:

Personal behavior patterns are not simply "free" choices about "lifestyle," isolated from their personal and economic context. Lifestyles are, rather, patterns of choices made from the alternatives that are available to people according to their socioeconomic circumstances and the ease with which they are able to choose certain ones over others.[11(p76)]

Milio is critical of many traditional approaches to health education that emphasize knowledge acquisition and consequently expect behavior change. In addressing the role of public health in primary care, Milio voices concern that "health damage accumulates in societies too, vitiating their vitality . . . [and charges nurses to redirect energies] so as to foster conditions that help people to retain a self-sustaining physiological and social balance."[12(pp188,189)]

One cannot help but note the similarities between Milio's health resources and the concepts in the health belief model. The health belief model is more comprehensive than Milio's framework in examining the internal dynamics of health decision making. However, Milio offers a different set of insights into the arena of health behaviors by proposing that many low-income individuals are acting within the constraints of their limited resources. Furthermore, she goes beyond the individual focus and addresses changes in the health of populations as a result of shifts in decision making by significant numbers of people within a population.

Critical Social Theory

Just as Milio uses societal awareness as an aid to understanding health behaviors, critical social theory employs similar means to expose social inequities that prohibit people from reaching their full potential. This theoretic approach is based on the belief that life is structured by social meanings that are determined, rather one-sidedly, through social domination.[13] In contrast to the assumptions of analytic empiricism, critical theory maintains that standards of truth are socially determined and that no form of scientific inquiry is value free.[13,15] Proponents of this theoretic approach posit that social discourse that is not distorted from power imbalances will stimulate the evolution of a more rational society. The interests of truth are served only when people are able to voice their beliefs without fear of authority or retribution.[13]

Allen[14] discusses how nursing practice can be enriched by enabling clients to remove the conscious and unconscious constraints in their everyday lives. He states that women and the economically impoverished are especially vulnerable to being labeled by pseudodiseases that are rooted in social formations, such as hysteria and depression. Health-care providers often frame such problems only within the context of the individual or, at best, the family. But critical social theory can enable a nurse to reframe such an interpretation to gain an understanding of the historical play of social forces that have limited the choices truly available to the involved parties. Through exploration of the societal forces, traditions, and roles that have created the meanings of health and illness, clients may be freed of the isolation and alienation that accompany individual problem ownership.

At the collective level, Waitzkin asserts that the current emphasis on lifestyle diverts attention from important sources of illness in the capitalist industrial environment; "it also puts the burden of health squarely on the individual rather than seeking collective solutions to health problems."[16(p664)] Salmon[17] supports this position by noting that the basic tenets of Western medicine promote the delineation of individual factors of health and illness, while obscuring the exploration of their social and economic roots. He states that critical social theory "can aid in uncovering larger dimensions impacting health that are usually unseen or misrepresented by ideological biases. Thus, the social reality of health conditions can be both understood and changed."[17(p75)]

Because the theory holds that each person is responsible for creating social conditions in which all members of society are able to speak freely, the nurse is challenged, as an individual and as a member of the profession, to expose power imbalances that prohibit people from achieving their full potential. Nurses versed in critical theory are equipped to see beyond the perpetuation of status quo ideas and may be able to generate unique ideas that are unencumbered by previous stereotypes.[14]

Other Examples of Upstream Thinking

Recent nursing literature provides several other examples of upstream thinking. In a thought-provoking commentary on an intervention program for middle-aged women experiencing subclinical depression, Davis[18] (cited in Gordon and Ledray) notes a lack of congruence between the study's portrayal of depression as a problem with societal roots and its instruction in coping strategies as the intervention program. While recognizing the merits of the intervention program, she comments that, "if our principal task as progressive nurses is to develop and utilize interventions that will ameliorate these social problems, then the emphasis in nursing education and practice might well be on those social actions that aim to change basic social factors such as ageism and sexism."[18(p277)]

Chopoorian[19] takes a different tack, emphasizing the concept of environment and suggesting that nurses develop a consciousness of the social, political, and economic aspects of environment. She maintains that a static portrayal of the environment precludes nurses from acting as advocates for people who lack adequate housing and health care and live in intolerable circumstances. She charges nurses to move beyond a psychosocial conceptualization of the environment into a sociopolitical-economic conceptualization. Through this reconceptualization, nurses will see that human responses to health and illnesses "are related to the structure of the social world, the economic and political policies that govern that structure, and the human, social relationships that are produced by the structure and the policies."[19(p46)]

THE NEED FOR ALTERNATIVE PERSPECTIVES

The danger of the conservative perspective lies not within its content, but rather in the omission of other, larger theories that enable nurses to view situations from both a microscopic and a macroscopic perspective. In discussing the dilemmas of "studying health behavior as an individual phenomena [sic], rather than in the context of a broader social change phenomena [sic]," Cummings[20(p93)] reminds us that the approaches are complementary, and both are necessary to a comprehensive understanding of health promotion. The strengths and utility of each theoretic approach are most clearly revealed through an understanding of alternative approaches.

Nursing needs conceptual foundations that enable its practitioners to understand health problems manifested at community, national, and international levels as well as those at the individual and family levels. The continued bias in favor of individual-focused theories robs nurses of an understanding of the richness and complexity of forces that shape the behavior of populations. The omission of theories that relate nursing to the social context of behavior may leave nurses with a minimal understanding of their responsibilities to facilitate change at this level and without the tools to promote such change in an effective and systematic manner.

Maglacas[21] provides a global perspective on the health conditions of societies throughout the world and draws attention to the gaps in service access between the rich and the poor. She then charges nurses within each society and culture to act in response to the inequities in health within that society. If nurses are to be able to enact change at the societal level, they need to be provided with theoretic frameworks that are consistent with such ends and with theoretic perspectives in which social, economic, and political forces are given equal weight with the interpersonal aspects of nursing. Through these means, nurses gain insight into the social precursors of poor health and restricted opportunities and learn rationales for engaging in social action. By tipping the scales of nursing back toward consideration of theories that address health from a societal perspective, nurses can receive not only a richness of understanding but also the means by which to enact this kind of change.

REFERENCES

1. Dreher MC. The conflict of conservatism in public health nursing education. *Nurs Outlook.* 1982;30:504-509.

2. McKinlay JB. A case for refocussing upstream: The political economy of illness. In: Jaco EG, ed. *Patients, Physicians, and Illness.* 3rd ed. New York, NY: Free Press; 1979:9-25.

3. American Nurses' Association. *Nursing: A Social Policy Statement.* Kansas City, Mo: American Nurses' Association; 1980.

4. White CM. A critique of the ANA social policy statement. *Nurs Outlook.* 1984;32:328-331.

5. Rosenstock IM. Historical origins of the health belief model. In: Becker MH, ed. *The Health Be-*

lief Model and Personal Health Behavior. Thorofare, NJ: Charles B. Slack; 1974:1-8.

6. Becker MH, Maiman LA. Models of health-related behavior. In: Mechanic D, ed. *Handbook of Health, Health Care, and the Health Professions.* New York, NY: Free Press; 1983:539-568.

7. Jones PK, Jones SL, Katz J. Improving follow-up among hypertensive patients using a health belief model intervention. *Arch Intern Med.* 1987; 147:1557-1560.

8. Janz NK, Becker MH. The health belief model: A decade later. *Health Educ Q.* 1984;11:1-47.

9. Melnyk KM. Barriers: A critical review of recent literature. *Nurs Res.* 1988;37:196-201.

10. Milio N. A framework for prevention: Changing health-damaging to health-generating life patterns. *Am J Public Health.* 1976;66:435-439.

11. Milio N. *Promoting Health Through Public Policy.* Philadelphia, Penn: F.A. Davis; 1981.

12. Milio N. *Primary Care and the Public's Health.* Lexington, Mass: Lexington Books; 1983.

13. Allen D, Diekelmann N, Bennet P. Three paradigms for nursing research. In: Chinn P, ed. *Nursing Research Methodology: Issues & Implementation.* Rockville, Md: Aspen Publishers; 1986:23-28.

14. Allen DG. Nursing research and social control: Alternate models of science that emphasize understanding and emancipation. *Image: The Journal of Nursing Scholarship.* 1985;17:58-64.

15. Allen DG. Critical social theory as a model for analyzing ethical issues in family and community health. *Fam Commun Health.* 1987;10: 63-72.

16. Waitzkin H. A Marxist view of health and health care. In: Mechanic D, ed. *Handbook of Health, Health Care, and the Health Professions.* New York, NY: Free Press; 1983:657-682.

17. Salmon JW. Dilemmas in studying social change versus individual change: Considerations from political economy. In: Duffy ME, Pender NJ, eds. *Conceptual Issues in Health Promotion—A Report of Proceedings of a Wingspread Conference.* Indianapolis, Ind: Sigma Theta Tau; 1987:70-81.

18. Davis AJ. Cited by Gordon VC, Ledray LE. Growth-support intervention for the treatment of depression in women of middle years. *West J Nurs Res.* 1986;8:263-283.

19. Chopoorian TJ. Reconceptualizing the environment. In: Moccia P, ed. *New Approaches to*

Theory Development. New York, NY: National League for Nursing; 1986: 39-54. Publication 15-1992.

20. Cummings KM. Dilemmas in studying health as an individual phenomenon. In: Duffy ME, Pender NJ, eds. *Conceptual Issues in Health Promotion—A Report of Proceedings of a Wingspread Conference.* Indianapolis, Ind: Sigma Theta Tau; 1987:91-96.

21. Maglacas AM. Health for all: Nursing's role. *Nurs Outlook.* 1988;36:66-71.

18

Environmental Paradigms: Moving Toward an Ecocentric Perspective

DOROTHY KLEFFEL, RN, MPH, DNSc

This article examines a taxonomy of three environmental paradigms. The egocentric paradigm is grounded in the person and is based on the assumption that what is good for the individual is good for society. The homocentric paradigm is grounded in society and reflects the utilitarian ethic of the greatest good for the greatest number of people. The ecocentric paradigm is grounded in the cosmos, and the environment is considered whole, living, and interconnected. Historically, nurses have adhered primarily to the egocentric paradigm and to a lesser extent to the homocentric paradigm. However, because the world has become a global community, contemporary nurse scholars are shifting to the ecocentric paradigm. [Keywords: Ecocentric, Environment, Paradigm, Philosophy]

The environmental focus of nursing has traditionally been centered on clients' immediate surroundings in the hospital or other institution, home, or community. This circumscribed environmental worldview of nursing is undergoing change as nurses become aware of the adverse effects of environmental disasters and degradation on human health. Regional catastrophic environmental events like the Bhopal chemical leak, the Chernobyl nuclear disaster, and the Exxon Valdez oil spill have had immediate and lasting consequences. Global dimensions of the decline of the planet's environment include worldwide temperature rise, ozone depletion, destruction of the world's forests, human overpopulation, depleted fish populations, soil erosion, worldwide hunger, homelessness, and massive species extinction.[1,2] These are not isolated environmental problems that can be addressed by individual effort; they require the coordinated effort of people across the entire planet. Nurses are beginning to understand the scope of environmental threats that threaten everything that exists, living and nonliving. Nurses' enhanced consciousness of the environment has caused the profession to question its current assumptions about the environmental domain of nursing knowledge.

Nursing scholars are becoming cognizant that the existing environmental paradigm does not provide the knowledge and theoretical base to account for environmental conditions that compromise health promotion and interfere with optimum health. Nurses in general do not understand the interrelations between social, political, and economic struc-

Source: Kleffel, D. (1996). Environmental paradigms: Moving toward an ecocentric perspective *Adv Nurs Sci*, 18 (4): 1–10. Reprinted with permission by from and copyright © 1996 Aspen Publishers, Inc.

tures and the origins of health and illnesses.[3] Nursing theory does not adequately describe the concept of the environment. Almost all nursing research conducted in the domain of environment involves only the immediate milieu of the client, family, or nurse.[4] Nursing's care theories do not allow for nonhuman interchange of care or caring because of their anthropocentricity. Anthropocentrism results in the subjugation of nonhuman nature, which jeopardizes the quality of the physical world and causes other forms of oppression and domination.[5]

These critiques of nursing's environmental assumptions indicate that the profession is experiencing an environmental paradigm shift. A *paradigm* is the body of values, commitments, beliefs, and knowledge shared by members of a profession. Research guidelines, questions, and methodology emanate from the paradigm. When new knowledge is discovered that no longer fits the paradigm, or when the paradigm no longer provides model problems and solutions, an anomaly exists. When anomalies become so numerous and significant that they can no longer be ignored, investigations are initiated by the profession. Theories are explored and rejected until a new paradigm emerges that leads to a new basis for practice.[6]

Contemporary nursing scholars are exploring a variety of new environmental ideas and theories as the profession changes its environmental worldview. To contribute to this dialogue, I examine a taxonomy of three environmental paradigms—egocentric, homocentric, and ecocentric—that summarize the assumptions of Western culture regarding the natural world since the 17th century.[7,8] I propose the inclusion of the ecocentric environmental perspective into a central position in nursing's body of knowledge. This mainstreaming of a global view would encourage and support nurses to act with others in averting worldwide environmental disaster.

EGOCENTRIC APPROACH

The egocentric approach is grounded at the personal level and assumes that what is best for the individual is best for society. It is concerned with liberty, rights, and independent action of the individual. It is the dominant Western worldview. Its philosophical foundation is individualistic and mechanistic and includes the thought of Plato, mainstream Christianity, Descartes, Hegel, George Berkeley, Hobbes, Locke, Adam Smith, Malthus, and Garrett Hardin.[8] The egocentric approach is a mechanistic paradigm and assumes that matter is composed of atomic parts, the whole is equal to the sum of the parts, causation is a matter of external action on inactive parts, quantitative change is more important than qualitative change, and there is dualistic separation of mind–body and matter–spirit.[7] In the egocentric approach, the individual is the focus of change.

Most practicing nurses adhere to the egocentric worldview. Their approach is individualistic. They regard the environment as the immediate surroundings or circumstances of the individual or as an interactional field that individuals adapt to, adjust to, or control.[3] The environment is defined in relation to the individual person rather than in terms of its own essence and intrinsic value.

Because the egocentric approach has been the dominant perspective in the Western world, many nurse theorists incorporated those ideas into their theories. An example of a nurse theorist who adhered to the egocentric paradigm was Roy.[9] She defined the environment as all internal and external conditions, circumstances, and influences surrounding and affecting the development and behavior of individuals and groups. Stimuli emanate from the environment and are categorized as focal (immediately confronting the person), contextual (all other stimuli present), and residual (beliefs and attitudes that impinge on the situation). The purpose of nursing is to enhance the adaptation of the patient to environmental stimuli. Roy[10] believed that the science of nursing focuses on human life processes as the core knowledge to be developed. Roy's theory is considered egocentric because of its emphasis on individual adaptation to the environment and on human beings to the exclusion of the rest of nature.

Egocentrism has been the guiding ethic of private entrepreneurs and corporations whose goal is maximization of profit from the development of natural resources. The egocentric approach is limited because of its assumption that the individual good is the highest good that will ultimately benefit society as a whole and that humans are fundamentally different from other creatures, which they are to dominate and control.[7]

HOMOCENTRIC APPROACH

The homocentric approach is the utilitarian ethic and is grounded at the social level.[7,8] Social justice, rather than individual progress, is the key value. Decisions are made based on the common good, which is the greatest good for the largest number of people. Humans are considered stewards and caretakers of the natural world. The philosophical foundations of homocentrism are both materialism and positivism. Its assumptions are that humans have a cultural heritage in addition to their genetic inheritance that results in their being qualitatively different from animals, that the determinants of human affairs are social rather than individual, and that culture is a cumulative progress that can continue indefinitely. All social problems are viewed as ultimately solvable. Exponents of the homocentric approach include John S. Mill and Jeremy Bentham

(utilitarian theorists), Barry Commoner (socialist ecology), Karl Marx and Mao Tse Tung (political theorists), and Jørgen Randers and Donella and Dennis Meadows (limits-to-growth theorists).

The body of knowledge derived from epidemiology serves as an information base for the practice of public health nursing. Public health nurses use epidemiology in diagnosing, planning, treating, and evaluating community health problems. The nurse who interacts with individual clients and families uses the information for assessing, planning, intervening, and evaluating at the community level.[11] Epidemiology is considered homocentric because of its emphasis on the health of populations rather than individuals.

In the homocentric view, the environment is the focus of change rather than the individual. The homocentric approach to the environment is basically anthropocentric in that humans are to manage nature for the benefit of humans. The management of nature for the intrinsic benefit of other species is not considered in this paradigm.[7]

ECOCENTRIC APPROACH

The ecocentric approach is grounded in the cosmos. The whole environment, including inanimate elements such as rocks and minerals, along with animate animals and plants, is assigned intrinsic value. It is rooted in holistic rather than mechanistic metaphysics. It assumes that everything is connected to everything else, that the whole is greater than the sum of its parts, that meaning is dependent on context, that biological and social systems are open, and that humans and nonhumans are one within the same organic system. Exponents of the ecocentric approach include most traditional Eastern systems of thought, traditional Native American philosophies, Thoreau, Gary Snyder, Theodore Rozak, Aldo Leopold,

Rachel Carson, Fritjof Capra, deep ecology, the holographic model, and ecofeminism.[7,8]

Within the ecocentric paradigm are four contemporary nursing theorists. Sarter[12] compared the philosophical perspectives of fellow nursing theorists Rogers, Neuman, Watson, and Parse and found common shared holistic themes of process, evolution of consciousness, self-transcendence, open systems, harmony, relativity of space and time, pattern, and holism. *Process* is the evolutionary change of human consciousness; *self-transcendence* is the method of the evolution of human consciousness through higher and higher levels toward unity with the universe. *Open systems* are the dynamic and continuous interactions between the person and the world and are essential for the evolution of human consciousness. *Harmony* is considered to exist both within the person and between the person and the environment. Space and time are considered nonlinear, relative, and fluid, with the past and future merging into the present. *Pattern* is information that represents the whole. Pattern recognition is nursing action that looks for patterns representing the whole rather than parts of the whole. Sarter noted that each of these theorists has been influenced, either directly or indirectly, by Eastern philosophies. She believed that the foundation of a commonly held nursing worldview has been laid.

Watson[13] has continued to develop her ecocentric perspectives, moving toward a unitary–transformative viewpoint. This model has eliminated the subject–object and mind–body duality. It acknowledges unity and integrality between humans and the environment; thus conceptualized, human beings and their worlds are not separated.

Other modern nursing scholars also adhere to the ecocentric paradigm. Schuster[14] advocated for a conscious choice of earth dwelling through self-identification and interconnectedness with all beings, which lead one naturally to care for the world in day-to-day living.

It is a way of being in the world that allows for all of creation, not just humans, to emerge.

Kleffel,[15] during a qualitative research study, identified 17 distinguished scholars whose work has addressed broad environmental dimensions related to nursing. All except two explicitly reflected the ecocentric paradigm and perceived the environment to be alive, whole, interconnected, and interacting. These scholars add strength to the idea of the united nursing worldview described by Sarter.[12]

The ecocentric approach has some philosophical difficulties. The central problem is finding a philosophically adequate justification for the intrinsic value of nonhuman nature. In mainstream Western thought, only humans have intrinsic worth, while the rest of nature has instrumental value as a resource for humans. It is not considered wrong to kill the last of a species or use the last mineral if human survival is at stake.[7]

ECOCENTRISM IN THE WORLD'S TRADITIONS

The egocentric paradigm has been the dominant worldview of most practicing nurses working in hospitals and other health institutions and is ascribed to by the greatest number of nurses in the profession. The homocentric perspective has influenced far fewer nurses, traditionally those practicing in the field of public health nursing, although there are signs of a shifting of the profession toward the homocentric approach in the form of aggregate and population-based nursing.[16] The ecocentric view is only beginning to inform the profession and has not yet achieved significant prominence in nursing scholarship or practice.

Embracing an ecocentric viewpoint has exhilarating potential for transforming nursing scholarship and practice beyond its traditional boundaries. We are now living in a global culture that is united by economic interdependence, international air transportation, and worldwide communications networks. Contemporary environmental degradation and disasters that adversely affect humans have moved into the global arena. Actions stem from worldviews, and the worldview of nursing has been mostly egocentric. Moving to the ecocentric paradigm will encourage nurses to address worldwide environmental problems that affect the health of everything that exists.

Solving global environmental problems will entail international efforts from a variety of disciplines and from many cultures. Such an approach will entail collaborative problem solving by people with differing traditions and cultural backgrounds. To work together, a common global environmental worldview that can incorporate these diverse perspectives is needed. The ecocentric paradigm, which is compatible with elements of Native American traditional ideas, Eastern philosophies, and contemporary Western thought, holds great promise for a unified worldview to which all humans can subscribe.

Native American Tradition

There are difficulties in universalizing the Native American belief system because it comprises so many different cultures. However, some generalizations can be made.[17] The Native American attitude was to regard all entities in the environment as having consciousness, reason, and volition as intense and complete as humans. These entities included the earth itself, the sky, the winds, rocks, streams, trees, insects, birds, and animals. This pervasive spirit in everything was considered a part of the Great Spirit, which fostered the perception of humans and nature as being unified and akin. The Native American's social circle or community included all nonhuman natural entities as well as other humans.

The consequences of the Native American inspired worldview of nature produced a harmony between them and their environment that restrained their killing of animals and gathering of plants to what was necessary for survival. Although there were occasional examples of destruction of nature during periods of enormous cultural stress, the overall and usual effort was conservation of resources. The Native American cultural traditions were not altruistic; they considered it in their own self-interest to defer to nature, which they believed would withhold its sustenance or actively retaliate if provoked.[17]

Eastern Systems of Thought

Similar themes of a unified, living, conscious, and interacting world are found in almost all Eastern systems of thought. With the exception of Islam, these systems are antihierarchal and anthropocentric. Although Islam maintains that humans are dominant over nature, a view similar to the Judeo-Christian tradition, it instructs its adherents to prevent environmental deterioration because the world is God's creation.[18] Other Eastern philosophies emphasize harmony and balance. All aspects of the environment interact, with the parts being within the whole and the whole being within the parts. Humans are a part of the whole and admonished to live in equilibrium with all other parts of the planet.[19]

Some examples of Eastern thought include the law of Karma of the Advita Vedanta, which binds humans together in continuity with the natural world.[20] The *wu wei* of Taoism is an awareness that allows one to maximize creative possibilities of oneself as a dimension of the environment.[21] The *Chi* of Chinese thought is a vital force that is the basic structure of the cosmos and exists in all things. Nature is the result of fusion and merging of vital forces to form the "great harmony."[22]

A popular image for portraying the manner in which things exist is described from the *Hua-yen* school of Buddhism.[23] From the great god Indra there hangs a marvelous net that stretches out infinitely in all directions. There is a jewel in each eye of the net. Since the net is infinite in dimension, the jewels are infinite in number. When one jewel is selected and carefully looked at, all of the other jewels in the net are reflected. In addition, each of the jewels reflected is also reflecting all of the other jewels, so that an infinite reflecting process occurs.

This image symbolizes the cosmos, in which there is an infinitely repeated interrelationship among all of the members of the cosmos. Thus, the part and the whole are one and the same, for what we identify as a part is merely an abstraction from a unitary whole. There is no part-and-whole duality as in Western thought. This totalistic world is a living body in which each cell derives its life from the other cells and in return gives life to the others.

Western Approaches

The ecocentric environmental themes found in Eastern and traditional Native American worldviews originated in ancient times. Several modern Western ecocentric environmental approaches reflect these ideas. The science of ecology, along with relativity and quantum theory, is creating a postmodern scientific worldview. This emerging worldview is in congruence with the traditional and indigenous environmental paradigms of preindustrial cultures.[24] Naess criticized traditional ecology (an egocentric approach), which he dubbed "shallow ecology,"[25(p95)] as being concerned only with pollution control and resource conservation in the interests of people in developed countries. He argued that there are deeper concerns (hence the phrase "deep ecology," also called "radical environmental-

ism") that touch on the principles of diversity, complexity, autonomy, decentralization, symbiosis, egalitarianism, and classlessness. Deep ecology derives its essence from some Eastern and Native American ideas as well as from feminism, John Muir, and other naturalist literature.[26]

The modern Gaia hypothesis is reminiscent of the ancient living organic theory. This view of the environment was proposed by Lovelock,[27,28] an atmospheric chemist. Lovelock saw the evolution of the species of living organisms as being so closely coupled with the evolution of their physical and chemical environment that together they constitute a single and indivisible evolutionary process. No clear distinction is made between living and nonliving material. The planet's organisms act together as a unity to regulate the global environment by adjusting the rates at which gases are produced and removed from the atmosphere. Lovelock warned that the earth's ability to self-regulate is affected by natural or human activity, which could force the climate into a new and different stable state that would result in the elimination of all living organisms.

The idea of the planet's stable state in the modern Gaia hypothesis reflects the idea of harmony in ancient Taoist thought. In both notions, the balance of the environment of the planet must be maintained, or ecological disaster will result.

Bohm,[29] a physicist and one of the early pioneers of the holographic model, believed that the universe is organized along holographic principles. Everything in the universe is part of a continuum, a seamless extension of everything else. There are no separate parts, just as a geyser in a fountain is not separated from the water from which it flows. However, the universe is not an undifferentiated mass. Things can have their own unique qualities and still be part of an undivided whole. Similarly, consciousness is present in all matter in various degrees. The universe cannot be divided into living and nonliving things. All things are interconnected; like a hologram, every portion of the universe contains the whole.

There are similarities of imagery between the holographic model and Indra's net. The giant hologram and Indra's net symbolize the cosmos. All parts of the hologram are interconnected; each jewel in Indra's net is connected with every other jewel. The parts of the hologram and each jewel of Indra's net reflect the whole. The whole of the hologram and the whole of Indra's net reflect each part or jewel. Bohm believed that fragmentation is the cause of most present-day problems. Applied to the environment, one portion of the planet cannot be harmed without resulting damage to the entire planet.

Another modern Western ecocentric view is ecofeminism. Ecofeminism is a theory that women and the environment are interconnected as both share and have been subjected to the same patriarchal domination.[30] A failure to understand these connections will result in the continued exploitation of both women and environment at the theory, policy, and practice levels. Ecofeminists recognize the interconnectedness of women and the environment and recognize the necessity of uniting feminism and ecology. However, feminist theory is not environmentally sensitive. Deep ecology and the Gaia hypothesis share themes of unity and wholeness to which ecofeminists can subscribe; however, both are oriented toward a patriarchal culture. Ecofeminists hold the view that the connections between the twin dominations of women and nature require a feminist theory and practice informed by an ecological perspective and an environmentalism informed by a feminist perspective.[31]

Ecofeminism is against domination of all kinds, including ageism, sexism, and the exploitation of nature. It is contextual and relational and includes consideration of nonhuman relationships with each other, humans, and the community. Ecofeminism identifies human nature within the historical context. It is antireductionist and pluralistic, centralizing on diversity of humans and nonhumans, yet affirming that humans are a part of the ecological community. Ecofeminism provides a central place for values that are typically underrepresented or ignored in our society such as care, love, friendship, and appropriate trust. Ecofeminism views theory building, objectivity, and knowledge as historically and contextually situated and as changing over time.[31,32]

IMPLEMENTING THE ECOCENTRIC PARADIGM

Understanding that the environment is alive, whole, interconnected, and interacting and that humans are one with the environment will encourage nurses to practice in an environmentally sensitive manner in whatever setting they work. Nurses working in local settings will understand the relationships between organizational resource use and the worldwide environment. Using the adage "think globally, act locally," they will act within their sphere by doing such things as calling for institutional audits of their work environment, taking client environmental histories, counseling clients regarding the effects of ozone depletion on the incidence of skin cancers and cataracts, reducing the use of toxic materials, purchasing recycled materials and supplies, using products with environmentally friendly packaging, saving water, managing waste safely, using both sides of the paper when copying reports and forms, using reusable products, reducing the use of disposable items, buying rechargeable batteries,[33] and questioning animal experimentation.[34]

Moving to the ecocentric paradigm will mean extending the concept of the nursing client to include the planetary environment. Some nurses will choose to work in the global environmental arena and address international environmental causes of illnesses. For instance, the alarming increase of breast cancer worldwide is an area where nurses could make a difference. In the United States the risk of breast cancer has increased from 1 in 20 in 1960 to 1 in 8 today. Other industrial countries have similar rates. The incidence in developing countries is also rising, but at a slower rate. Risk factors and lifestyle account for only 20% to 30% of breast cancer cases. Some experts believe that pollutants and chemicals that duplicate or interfere with the effects of estrogen are a possible cause. They point to the fact that in Israel, breast cancer mortality in premenopausal women declined by 30 percent following regulations to reduce levels of DDT and carcinogenic pesticides in dietary fat.[35] Other experts believe that low-level radiation and synthetic chemicals such as chlorines are responsible for the increase in breast cancer in women.[36]

Mainstream medicine and science have ignored the possible environmental causes of breast cancer, focusing on the identification of women with risk factors, early case finding through breast self-examination, routine mammograms, and changing lifestyles (smoking cessation, exercise, and lowering dietary fat intake). By contrast, groups like the Women's Environment and Development Organization and Greenpeace are advocating for public attention to the possible links between the environment and breast cancer.[37] Nurses have followed medicine's lead by emphasizing compliance with breast self-examination, counseling women with risk factors associated with breast cancer, and providing education regarding healthy lifestyles. However, they have not directed their attention toward the relationships between breast cancer and the environment, which are being ignored by most research organizations. Using a global, multidisciplinary perspective, nurses could network with other researchers throughout the world to coordinate investigative efforts to identify environmental causes of breast cancer.

Emerging strains of recurring infectious diseases is another area where nurses could make a difference. AIDS, Lyme disease, the Hanta virus, the deadly Ebola virus, the recurrence of plague in India, and the increases in cholera, tuberculosis, and malaria worldwide are examples of conditions related to environmental alterations, climate changes, rapid international travel, and other human activity.[38] Although these diseases are causing illnesses and the deaths of millions of people, nurses generally do not regard scholarship or action in this arena as part of their domain. It is predicted that the epidemics will get worse as the displacement of wild populations and their habitats caused by development activities continue. International multidisciplinary efforts are required to keep ecosystems intact, minimize habitat alterations, require planners to prepare for unanticipated consequences of development, and establish a reliable global surveillance system. Acting internationally in concert with other nurses, other disciplines, and other organizations, nurses could, if they had a global vision, bring their unique skills and perspectives to addressing this type of global environmental phenomenon.

Moving toward an ecocentric perspective will give nurses a common worldview, already held by a great proportion of the world's peoples, of oneness with a living planet, harmony, balance, interconnectedness, and transcendence. It will empower nurses to move beyond their present domain boundaries to align their efforts with other disciplines and organizations worldwide to address the devastating environmental problems affecting the earth and threatening all of existence.

REFERENCES

1. Brown LR, Flavin, French H. *State of the World 1995: A Worldwatch Institute Report on Progress Toward a Sustainable Society*. New York, NY: Norton; 1995.

2. Brown LR, Nicholas L, Kane H. *Vital Signs 1995: The Trends That Are Shaping Our Future*. New York, NY: Norton; 1995.

3. Chopoorian TJ. Reconceptualizing the environment. In: Moccia P, ed. *New Approaches to Theory Development*. New York, NY: National League for Nursing; 1986.

4. Kleffel D. Rethinking the environment as a domain of nursing knowledge. *ANS*. 1991; 14(1):40–51.

5. Schuster EA. Earth caring. *ANS*. 1990; 13(1):25–30.

6. Kuhn TS. *The Structure of Scientific Revolutions*. Chicago, Ill: University of Chicago; 1970.

7. Merchant C. Environmental ethics and political conflict: A view from California. *Environ Ethics*. 1990;12(1):45–68.

8. Miller AS. *Gaia Connections: An Introduction to Ecology, Ecoethics, and Economics*. Savage, Md: Rowman & Littlefield; 1991.

9. Roy C. Roy's adaptation model. In: Parse R, ed. *Nursing Science: Major Paradigms, Theories, and Critiques*. Philadelphia, Penn: W.B. Saunders; 1987.

10. Roy C. An explication of the philosophical assumptions of the Roy Adaptation Model. *Nurs Sci Q*. 1988;1(1):26–34.

11. Shortridge L, Valanis B. The epidemiological model applied in community health nursing. In: Stanhope M, Lancaster J. *Community Health Nursing: Process and Practice for Promoting Health*. 3rd ed. Chicago, Ill: Mosby/Year-Book; 1992.

12. Sarter B. Philosophical sources of nursing theory. *Nurs Sci Q*. 1988;1(2):52–59.

13. Watson J. Nursing's caring–healing paradigm as exemplar for alternative medicine? *Altern Therapies*. 1995;1(3):64–69.

14. Schuster EA. Earth dwelling. *Holistic Nurs Pract*. 1992;6(4):1–9.

15. Kleffel D. *The Environment: Alive, Whole, Interacting, and Interconnected*. San Diego, Calif: University of California, San Diego; 1994. Dissertation.

16. Moccia P. *A Vision for Nursing Education*. New York, NY: National League for Nursing; 1993.

17. Callicott JB. Traditional American Indian and Western European attitudes toward nature: An overview. *Environ Ethics*. 1982;4(4):293–318.

18. Zaidi IH. On the ethics of man's interaction with the environment: An Islamic approach. *Environ Ethics*. 1981; 2(1):35–47.

19. Callicott JB. Toward a global environmental ethic. In: Tucker ME, Grim JA, eds. *Worldviews and Ecology: Religion, Philosophy, and the Environment*. Maryknoll, NY: Orbis Books; 1994.

20. Deutsch E. A metaphysical grounding for natural reverence: East-West. *Environ Ethics*. 1986;8(4):283–299.

21. Ames RT. Taoism and the nature of nature. *Environ Ethics*. 1986;8(4):317–350.

22. Wei-Ming T. The continuity of being: Chinese visions of nature. In Callicott JB, Ames RT, eds. *Nature in Asian Traditions of Thought: Essays in Environmental Philosophy*. New York, NY: State University of New York Press; 1989.

23. Cook FH. The jewel net of Indra. In: Callicott JB, Ames RT, eds. *Nature in Asian Traditions of Thought: Essays in Environmental Philosophy*. New York, NY: State University of New York Press; 1989.

24. Callicott JB. *Earth's Insights: A Survey of Ecological Ethics from the Mediterranean Basin to the Australian Outback*. Los Angeles, Calif: University of California Press; 1994.

25. Naess A. The shallow and the deep, long-range ecology movement: A summary. *Inquiry*. 1973;16:95–100.

26. Devall B, Sessions G. *Deep Ecology*. Salt Lake, Colo: Perigrine Smith; 1985.

27. Lovelock J. *Gaia: A New Look at Life on Earth*. New York, NY: Oxford University Press; 1979.

28. Lovelock J. *The Ages of Gaia: A Biography of Our Living Earth*. New York, NY: Norton; 1988.

29. Bohm D. *Wholeness and the Implicate Order*. London, England: Routledge & Kegan Paul; 1980.

30. Cheney J. Ecofeminism and deep ecology. *Environ Ethics*. 1987;9(2):115–144.

31. Warren KJ. Feminism and ecology: Making connections. *Environ Ethics*. 1987;9(1):3–20.

32. Warren KJ, Cheney J. Ecological feminism and ecosystem ecology. *Hypatia*. 1991;6(1):179–197.

33. Shaner H. Environmentally responsible clinical practice. In: Schuster EA, Brown CL, eds. *Exploring Our Environmental Connections*. New York, NY: National League for Nursing Press; 1994.

34. Todd B. An ecofeminist look at animal research. In: Schuster EA, Brown CL, eds. *Explor-*

ing Our Environmental Connections. New York, NY: National League for Nursing Press; 1994.

35. Platt A. Breast and prostate cancer rising. In: *Vital Signs 1995: The Trends That Are Shaping Our Future*. New York, NY: Norton; 1995.

36. Women's Environment and Development Organization. Does the breast cancer epidemic have environmental links? *News & Views*. 1992;6(1):1,9.

37. Women's Environment and Development Organization. Women's coalitions battle breast cancer and other environmental health problems. *News & Views*. 1995;8(1–2):2.

38. Platt A. The resurgence of infectious diseases. *World Watch: Working for a Sustainable Future*. 1995;8(4):26–32.

Part V

CONTEMPORARY
PERSPECTIVES OF
NURSING

Since the 1980s, several nurse scholars and theorists have shifted from a traditional, logical positivistic worldview of nursing science to a simultaniety perspective, which is often labeled the 'human science paradigm' in nursing. Dr. Martha Rogers' work and theory of unitary man provided the impetus for this philosophical shift, and her followers or proteges developed their own theories based on the belief that humans are intentional, free-willed persons continuously engaging in a dynamic, interactive process with others and their environment. With this new perspective, the focus of nursing is to guide clients to reflect on their lived experiences from their perspective, and explore the meanings of their past, present, and future life in relation to their desired being and becoming toward life and health. Some renown theorists whose work is based on the human science paradigm are Rogers, Newman, Parse, and Watson.

Before discussing new perspectives, Jacqueline Fawcett's article, entitled "The State of Nursing Science: Hallmark of the 20th and 21st Century," examines nurses' success in achieving specific hallmarks in nursing theory development, nursing research and practice, that she published in three articles in the 1980s. Dr. Fawcett states that she has not seen any evidence of movement toward achieving those earlier criteria, and she expresses concern for the continued existence of the nursing discipline. As for nursing research, Dr. Fawcett decries the paucity of published studies guided by nursing theories or models, or based on nursing methodologies, which she feels must be empirically tested. In nursing practice, she compared advanced practice nurses to junior doctors or physician assistants, whose practice is based on medical, not nursing science. Dr. Fawcett advocates that all nurses should be prepared at the doctoral level, and become scholar researchers, with a base in nursing practice. This controversial article may stimulate much discussion about her views on the future of nursing and the potential demise of the profession.

Humanistic nursing science is based on understanding, valuing, and analyzing the changing life patterns of humans as an ongoing process reflected in the unity of the 'lived experience.' In their article, "Nursing Knowledge and Human Science: Ontological and Epistemolocial Considerations," Drs. Gail Mitchell and William Cody describe the meaning of human science proposed by Wilhelm Dilthey. They critique the work of several nurse theorists—Paterson and Zderad, Newman, Parse, and Watson, as to the 'goodness of fit' of these nursing theories with a human science for nursing. This chapter will assist graduate nurses to understand the foundation of contemporary nursing theories, and hopefully help them apply the theories in practice.

In an effort to link humanistic nursing science with Carper's 'ways of knowing,' Dianne Raymond wrote the article, "Esthetic and Personal Knowing Through Humanistic Nursing." She begins with a description and critique of Paterson and Zderad's humanistic nursing model, followed by a clinical example. Next she explains how the phases in a therapeutic nursing relationship are applied as the patient's lived experience unfolds. The shift in nursing's philosophy of science, and the concomitant changes in research methodology are described and advocated to expand humanistic nursing science and practice.

The controversy about whether the nursing discipline should have a single, unitary theory or multiple paradigms has gone on for several decades. Joan Engebretson's article, "A Multiparadigm Approach to Nursing," adds another dimension to the discussion. Dr. Engebretson begins by identifying some discrepancies between biomedical nursing practice, which is commonly seen today, and holistic nursing theories. She discusses some contemporary controversies related to the development and use of current nursing theories, and compares cultural differences in holism and healing. Then, based on her ethnographic work and research, she develops a multiparadigm model representing a cross-cultural, holistic approach to health and healing. Her model consists of four paradigms for healing—mechanical, purification, balance, and supranormal, which are applied by five types of healing modalities—physical manipulation, applied and ingested substances, energy, psychological, and spiritual methods. Her model provides a variety of means for healing from the physical to the spiritual modalities, and also demonstrates movement from empiric based knowledge to metaphysical sciences. Since many consumers are turning to nontraditional or complementary methods for healing, nurse practitioners should acquire more knowledge of these modalities and consider their value as we move toward using more Eastern ways of healing.

19

The State of Nursing Science: Hallmarks of the 20th and 21st Centuries

JACQUELINE FAWCETT, RN, PHD, FAAN

Science generally is regarded as the systematic, controlled, empirical, and critical activities undertaken to generate and test theories. Nursing science, therefore, comprises those systematic, controlled, empirical, and critical activities undertaken to generate and test nursing theories. This column focuses on my view of the state of nursing science circa 1999. My comments reflect countless hours of solitary thought, as well as 35 years of dialogue with colleagues and students in classrooms and at local, regional, national, and international workshops and conferences. I have become increasingly troubled by the state of our science but have retained sufficient optimism to accept the invitation to write this column and share my vision of what we can do if we want to save our discipline and advance our science.

HALLMARKS OF 20TH-CENTURY NURSING

During the 1980s, I published a trilogy of articles that reflected my excitement with the state of nursing science and my optimism for the future of the discipline of nursing. In the first article, I identified four hallmarks of success in nursing theory development (Fawcett, 1983). In the second article, I identified three hallmarks of success in nursing research (Fawcett, 1984). In the third article, a colleague and I identified four hallmarks of success in nursing practice (Fawcett & Carino, 1989).

The four hallmarks of success in nursing theory development that I identified were specification of a metaparadigm for nursing, explication of conceptual models of nursing, explication of unique nursing theories, and theories shared with other disciplines. The meaning and content of the nursing metaparadigm, conceptual models, and unique nursing theories most likely are well known to readers. Shared theories may require some explanation. Simply put, a shared theory is one that has been borrowed from another discipline and then tested to determine its empirical adequacy in nursing situations. If the theory is found to be empirically adequate in legitimate nursing situations, it may be considered to be a shared theory.

The three hallmarks of success in nursing research that I identified were specification of the boundaries of nursing research, explication of the types of research needed by the professional discipline of nursing, and delineation of research activities appropriate for

Source: Fawcett, J. (1999). The state of nursing science: hallmarks of the 20th and 21st centuries. *Nursing Science Quarterly*, 12 (4): 311 – 315. Reprinted by permission of and copyright © 1999 Sage Publications, Inc.

nurses according to educational preparation. The boundaries of nursing research were, I maintained, set by the metaparadigm of nursing and by the rules of research that are inherent in each conceptual model of nursing. The metaparadigm sets the global boundary for research as examination of nursing's efforts to facilitate person-environment interactions having to do with health. Each conceptual model of nursing provides an interpretation of that boundary and presents more circumscribed boundaries in the form of a set of conceptual and methodologic rules for research.

Drawing from the notion that nursing is a professional rather than an academic discipline, I maintained that basic, applied, and clinical types of research are required. An academic discipline has as its mission only the development and dissemination of knowledge. A professional discipline, in contrast, has as its mission the development, dissemination, and utilization of knowledge. Basic research focuses only on development of knowledge, without regard to its later use; this type of research is conducted by the members of both academic and professional disciplines. Applied research focuses on determination of the practical limits of knowledge, that is, determination of the range of practical situations in which each theory is empirically adequate. Applied research also is conducted by members of both academic and professional disciplines. Clinical research focuses on the effects of actual implementation of theories in clinical practice situations; this type of research is conducted only by members of professional disciplines.

For the third hallmark of success in nursing research, delineation of research activities appropriate for nurses according to educational preparation, I drew from the American Nurses' Association Commission on Nursing Research 1981 statement of guidelines for the investigative functions of nurses. The commission issued guidelines for participation in a wide range of research-related activities that took into account distinct differences in research capabilities between the graduates of associate degree nursing programs, baccalaureate nursing programs, master's degree nursing programs, practice-oriented doctoral programs (DNSc), and research-oriented programs (PhD).

The four hallmarks of success in nursing practice that Carino and I identified were use of conceptual models of nursing to guide nursing practice, development of classification systems, establishment of formal linkages between nursing education and nursing service, and recognition of clinical scholars and clinical scholarship. The first three hallmarks are self-explanatory. The fourth hallmark characterizes clinical scholarship as a professional imperative and the consequent emergence of nurse clinicians as clinical scholars. Clinical scholarship takes many forms, including the development and testing of assessment formats and intervention protocols and the application of clinical nursing research findings in daily clinical practice. Clinical scholars are nurse clinicians who practice nursing in an increasingly thoughtful manner. "They continually contemplate situations and stretch their minds toward insights into nursing practice and helping people to improve their health. Nurses who are true clinical scholars are noted for their ability to make novel connections between things or ideas—mental leaps and intuitive lunges that improve nursing practice and, therefore, enhance the well-being of their patients" (Fawcett & Carino, 1989, p. 6).

CURRENT TRENDS IN NURSING SCIENCE

Throughout the 1990s, my excitement about the advances in nursing science that led to the trilogy of hallmark articles has been progressively dampened. I have been particularly discouraged because I have seen little that might indicate a need for updates in those hallmark works. That is, although I do not see any evidence of a loss of ground for the existing hallmarks, I do not see any progress either. Even more to the point, I have seen nothing that might qualify as a new hallmark of success in nursing theory development, nursing research, or nursing practice. Moreover, my early optimism has turned to pessimism, reflecting a very real concern for the continued existence of the discipline of nursing.

Research conducted by nurses has increased in quantity and, some might argue, in quality in recent years. But I can no longer support the maxim that research conducted by nurses is, by definition, nursing research. That is because the current trend in research by nurses signals a major threat to the very survival of our discipline. More specifically, much of the research conducted by contemporary nurse researchers (i.e., those nurses who are academically qualified to advance science through research) has not been nursing research and has done nothing to advance nursing science. Instead, much of the research has employed nonnursing methodologies to generate new theories guided by nonnursing conceptual frameworks and to test theories developed by members of other disciplines. Note, for example, that just 6 (8%) of the 73 studies reported in Nursing Research and Research in Nursing and Health in 1998 involved the generation or testing of nursing theories using nursing methodologies. However, 2 of the 6 studies were designed to test ad hoc theories that combined concepts from nursing and some other discipline, and another 2 of the 6 tested ad hoc nursing theories developed from an interdisciplinary literature exclusive of nursing. Thus, just 2 (3%) of the 73 studies were guided by widely recognized nursing theories, namely, Leininger's theory of culture care diversity and universality and Pender's

theory of health promotion. Clearly, much science was produced in 1998, but very little nursing science.

The argument could be advanced that the studies that were guided by nonnursing conceptual frameworks and theories were focused on the development of shared nursing theories, which I previously identified as a hallmark of success in nursing theory development (Fawcett, 1983). However, the investigators who reported those studies did not identify the development of shared theory as a goal, nor did they explicitly discuss any modifications in the original theories that might be required for their use in legitimate nursing situations.

Turning to practice, services offered by nurses have become seemingly more comprehensive and sophisticated. But I can no longer support the maxim that practice by nurses is, by definition, nursing practice. That is because the current trend in practice by nurses, especially by so-called advanced practice nurses, signals another major threat to the survival of our discipline. More specifically, many of the services offered by contemporary nurse practitioners (i.e., those nurses academically and professionally qualified to utilize science through practice) have not been based on nursing science and have done nothing to inform nursing science. Instead, nurse practitioners increasingly base their practice on medical science and perform tasks "traditionally within the domain of medical practice" (Orem, 1995, p. 41). Note, for example, that nurse practitioners are said to resemble physicians' assistants (Martha Rogers, cited in Huch, 1995), junior doctors (Meleis, 1993), or pseudodoctors (Kendrick, 1997) engaged in nursing qua medicine (Watson, 1996).

The reasons for the current trends in research and practice most likely are many and complex. With regard to research, perhaps editors and peer reviewers think that the use and testing of nonnursing conceptual frameworks and theories will increase the visibility of research conducted by nurses among members of other disciplines and the public. Perhaps researchers who base their studies on conceptual models of nursing and nursing theories do not submit their reports to the two journals cited here because they think that such studies are not published in those journals. I would be remiss, then, if I did not mention that almost every report of research based on an explicit conceptual model of nursing that I have submitted to either journal has been published. Thus, it is unlikely that systematic bias against nursing science is operating. However, in contrast to Nursing Science Quarterly and Visions: The Journal of Rogerian Nursing Science, neither of the other two journals cited requires research to reflect advances in nursing science through the testing of a conceptual model of nursing or a nursing theory.

With regard to practice, perhaps practitioners think that if they emulate medical practice, their services will be more highly valued by the public and other health professionals. Or, perhaps many nurses feel so oppressed by physicians that they, like virtually all oppressed persons, have a disdain for the science of their own discipline and identify with the science of the perceived oppressor, medicine.

THE HALLMARK OF 21ST-CENTURY NURSING: A PREDICTION

While in the depths of pessimism, I began to think of a way to save our discipline. It has become increasingly clear to me that the discipline of nursing can survive if, and only if, we end our romance with medical science and the conceptual frameworks, theories, and methodologies of nonnursing disciplines. We see evidence of that romance every day in the reports of studies conducted by nurses but guided by nonnursing conceptual frameworks, theories, and methodologies. We also see evidence of that romance in advertisements for either a nurse practitioner or a physician's assistant—as if they were interchangeable professions. And, perhaps most disturbing, we see evidence of that romance every time that nurse practitioners are featured in the news media, including the nursing media, and talk about how they provide the same services as primary care physicians and receive—or hope to soon receive—the same reimbursement as physicians for those services from third-party payers. No wonder, then, that physicians claim that nurses are infringing on medical turf. No wonder, then, that we tolerate and even support Nurse Practice Acts that require supervision of nurse practitioners by a licensed physician.

If we do not end the romance with nonnursing disciplines. I predict that we will not survive as a distinct discipline. If, however, we do end the romance, we have a chance at survival but only under certain conditions. Those conditions, I believe, involve embracing nursing science through the integration of research and practice, which will require a change in the educational preparation of all nurses and will mandate a change in the employment conditions of nurses. More specifically, I believe that our discipline will not only survive but flourish through rapid advances in nursing science if all nurses become nurse scholars. I envision nurse scholars as nurses who integrate nursing science versions of the roles of nurse researcher and nurse practitioner. Today's separate roles of nurse researcher and nurse practitioner will no longer exist. Rather, all nurses will perform a single role—that of nurse scholar. The immediate and obvious advantage of a single role is the elimination of the so-called research-practice gap. If actualized, I predict that the single role of nurse scholar will become the one hallmark of the success of 21st-century nursing.

I envision nurse scholars as academically and professionally qualified to develop and utilize nursing science. More specifically, I envision nurse scholars as qualified to conduct nursing discipline-specific research and to practice from a nursing discipline-specific perspective. Nurses will focus on discipline-specific research and practice and employ nursing methodologies to generate, test, and apply nursing theories within the context of conceptual models of nursing. Only when that occurs can the research and practice activities of nurses be said to advance nursing science, and only then can research and practice be said to contribute to the discipline of nursing.

All nurse scholars will actively engage in integrated research-practice activities, using nursing methodologies to test and apply conceptual models of nursing and nursing theories in the provision of nursing services to people. Clearly, nurse scholars are not the nurse researchers or nurse practitioners of today but, rather, are nursing practitioners (Orem, 1995) or senior nurses (Meleis, 1993) who are engaged in nursing qua nursing (Watson, 1997). Inasmuch as nurse scholars constantly conduct nursing discipline-specific research and engage in nursing discipline-specific practice, they advance nursing science continuously.

Nurse scholars are initially prepared for their integrated role responsibilities in post-baccalaureate doctorate of nursing (ND) programs. I believe that today's diversity in entry levels cannot continue to exist if our discipline is to survive. Thus, I envision the ND as the entry level for all nursing. Moreover, given the holistic, comprehensive nature of nursing discipline-specific practice, I envision no need for unlicensed assistive nursing personnel. ND-prepared nurse scholars want to be at the patient's side, which is the only place where they can perform integrated research and practice role activities.

ND-prepared nurse scholars use nursing methodologies, which are derived from ex-plicit conceptual models of nursing and nursing theories, to guide their integrated research and practice activities. The integration of research and practice is evident as ND-prepared nurse scholars use the data obtained from every encounter with a patient for nursing research purposes. Every nurse-patient encounter, then, becomes a case study, with an individual patient serving as his or her own control (Wood, 1978). Thus, each case study is an experiment that tests the efficacy of the conceptual model and theories used to guide the nurse-patient encounter. In other words, ND-prepared nurse scholars use the clinical data available to them in every patient situation to determine the credibility of existing conceptual models of nursing and the empirical adequacy of existing nursing theories, thereby contributing constantly to nursing science.

Rather, their area of expertise or specialization is in a particular conceptual model of nursing or nursing theory. These scholars carry out their role responsibilities with the individuals, families, and/or communities regarded as legitimate patients within the context of that particular conceptual model of nursing or nursing theory. In addition, they apply the relevant nursing methodology to the full range of conditions and situations encompassed by the conceptual model or theory.

ND-prepared nurse scholars receive advanced preparation in doctor of philosophy (PhD) programs. The focus of PhD programs in nursing science is on the use of nursing methodologies, derived from conceptual models of nursing and nursing theories, with groups of patients rather than with individual patients. More specifically, PhD-prepared nurse scholars use aggregate data obtained from multiple encounters with patients to determine the credibility of various existing conceptual models of nursing and the empirical adequacy of various existing nursing theories. They also use those data to develop new conceptual models of nursing, nursing theories, and nursing methodologies. In other words, they combine single case studies to advance nursing science.

Rather than specialize in a particular conceptual model of nursing or nursing theory, PhD-prepared nurse scholars are generalists who examine the differential efficacy of two or more conceptual models of nursing or nursing theories with diverse patients with diverse conditions in diverse situations. The results of such examinations ultimately will lead to a better understanding of the "fit" of a particular intellectual perspective with a particular patient and, therefore, a substantial advance in nursing science.

ND- and PhD-prepared nurse scholars function as "attending nurses," that is, nurses who are with patients continuously wherever they are: "in and outside of institutions, schools, homes, clinics, and community settings" (Watson, 1996, p. 163). Thus, each patient always has his or her own nurse scholar, who collaborates with other health professionals when the patient requires services from others. Attending nurses, of course, carry out integrated research and practice role responsibilities. As attending nurses, ND- and PhD-prepared nurse scholars may work in nurse corporations, which are made up of nurse scholars in equal partnership with one another, or they may elect to be self-employed. Nurse corporations contract with individuals, families, communities, medical centers, community and specialty hospitals, home care agencies, hospices, and other agencies and organizations for the provision of distinctively nursing services guided by conceptual models of nursing, nursing theories, and nursing methodologies. The idea of nurse corporations was proposed by Sills (1983), who explained:

> The conceptual key to the corporation proposal is that it changes the fundamental nature of the social contract. The professional nurse would no longer be an employee of the hospital or agency, but rather a member of a professional corporation that provides nursing services to patients and clients on a fee-for-service basis. . . . Such a change in the nature of the social contract is, it seems to me, fundamentally necessary for the survival of nursing as a profession rather than an occupational group of workers employed by other organizations. p. 573

Sills viewed nurse corporations as a solution to the problem of collective bargaining by nurses and an organizational way to address the economics of nursing practice.

I envision nurse corporations as extending beyond the provision of nursing services to the provision of programs of nursing education. In this case, nurse corporations contract with universities to design and implement ND and PhD programs. Universities, of course, have the right and responsibility to appoint only those partners in the nurse corporation who meet the university's criteria for faculty. Furthermore, universities, as well as clinical agencies, might elect to contract with more than one nurse corporation. Self-employed nurse scholars are entrepreneurs who contract directly with universities for appointment to the faculty and with clinical agencies for practice and research privileges. Alternatively, they engage in private practice, contracting directly with patients for certain nursing services, with students for such educational services as tutoring and mentoring, and with nurse corporations for the continuing education of the partners.

CONCLUSION

Achievement of the proposed hallmark of 21st-century nursing depends on our individual and collective willingness to take potentially enormous risks and "have the courage to take a position about why people need nursing and about what nursing can and should be" (Orem, 1995, p. 414). Clearly, if we want to ensure the survival of our discipline, all of us must fall in love with nursing science now and develop a passion for the destiny of the discipline of nursing.

REFERENCES

Fawcett, J. (1983). Hallmarks of success in nursing theory development. In P. L. Chinn (Ed.), *Advances in nursing theory development* (pp. 3–17). Rockville, MD: Aspen.

Fawcett, J. (1984). Hallmarks of success in nursing research. *Advances in Nursing Science*, 7(1), 1–11.

Fawcett, J., & Carino, C. (1989). Hallmarks of success in nursing practice. *Advances in Nursing Science*, 11(4), 1–8.

Huch, M. H. (1995). Nursing and the next millennium. *Nursing Science Quarterly*, 8, 38–44.

Kendrick, K. (1997). What is advanced nursing? *Professional Nurse*, 12(10), 689.

Meieis, A. I. (1993, April). *Nursing research and the Neuman model: Directions for the future.* Panel discussion at the Fourth Biennial International Neuman Systems Model Symposium, Rochester, NY.

Orem, D. E. (1995). *Nursing: Concepts of practice* (5th ed.). St. Louis, MO: C. V. Mosby.

Sills, G. M. (1983). The role and function of the clinical nurse specialist, In N. L. Chaska (Ed.), *The nursing profession: A time to speak* (pp. 563–579). New York: McGraw-Hill.

Watson, J. (1997). The theory of human caring: Retrospective and prospective. *Nursing Science Quarterly*, 10, 49–52.

Watson, M. J. (1996). Watson's theory of transpersonal caring. In P. H. Walker & B. Neuman (Eds.), *Blueprint for use of nursing models: Education, research, practice, and administration* (pp. 141–184). New York: NLN Press.

Wood, K. W. (1978). Casework effectiveness: A new look at the research evidence. *Social Work*, 23, 437–458.

20

Nursing Knowledge and Human Science: Ontological and Epistemological Considerations

GAIL J. MITCHELL, RN, MScN

WILLIAM K. CODY, RN, MSN

This chapter examines the meaning of human science in relation to extant nursing knowledge. The origins of the human science tradition are traced to the philosopher Wilhelm Dilthey, who challenged the dominance of the positivist perspective for generating knowledge of the human lifeworld. Specific ontological and epistemological criteria for human science are proposed. Four nursing frameworks, Paterson and Zderad's humanistic nursing, Newman's model of health as expanding consciousness, Watson's human science and human care, and Parse's theory of human becoming, are found to have consistencies and inconsistencies with the human science tradition. It is proposed that the human science perspective is present in and will continue to be reflected in the evolution of nursing science.

Increasingly, nursing is being referred to as a human science (Connors, 1988; Gortner & Schultz, 1988; Meleis, 1990; Munhall, 1989; Parse, 1981, 1987; Watson, 1985). The meaning of this term as it is used in the literature, however, is not clear. Munhall (1989), Parse (1981) and Watson (1985) refer to human science as distinct from natural science and as bearing specific views, concepts, and methods. Contrary to this position, Connors (1988) and Gortner and Schultz (1988) refer to human science as the fields of biology, psychology, anthropology, and sociology. Is human science inclusive of any inquiry about human beings, or

is it a distinctive philosophical foundation for science? Is nursing currently a human science or is this an ideal to be esteemed and aspired to? The purpose of this chapter is to examine the meaning of human science as originated by Dilthey (1961, 1976, 1977a, 1977b, 1988) and explicated by Giorgi (1970, 1971, 1985) and to compare selected works from nursing's extant theoretical base to the explicit attributes that constitute "human" science.

DEFINING HUMAN SCIENCE

The origins of the term *human science* can be traced to the philosopher Wilhelm Dilthey

Source: Mitchell, G. J., & Cody, W. K. (1992). Nursing knowledge and human science: Ontological and epistemological considerations. *Nursing Science Quarterly*, 5 (2): 54-61. Reprinted by permission of and copyright © (1992) Sage Publications, Inc.

(1833-1911). The German term for human science, *Geisteswissenschaften*, has also been translated as "human studies." Translators frequently note the linguistic challenge involved in capturing the meaning of freshly coined and esoteric German expressions in English. Also noted in Dilthey's works is his tendency to refer to "psychic" life in a nineteenth-century fashion while writing of the coherent whole of lived experience. Dilthey did, however, describe life as unity, a living nexus. And he consistently referred to individuals as wholes and to human life as interconnected with others and history. The intent of the authors here is to offer an admittedly hermeneutical interpretation of Dilthey's view, in what is believed to be the unitary perspective of human beings that he intended.

Dilthey in the late 1800s was very concerned about what he called a "crisis in science," a crisis of modern consciousness, thought, and values (Ermath, 1978). The industrial society had already concretized the successes of the natural sciences, and the developing science of *Anthropologie*, with no other model, was rapidly abandoning any interest in human consciousness in favor of a crude "mindless" naturalism (Ermath, 1978). Dilthey (1977a) described what he saw as a sterile empiricism that disconnected life from knowledge. His fears were stoked by the growing trend to regard human behavior and culture as susceptible to the methods of natural science, which, he thought, stripped life of human meaning and purpose (Dilthey, 1977a). He proposed that "the deepest problem of modern thought and culture is to understand life as it is lived by man" (Ermath, 1978, p. 17).

Dilthey (1977a, 1977b, 1988) believed that the development of a human science held the only hope for understanding life as it is humanly lived. He proposed that the human sciences required concepts, methods, and theories which were fundamentally different from those of the natural sciences (Dilthey, 1977a, 1988). Dilthey viewed human beings as the preeminent source of knowledge. His philosophy took as its basis the whole of lived experience, the coherent nexus of life as it is humanly lived (Dilthey, 1977a). He wrote about "living" knowledge and "reflective" life. History and culture were, for Dilthey, manifestations of patterns of human life, pervaded with meaning. The natural sciences, concerned with the elaboration of physical laws from observation and experimentation, were, for Dilthey, very different from the concerns a true human science would focus on: meaning, values, and relationships within the coherent texture of humanly lived experience. The subject matter of the human sciences is "the interrelation of life, expression, and understanding" (Dilthey, 1976, p. 175).

Dilthey proposed that the lived experience should be "the basic empirical datum of the human sciences" (Ermath, 1978, p. 97). Further, the researcher, a living being too, is inexorably and unequivocally "in" and "of" what is investigated. There could be no meaningful objective/subjective dichotomy and no analytic reduction beyond experience as humanly lived. Human experience is a coherent whole to which subjectivity is fundamental; objectivity is a human creation. Dilthey maintained that life is a process, a continuous becoming which manifests itself in the dynamic unity of experience (Dilthey, 1976). Human beings were described as individual wholes with intrinsic value (Dilthey, 1977b). Dilthey (1977b) referred to the self as a "life-unity" that is free yet also determined by history. The concept of free will is a fundamental assumption of human science. On free will, Dilthey (1988) wrote, "This is an immediately given actuality. *It cannot be denied* . . . [O]ne *cannot explain* the fact of free will, for it is precisely its hallmark that we cannot break it down in a conceptual system" (p. 270).

More recently, the psychologist Giorgi (1970, 1971, 1985) has reasserted the need for an approach to the human sciences fundamentally different from conventional empirical methods. He proposed to study human beings as persons, as experiencing participants. He challenged the prevailing positivistic methods of psychology, contending that human experience must be understood in the way that it reveals itself, and he maintained that the study of lived experience could be done scientifically (Giorgi, 1985).

According to Giorgi, understanding life experiences requires a focus on meaning within the context of the person's experience of the phenomenon. Human beings cannot be known as objects, nor as separate from their lives. Echoing Dilthey, Giorgi maintained that a person is not "a passive receiver of physical energies, but rather his or her behavior reflects intentionality" (Giorgi, 1971, p. 23). Giorgi also addressed the influence of the researcher in conceptualizing research and the impact of the researcher on study findings. For Giorgi, the most important variable in the human sciences is the meaning of the lived experience for the subject. An exposition of the major thinkers and scholars, such as Gadamer (1976), Geertz (1973), Heidegger (1962), Ricoeur (1974), Schutz (1967), and Winch (1958), who have built on the tradition of which Dilthey is the foremost progenitor, is beyond the scope of this article.

The domination of twentieth-century social science by positivistic approaches in stark contrast to human science philosophy has been well documented (Polkinghorne, 1983) and contributes to the contextual situation in which this article emerges. The philosophical stance of human science outlined here has underpinned or strongly influenced the works of the six seminal scholars mentioned above and many others in the tradition of human science. These scholars have recognized the manifest necessity for the human sciences to explore and understand lived experience, the full complexity of human meanings and values, with no more fundamental reference than the human lives which are the phenomena of concern; indeed this formidable undertaking is the very mission of human science.

Based on the above explications of human science by Dilthey and Giorgi, specific ontological and epistemological attributes emerge as crucial to this approach for nursing science. Human science, in view of its origins and its philosophical foundations, cannot be viewed as a generic term for any and all disciplines studying human beings. It is proposed here that for a scientific discipline to be considered a "human science" logically it must incorporate the ontology and epistemology of its philosophical underpinnings, as described in Table 25.1.

A distinction must be made between a "humanistic" philosophy of science and "human science." According to Webster (1985), "humanism" entails a rejection of supernaturalism and asserts "the essential dignity and worth of man [*sic*] and his capacity to achieve self-realization through the use of reason and scientific method." Humanism thus is seen to acknowledge human values and potentialities without requiring a critique of "scientific method." Human science, in contrast, unequivocally rejects the methods of natural science (Dilthey, 1976, 1977a, 1988; Giorgi, 1985) and asserts from the outset that lived experience, the world as experienced, meaning, and understanding are all aspects of a unitary process of human life and cannot be adequately described, explained, or analyzed through objectification, measurement, or reduction.

SIGNIFICANCE OF HUMAN SCIENCE FOR NURSING

If nurses embrace the human science paradigm, activities in theory development, re-

TABLE 25.1.   Ontology and Epistemology of the Human Science Paradigm

Ontology	Epistemology
Human beings are unitary wholes in continuous interrelationship with their dynamic, temporal, historical, cultural worlds.	Research and practice focus on the coherent experience of the person's meanings, relations, values, patterns, and themes.
Human experience is preeminent and fundamental and reality is the whole complex of what is experienced and elaborated in thinking, feeling, and willing.	Lived experience is the basic empirical datum, as gleaned from the participant's description free of comparison to objective realities or predefined norms.
Human beings are intentional, free-willed beings who actively participate in life continuously.	The person's coparticipation in generating knowledge of lived experience is respected, and no more fundamental reference than what is disclosed by the person is sought.
The researcher is inextricably involved with any phenomenon investigated.	The researcher seeks knowledge and understanding of lived experience and is cognizant of the other's lived reality as a unitary whole.

Source: Synthesized and condensed from Dilthey, 1961, 1976, 1977a, 1977b, 1988; and Giorgi, 1970, 1971, 1985.

search, and practice will change to reflect the new philosophical perspective. An examination of nursing's philosophical and theoretical body of literature reveals that, in the past decade, such a change has already begun. In order to explore to what extent nurses are incorporating beliefs of the human science paradigm in theory, research, and practice, four nursing frameworks were selected for analysis. These frameworks are Paterson and Zderad's (1988) humanistic nursing, Newman's (1986a, 1990) model of health as expanding consciousness, Watson's (1985) human science and human care, and Parse's (1981, 1987, 1990a) theory of human becoming (formerly man-living-health, 1981). These frameworks were selected because all their authors claim a unitary conceptualization of human beings,

thereby evincing some degree of interfacing with the human science perspective. Further, these authors have publicly renounced the natural science approach and have called for new and different methods more congruent with nursing's philosophical foundations.

Critical to the development of nursing theories underpinned by the human sciences would be the acknowledgment of human beings as individual wholes who are situated in-the-world and who are respected as intentional, free-willed persons. Any theoretical principles and concepts used to structure a theory would need to incorporate these beliefs. Also essential would be approaches which view the individual's lived experience as the focus in both practice and research and which honor the person's lived experience as reality. Researchers and practitioners would be regarded as coparticipants with persons in inquiry and practice in a human science paradigm.

ANALYSIS OF THE NURSING FRAMEWORKS

Inquiry into the four frameworks above revealed a definite commitment to the human science paradigm. Parse's theory of human becoming was found not only to be consistent with the human science beliefs but to clarify, expand, and develop this approach. Consequently, an in-depth analysis of Parse's theory will be offered at a later point. Analysis of the works of Newman, Paterson and Zderad, and Watson illuminated consistencies and inconsistencies in relation to the beliefs of human science. Consistencies and commonalities included affirmation, to varying degrees, of the wholeness of the human being, the significance of subjective experience, and mutual participation in the creation of reality.

The inconsistencies took two main forms. In some instances, the author(s) acknowledged an inability to reconcile traditional objectivist beliefs with beliefs congruent with human science, and consequently they incorporated conflicting beliefs in theoretical conceptualizations. Alternately, the author(s) extended and elaborated on beliefs essential to the human science tradition, leading to significant dissidence with the core philosophy. These two inconsistencies are discussed with specific examples to illustrate logical incongruencies with the human science tradition. The intent here is not to rebuke the nursing theorists for their philosophical obscurities, for obscurity engenders clarification. Rather, the intent is to illuminate the inconsistencies in order to foster clarity and further the development of nursing science.

INCORPORATING DIVERGING BELIEFS

As previously noted, the nursing frameworks revealed both consistencies and inconsistencies with the foundational beliefs of the human science paradigm. Perhaps reflecting the evolutionary nature of knowledge and theory development, several of the authors incorporated diverging beliefs in their work, leaving the reader unclear as to their philosophical underpinnings. The inconsistencies arise in three main areas: the human being's wholeness, the intentionality and free will of the person, and the nature of reality. Each of these will be explored in relation to the works of Paterson and Zderad (1988), Newman (1986a, 1990), and Watson (1985).

Wholeness of Human Beings

Paterson and Zderad (1988) in their humanistic nursing practice propose that "the nurse sees the patient as a whole, a gestalt" (p. 25). Human beings are described as "in-the-world" and nurses are guided to recognize the complexity and uniqueness of each person's relating and experiencing. Paterson and Zderad note, however, that this view of the person as a whole conflicts with the evaluative stance of the conventional nursing process. They address this conflict by positing that "both subject-subject and subject-object relationships are essential for clinical nursing" (Paterson & Zderad, 1988, p. 27) in which focusing on discrete parts rather than the whole person is sometimes necessary. This attempt to incorporate human science beliefs with biomedical traditions leads to conceptual inconsistencies. It is suggested here that nurses cannot switch their very beliefs according to the nature of the practice situation. What seems to be overlooked by Paterson and Zderad is that nurses can live according to human science beliefs and still perform tasks related to the execution of medical orders. There need not be the subject-subject, subject-object dilemma as espoused by these authors. Though Paterson and Zderad reflect on the inadequacy of the labelling process for capturing lived experiences, they accept the linear, causal nursing process and the diagnosing of human responses as necessary evils, required for economic reasons. Paterson and Zderad maintain that the natural science tradition is inappropriate for nursing, yet they do not reconcile the inconsistencies between reductionistic and unitary approaches with human beings.

Newman explicitly expresses a belief in the unitary nature of human beings, yet she also discusses the human being as a "system" made up of physiological structures and functions, such as the immune system and the genetic code, reflecting a natural science orientation. The unity of the human "system," for Newman, is predicated on the idea that "mind and matter are made of the same basic stuff" (1986a, p. 37). It is apparently quite appropriate within Newman's model to discuss the physiological, psychological, and emotional processes of the "human system" in conventional terms, so long as one remembers that everything, from the atom to the human being and beyond, is a manifestation of the implicate order, or "absolute consciousness" (pp. 33-37). Similarly, Watson (1985) maintains that the person is conceptualized as an irreducible whole, yet she repeatedly refers to body, mind, spirit and soul, and physical, emotional, and spiritual spheres. Her definitions of health and illness are dependent on the harmony or disharmony within these aspects. Watson also refers to several selves; the "real self," the "inner self," and the "ideal self" are presented as distinct entities. She refers to the "I" and the "Me" of the person and the potential disharmony of these aspects. It is not consistent to maintain that a person is a unitary whole and then to define the person according

to these separate parts or spheres. Dilthey (1977a) maintained that "we continually experience a sense of connectedness and totality in ourselves" (p. 53). The authors' struggles to incorporate the concept of the unitary human being into nursing theory and practice parallel a long and complex tradition of discourse in the human sciences.

Intentional Free-Willed Beings

Human science conceptualizes human beings as intentional and inherently free-willed; therefore the nurse would seek no more fundamental reference than the lived experience of the person. Paterson and Zderad (1988) address the *nurse's* intention and free will to commit authentically to another. The authors also regard the human being as free-willed, yet they suggest, "The nurse is alert to opportunities for the patient to exercise his [*sic*] freedom of choice within the limits of safe and sound practice" (p. 17). The nurse is guided to monitor the patient's choices and to determine if they are responsible ones. To carry out this monitoring, the nurse would have to rely on some schema of normative standards or beliefs in order to judge what is "responsible," which is an inconsistent practice if the nurse wishes to respect the human science belief that the individual is an intentional being possessing free will.

Newman's (1986a) conceptualization of freedom describes an arclike progression as consciousness expands. Human beings first *lose* freedom as they "come into being," are "bound in time" and "find . . . identity in space," until they reach a stage in which choice is engendered through movement (p. 46). "Restriction of movement forces one into a realm beyond space and time" (p. 62). Thereafter one throws off self-concerns, recognizes one's own "boundarylessness" and "timelessness" and *gains* the freedom of returning to "absolute consciousness" (p. 46). It is essentially the movement toward spirituality that imbues the human being with freedom, which is relative to the extent that consciousness is expanded.

The notion that human freedom underpins human science is quite different, in that freedom is never "lost," and there is no requisite for expanding consciousness to "gain" it. Human beings are believed to be free to choose meaning and direction because they make such choices continuously in living everyday life (Dilthey, 1988). "It is true," writes Dilthey (1988), "that the will depends on intellect, but the will can choose or not choose what the intellect understands . . . in fact the will is free precisely inasmuch as in it the search for a reason ends" (p. 270). Newman's (1986b) proposal for "the diagnosis of pattern" would appear to be hinged on her notion of freedom as relative to expanded consciousness. She states, "The role of the nurse within a paradigm of pattern is to help clients recognize their own patterns," a process in which a "burst of insight" occurs that "opens up" a "pathway of action" (pp. 55-56). From a human science perspective, by contrast, the pathway of action is always open.

Watson (1985) says that human beings are free to self-determine and free to choose. Nurses are guided to hold nonpaternalistic values which respect human autonomy and freedom. Yet this belief is violated in two ways. First, there are references to the nurse's helping, integrating, and "correcting" the patient's condition to increase harmony and to try to find meaning in the situation. Second, Watson maintains that "*ideally* [italics added], a person should have the opportunity for self-determination of the meaning of a health-illness experience *before professionals make decisions* [italics added] about treatments and interventions" (1985, p. 66). Human science philosophy abdicates the position of science as the arbiter of truth; the human scientist is a seeker of truth, a seeker rather than a dispenser of wisdom. Dilthey maintained that "under-

standing constitutes the goal of the human studies in the way that explanation defines the natural sciences" (cited in Makkreel, 1977, p. 7). Knowledge is not used or applied to the person, but rather knowledge enhances understanding for participating with the person in the process of becoming. Dilthey (1976) proposed, "In everything there is the same limitation of possibilities and yet freedom to choose between them, and the beautiful feeling of being able to move forward and to realize new potentialities in one's own existence" (p. 245).

The Nature of Reality

In a human science ontology, human beings and their worlds as experienced cannot be separated. Human science does not distinguish between subjective and objective realities because the focus of scientific activities is the humanly lived experience of the world, in which subjectivity is primal. Paterson and Zderad suggest that "nurses are drawn toward two realities—the reality of the objective scientific world and the reality of the subjective-objective world" (p. 36). The authors' endorsement of the traditional nursing process automatically places the person in the position of object and the nurse in the role of arbiter of truth. Again this reflects the conflicting views proposed with respect to the nurse-patient relationship.

Newman's (1986a) view of the nature of reality draws on Bohm's (1980) theory of the implicate order. All humanly experienced phenomena comprising the explicate order are posited as manifestations of an unseen, unknowable implicate order which comprises the unity of all that is. According to this view, patterns of human experience are reflective of this underlying primary reality. Newman writes, "We need to remind ourselves that our manifest reality is a small portion of the total enfoldment of the pattern in time-space

(1986a, p. 15). Her model theoretically eliminates the subject-object duality, according to its ontology. However, Newman's (1986a, 1986b) view is that neither objectivity nor subjectivity has any validity, since the perspective adapted from Bohm says there are no boundaries to (physical) reality. From a human science perspective, this is still essentially an objectivist reality, founded on the basis of the speculations of physical scientists that the nature of reality is a complex, multidimensional whole. The human being in such a model is defined by what physical science says about matter and energy. By contrast, human science directly asserts that human reality as lived is itself a complex multidimensional whole (Dilthey, 1977a).

The preeminence of the human experience is ostensibly highly valued in Watson's theory. She speaks of developing knowledge about the lived world of human experience and contends that the phenomenological research method is most congruent with her theoretical perspective. However, Watson distinguishes the person's experience of the world (phenomenal field) from the world as it actually is. For example, she proposes that nurses "help integrate the person's subjective experience and emotions with the objective external view of the situation" (Watson, 1985, p. 65). Watson also suggests that there can be incongruencies between the person and nature (world). For example, she states, "If a person does not feel congruent with mind, body, and soul . . . or rejects the self . . . or is obsessed with an ideal self, the person will be dissatisfied and maladjusted" (p. 57). These distinctions reveal a belief in an objective reality separate from the person's experience of it. This essentially dichotomous view is inconsistent with human science philosophy, in which being human means participating in the creation of reality. Human consciousness already is the unity of the person's subjective-objective relationship with the world; it is not something to be aspired to (Dilthey, 1977a). The use of the conventional subjective-objective constructs speaks to the exigencies of traditional science but is inconsistent with the understanding of humanly lived reality that underpins human science.

EXTENDING ESSENTIAL BELIEFS

In several instances within the frameworks examined, departures from the human science tradition were noted in areas where some congruence might be expected based on the overall presentation and central concepts. Paterson and Zderad (1988) move from focusing on the human being's lived experience to focusing on nurses' lived experiences and their descriptions of human beings. Both Newman (1986a) and Watson (1985) go well beyond the lived experience as the primal foundation of human knowledge by assigning higher order importance to metaphysical concepts.

It is clear that the basic empirical datum in Paterson and Zderad's humanistic nursing is the nurse's experience, "the between" of existentially experienced nursing situations. The authors address the importance of meanings, patterns, values, and themes, but it is not clear whose experiences are paramount, the nurse's or the patient's. Paterson and Zderad contend that nursing must be described phenomenologically, that nurses' descriptions of nursing situations with patients will build the knowledge and "make explicit a science of nursing" (1988, p. 3). This is a description of the practice of nursing, however, not of a nursing science based on the health experience of human beings. Giorgi (1985) proposed that a discipline is not ready-made in the world and simply viewed and studied. Rather, it is created by a unique knowledge base that is housed within its theories. Thus, to study the nursing act phenomenologically as Paterson and Zderad suggest is to study the particular nurse's view of nursing. It is suggested in this article that nursing science focuses on the concepts of human-environment and health, not the nurse's views of the between. To be consistent with the human science approach nurses must rely on the person's description as it is given, and not on what that experience is assumed to be. Paterson and Zderad's focus on the practitioner's experience reflects a serious departure from beliefs related to the practice of a human science, which investigates lived experiences and life expressions of human beings.

Human consciousness is an important concept in human science; it is the origin of all knowledge about lived experience (Dilthey, 1988). The ontology of Newman's theory is largely metaphysical, in that the key concept of "absolute consciousness" is beyond the realm of lived experience. Newman (1986a) ascribes consciousness to atoms, rocks, plants, animals, and unspecified "astral" and "spiritual" entities (pp. 33-37). In human science philosophy there is no way of knowing a more fundamental ground behind or beyond the lived experience of the person. One wonders why Newman (1986a), whose central thesis is "health as expanding consciousness," has completely ignored continental European philosophy and theory on consciousness throughout her work. Instead, Newman cites works of speculative physics as underpinning her theory, even when addressing human experience. Dilthey (1977a) maintained that "consciousness cannot go behind itself" (p. 75). It is the structure of consciousness that sheds light on the coherent unity of human life.

In human science, humanly lived experiences elaborated in thinking, feeling, and willing are the complex whole of reality. Watson emphasizes the significance of human experience as it is lived. However, her emphasis on the metaphysical, spiritual realm clouds the issue of the primacy of lived experience. Watson (1985) states that "the human soul is more than physical, mental, emotional existence . . . the soul exists for something larger than physical life" (p. 45). She maintains, "The soul, inner self, spiritual self is tied to a higher degree of consciousness . . . that transcends time and space" (p. 46). This soul, which "may be underdeveloped and in need of reawakening" (p. 45), reflects a reality beyond that which is directly experienced by human beings and is in conflict with the purported human science origins of Watson's theory.

Watson explicitly presents her framework as emerging from the human science paradigm. Paterson and Zderad refer to their work as humanistic, a related term but not synonymous with human science. Although the concepts Newman uses are abundantly addressed in human science, the ontology underpinning her theory is derived instead from speculative physics. The selective extraction of inconsistencies with the human science paradigm in these authors' works is not intended to suggest a failing on their part but is intended to foster greater conceptual clarity and is offered in the spirit of scholarly questioning and debate. The purpose of this analysis was to determine to what extent the values and beliefs of the human science paradigm were currently evident in nursing's extant knowledge base. The authors conclude that the human science tradition is present to varying degrees in nursing science.

Of the four theories explored here, Parse's (1981, 1987, 1990a) theory of human becoming remained consistent with the fundamental ontology and epistemology of the human science tradition. The theory can be seen to have expanded and clarified major ideas of the human science tradition. Parse's (1981) work was the first publication in nursing to specify nursing as a human science in Dilthey's traditional sense. Parse's theory is analyzed here with regard to both its adherence to and expansion of the human science tradition.

PARSE'S THEORY OF HUMAN BECOMING

Parse's first chapter begins, "To posit the idea of nursing rooted in the human sciences is to make explicit an alternative to the traditional practice of nursing as a medical model grounded in the natural sciences" (1981, p. 3). Parse describes nursing as a human science focusing on the unitary human being's experience of living and creating health, and she cites Dilthey in her explication of the concepts of her theory. She states that the methodologies of human sciences focus on "uncovering the meaning of phenomena as humanly experienced" and "on understanding the connectedness of life itself," (1981, p. 11). Dilthey (1977b) suggested that explicating human interrelatedness connects that which is universally human with that which is individual.

Parse (1981) synthesized concepts from Rogers' (1970) science of unitary human beings and tenets of contemporary existential phenomenology in such a way that the fundamental notion of human science proposed by Dilthey was brought to fruition for nursing science in the theory of human becoming. The tenets of human subjectivity and intentionality, and the concepts of human coexistence, coconstitution, and situated freedom, drawn from existential phenomenology, reflect the development of ideas germinated by Dilthey and others in the philosophy of human science. The synthesis of concepts from Rogers' work with concepts from existential phenomenology to form a unique, coherent theory of nursing underscores the compelling fit between human science philosophy and nursing as a unique and autonomous discipline. Parse (1987) avoided conceptual inconsistencies by inventing nursing practice and research methodologies which flow directly from the ontological and epistemological foundations of her theory. In this way there is no need to reconcile human science beliefs with biomedical traditions. Parse's theory and her practice and research methodologies express and structure the beliefs which underpin human science in a new way specifically for nursing science.

Parse's (1981, 1987, 1990a) theory of human becoming has three central themes: meaning, rhythmicity, and cotranscendence. Her explication of these themes moves her theory beyond human science as described by Dilthey (1961). Parse describes the human being as an open unity who freely chooses meaning in situations, bears responsibility for choices, and co-constitutes with the environment rhythmical patterns of relating in the process of co-transcending with emerging possibilities. Health is described as a "process of becoming, a cocreated process of living value priorities" (1981, p. 31). Health is the day-to-day living of rhythmical patterns reflecting the person's unfolding and co-transcending with the possibles (the moving onward in life in a chosen way) (Parse, 1981).

The goal of practice in Parse's theory is the quality of life from the person's perspective (1987). Nurses in true presence with people live the practice method, which revolves around the all-at-once of illuminating meaning through "explicating," synchronizing rhythms through "dwelling with," and mobilizing transcendence through "moving beyond" (1987, p. 167). Parse's research method is rooted in phenomenology and is structured to be congruent with the assumptions and principles of the human becoming theory. It focuses on uncovering the structures of universal lived experiences in the human-universe-health interrelationship. The goal of the method is to enhance understanding of lived experiences of health.

CRITIQUE OF THE THEORY OF HUMAN BECOMING

Parse presents her theory as emerging from the human science paradigm and she remains congruent with those philosophical underpinnings throughout her work. The human being is viewed as unitary, mutually interrelating with environment, and there is no reference to human beings other than as living unities. The person's lived experience is clearly regarded as the preeminent ground of human health. The researcher explores universal lived experiences of health, with the goal of enhancing understanding. This is consistent with Dilthey's concern "to understand life as it is lived by man" (Ermath, 1978, p. 17). Both the research and practice methods focus on the lived experience of human beings. There is no subject-object dichotomy; reality is viewed as cocreated with the universe and others while experienced uniquely by the person. Nursing is seen as a scientific discipline in which the concepts of unitary human beings, mutual unfolding, human coexistence, intentionality, free will, and intersubjective sharing of meaning may at last be fully elaborated and incorporated in praxis. Dilthey consistently maintained that all theory was theory for praxis (Ermath, 1978).

Parse suggests that persons "unfold with contemporaries the ideas of predecessors . . . in a continuity that connects past with future" (1981, p. 26). The "way the person lives in interrelationship with others reflects chosen meanings and reveals cherished values" (1981, p. 48). Individuals freely choose the meaning of situations and freely live personal values by choosing ways of being/becoming from among possibilities. Again, this is consistent with Dilthey's (1961) view of human interconnectedness, yet it goes beyond his view.

Guided by Parse's theory, the nurse in true presence with the person focuses on the individual's own meaning without judging, labeling, or trying to change the person. The nurse goes with the person as he or she explores options, images consequences of choices, and plans to live hopes and dreams. In the true presence of the nurse the individual clarifies the meaning of the situation and new meanings are uncovered; new insights generate new possibles, the understanding of opportunities and limitations in light of what is truly valued. The nurse coparticipates with the person in the process of moving beyond the now moment, guided by the theory to understand that the person chooses his or her own way (Parse, 1987). Parse maintains that individuals know their own way, reflectively and prereflectively. The nurse in true presence bears witness to the person's unfolding and becoming (Parse, 1990b). In creating the theory of human becoming, Parse has uncovered the intrinsic relevance of the human science perspective, which is centrally concerned with what it means to be human for the discipline of nursing.

In Parse's (1987) research methodology, the researcher "lives" dialogical engagements with participants. This is described as "an intersubjective being with, in which the researcher and participant live the I-Thou process as they move through an unstructured discussion about the lived experience" (1987, p. 176). The researcher views the participant as the expert on the lived experience being explored and remains focused on the phenomenon as it is revealed by the person. The researcher participates in generating enhanced understanding of the phenomenon by creatively abstracting the structure of the lived experience in the language of science.

In summary, Parse's theory, intentionally structured as a human science theory of nursing, accurately reflects the ontology and epistemology of human science philosophy. Parse's theory lays a foundation for a nursing science that is grounded in the meaning of lived experiences in the human-universe process. The theory focuses on the lived experience of unitary human beings in continuous interrelationship with their worlds. Reality as perceived by the person is not compared to an "objective" reality but is respected, as is the free will of the person, in choosing ways of becoming. Parse's theory is thus congruent with yet goes beyond the ontology and epistemology of human science as posited in this article and is an emergent, a newly created theory for praxis that uncompromisingly incorporates the beliefs of human science into nursing research and practice.

CONCLUSION

Nursing science is currently undergoing change as new views emerge which challenge the traditional methods of natural science-based, biomedical nursing. The human science paradigm is one such view. This perspective is surfacing in nursing at a time when nurse scholars are questioning the precepts of the natural science paradigm and, in doing so, are expressing many of the concerns which led Dilthey to propose a different approach to human science over a hundred years ago. It has been suggested in this article that the human science tradition is not merely any study of human beings, but a particular way of studying human life which values the lived experience of unitary persons and seeks to understand life in all its interwoven patterns of meanings and values.

Nurse scientists are defining boundaries and seeking knowledge which is unique to nursing. This knowledge is currently organized in conceptual and theoretical frameworks, some of which reflect the values and beliefs of the human science paradigm. Of the four frameworks explored here, one, Parse's theory of human becoming. was found not only to be congruent with but to go beyond the human science perspective. The other three frameworks, Paterson and Zderad's humanistic nursing, Newman's model of expand-

ing consciousness, and Watson's human science and human care, demonstrated both consistencies and inconsistencies with the philosophy of human science. Continued explication of the assumptions, values, and beliefs which underpin different theoretical approaches is needed, so that nurses can understand with depth and clarity the foundations of the unique knowledge base of nursing. Only through contemplative consideration of the philosophical basis of the extant body of theory and through open critique and discourse can nurses choose which paths to follow in the quest for knowledge.

REFERENCES

Bohm, D. (1980). *Wholeness and the implicate order*. London: Routledge.

Connors, D. (1988). A continuum of researcher-participant relationships: An analysis and critique. *Advances in Nursing Science, 10*(4), 32-42.

Dilthey, W. (1961). *Pattern and meaning in history: Thoughts on history and society* (H.P. Rickman, Ed. and Trans.). New York: Harper & Row.

———. (1976). *Selected writings* (H.P. Rickman, Trans.). Cambridge: Cambridge University Press.

———. (1977a). Ideas concerning a descriptive and analytic psychology. (Original work published 1894). In R.M. Zaner & K.L. Heiges (Trans.), *Descriptive psychology and historical understanding* (pp. 23-120). The Hague. Netherlands: Nijhoff.

———. (1977b) The understanding of other persons and their expressions of life. (Original work published 1927). In R.M. Zaner & K.L. Heiges (Trans.), *Descriptive psychology and historical understanding* (pp. 123-144). The Hague, Netherlands: Nijhoff.

———. (1988). *Introduction to the human sciences* (R. J. Betanzos, Trans.). Detroit: Wayne State University Press. (Original work published 1883)

Ermath, M. (1978). *Wilhelm Dilthey: The critique of historical reason*. Chicago: University of Chicago Press.

Gadamer, H.G. (1976). *Philosophical hermeneutics* (D.E. Linge. Trans.). Berkeley: University of California Press.

Geertz, C. (1973). *The interpretation of cultures*. New York: Basic Books.

Giorgi, A. (1970). *Psychology as a human science*. New York: Harper & Row.

———. (1971). Phenomenology and experimental psychology: II. In A. Giorgi. W. Fischer & R. von Eckartsberg (Eds.), *Duquesne studies in phenomenological psychology*, (Vol. l, pp. 3-29). Pittsburgh, PA: Duquesne University Press.

———. (1985). Sketch of a psychological phenomenological method. In A. Giorgi (Ed.), *Phenomenology and psychological research* (pp. 8-22). Pittsburgh: Duquesne University Press.

Gortner, S.R., & Schultz, P.R. (1988). Approaches to nursing science methods. *Image: Journal of Nursing Scholarship, 20*, 22-24.

Heidegger, M. (1962). *Being and time* (J. Macquarrie & E. Robinson, Trans.). New York: Harper & Row.

Makkreel, R.A. (1977). Introduction. In R.M. Zaner & K.L. Heiges (Trans.), *Descriptive psychology and historical understanding* (pp. 1-20). The Hague. Netherlands: Nijhoff.

Meleis, A. (1990, September). *Directions for nursing theory development*. Paper presented at the National Nursing Theory Conference, Los Angeles, CA.

Munhall, P. (1989). Philosophical ponderings on qualitative research methods in nursing. *Nursing Science Quarterly, 2*, 20-28.

Newman, M. (1986a). *Health as expanding consciousness*. St. Louis: Mosby.

———. (1986b). Nursing's emerging paradigm: The diagnosis of pattern. In A. M. McLane (Ed.), *Classification of nursing diagnoses: Proceedings of the seventh conference*. St. Louis: Mosby.

———. (1990). Newman's theory of health as praxis. *Nursing Science Quarterly, 3*, 37-41.

Parse, R.R (1981). *Man-living-health: A theory of nursing*. New York: Wiley.

———. (1987). *Nursing science: Major paradigms, theories and critiques*. Philadelphia: Saunders.

———. (1990a, September). [Speaker on] *Panel of nursing theorists*. National Nursing Theory Conference, Los Angeles, CA.

———. (1990b). Health: A personal commitment. *Nursing Science Quarterly, 3*, 136-l40.

Paterson, J.G., & Zderad, L.T. (1988). *Humanistic nursing*. New York: National League for Nursing.

Polkinghorne, D. (1983). *Methodology for the human sciences: Systems of inquiry*. Albany: State University of New York Press.

Ricoeur, P. (1974). *The conflict of interpretations: Essays in hermeneutics* (W. Domingo et al., Trans.). Evanston, IL: Northwestern University Press.

Rogers, M.E. (1970). *An introduction to the theoretical basis of nursing*. Philadelphia: Davis.

Schutz, A. (1967). *The phenomenology of the social world* (G. Walsh & F. Lehnert, Trans.). Evanston, IL: Northwestern University Press.

Watson, J. (1985). *Nursing: Human science and human care*. Norwalk, CT: Appleton-Century-Crofts.

Webster's ninth new collegiate dictionary. (1985). Springfield, MA: Merriam-Webster.

Winch, P. (1958). *The idea of a social science and its relation to philosophy*. London: Routledge & Kegan Paul.

21

Esthetic and Personal Knowing through Humanistic Nursing

DIANNE PELLETIER RAYMOND

Carper (1978) discussed four fundamental patterns of knowing in nursing:

1. empirics, the science of nursing;
2. ethics;
3. personal knowledge; and
4. esthetics, the art of nursing.

Paterson and Zderad's (1976) humanistic nursing model offers a methodology for fostering the development of knowledge through personal and esthetic patterns. Empirical science cannot adequately address all phenomena encountered in nursing. Nursing is concerned with such human experiences as suffering, guilt, anger, hopelessness, and fear. The phenomenological approach proposed by Paterson and Zderad (1976) provides the nurse with a method to attend to lived experiences such as these. Phenomenology, however, can neither replace other measures of inquiry in nursing nor account for all its goals (Oiler, 1982). The purpose of this paper is to briefly describe Paterson and Zderad's phenomenological approach, to offer a commentary on McKinnon's 1991 article related to humanistic nursing, to explore a specific nursing situation utilizing the hu-

manistic nursing paradigm, and to advocate use of the model in qualitative research and theory development.

HUMANISTIC NURSING MODEL DESCRIBES LIVED EXPERIENCES

The humanistic nursing model (depicted in the figure "Humanistic Nursing Model"), as proposed by Paterson and Zderad (1976), has its own phenomenological methodology for describing lived experiences. The authors call their approach phenomenological nursology. According to Paterson and Zderad (1976), phenomenological nursology is a medium through which concept and theory development can take place.

Phenomenologic nursology is comprised of five phases. The first four phases involve assessment and the final phase is analogous to the nursing diagnosis. The lived experience as viewed by the patient unfolds through the therapeutic relationship itself. The phases are identified as follows (Paterson & Zderad, 1976):

- Phase I: Preparation of the nurse knower for coming to know (the patient).

Source: Raymond, D. P., (1995) Esthetic and personal knowing through humanistic nursing. *N&HC: Perspectives on community* 16 (6): 332–336. Reprinted with permission by from the National League for Nursing

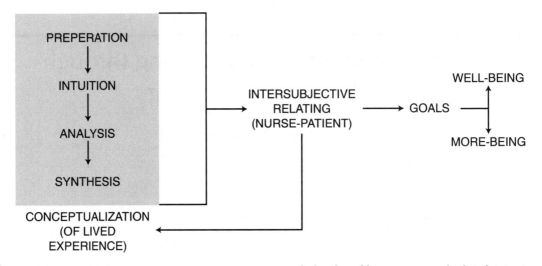

Figure 26.1. Model depicts Humanistic Nursing Framework developed by Paterson and Zderad (1976) as viewed by author.

- Phase II: Nurse knowing the other (the patient) intuitively.
- Phase III: Nurse knowing the other (the patient) scientifically.
- Phase IV: Nurse complementarily synthesizing known others.
- Phase V: Succession within the nurse from the many to the paradoxical one (conclusion).

McKinnon (1991) contended that Paterson and Zderad's model offered neither guidelines for administering patient care nor a means of evaluating its effectiveness. Further, the author stated that a main weakness of the model is its failure to hold the nurse accountable for the quality of patient care. One may argue that the nurse who does not also consider the lived experience of the patient in approach to care may not be totally accountable to the patient. Without a consideration of needs as the patient views it, there is a danger of addressing needs only from an outsider's perspective, which may be narrow or inaccurate. Further, one may argue that fostering the kind of relationship necessary for understanding the world view of

the patient may potentially enhance the quality of patient care delivered. The ethical dictum of phenomenology is the imperative to turn to the people who actually live the experience (Swanson-Kauffman & Schonwald, 1988).

It is important to note that the humanistic model is at a descriptive level in theory development (Brouse & Laffrey, 1989). The aim of the model is to describe the human experience as it is lived by the patient. The model does not attempt to predict or to control nursing phenomena. In other words, the model does not claim to provide all of the guidelines necessary in administering nursing care. According to Brouse and Laffrey (1989), "The phenomenological method is complementary to but operates at qualitatively different levels from empirical science" (p. 207). Empirical science provides a view which is logically deduced, while phenomenology emphasizes the view of the subject (the lived experience). One view should not necessarily discount the other, but may be seen as a complement to the other. Thus, the phenomenological approach attempts to address questions that cannot be answered by empirical science.

The following paragraphs illustrate the application of the humanistic nursing model to a clinical situation in order to demonstrate its usefulness in practice. "Elise" was a patient who I encountered while working as a staff nurse on a psychiatric unit.

CLINICAL SITUATION AS LIVED BY "ELISE"

Elise was a 17-year-old woman of Acadian descent living in a rural community. Elise was referred to the psychiatric unit via the helpline by her mother, who had noted progressive withdrawal in Elise and failing grades in school. Elise lived at home with her mother and her brothers. Her father had died five years prior to the admission. She had been very close to her father. Elise's conversations with her mother were obsessed with thoughts of her father's death and God. She was described as reclusive to her room. Upon admission, Elise made it obvious to all staff that she did not want to be there with much crying and expressions of anger. She experienced auditory hallucinations. Her affect was flat with a mask-like expression on her face. She would sit for hours at a time looking straight ahead, immersed in her own world. Elise was tried on antipsychotic medication with little initial response. After one week on the psychiatric unit, she began to verbalize paranoid delusions of staff wishing to "lock" her up forever and the food being "poisoned." She began to gag on her food and medication and reported nausea. Her appearance further deteriorated.

PHASE I: PREPARATION OF THE NURSE FOR COMING TO KNOW

Through my years of nursing experience and years of education, as well as life experiences, I have prepared myself for coming to know the human condition. Through these experiences, I have developed the ability to empathize—to experience the feelings of another. The key to practice utilizing phenomenology is to have a nurse who is willing to operate in a methodology that mandates an investment of the personal self (Swanson-Kauffman & Schonwald, 1988). The outcome depends on the nurse's ability to engage in another's reality in an empathic sense. I had attended a case review where all the disciplines involved in Elise's care discussed her lack of progress. I was assigned to work with Elise. The most recent subjective data from her chart contained statements such as "I want to go home now!" and "I'm not getting better here." The chart noted that she was only sleeping two or three hours per night. I chose a time when Elise was sitting quietly in the solarium to approach her, respecting her need to maintain the distance between us. I approached her openly, leaving all of the accumulated data base behind—e.g., DSM-III-R diagnosis and increasing distrustful and aggressive behavior. A nurse that can be open provides a model for the patient (Berger, 1977). By approaching Elise openly, I encouraged her to be open with me. I introduced myself to Elise as her staff person for the day.

PHASE II: NURSE KNOWING OTHER INTUITIVELY

After a few superficial exchanges, Elise identified me as an authority figure on the unit and as a person who gave her medication. She proceeded to tell me that she felt that staff was deceiving her. She stated, "They tell me that if I take the medication that I'll get better and then I can go home. I think they tell me that so I'll take it. I don't want to take the medication. It will make me sick." I responded by providing Elise with a brief explanation of her medication and the symptoms that needed to be controlled before discharge was possible.

This was the beginning of an intersubjective relationship with Elise. I intuitively grasped her situation—allowed myself to feel what she must be feeling. Elise was losing her sense of contact with the people and the things in her world. She felt that she was forced into the hospital and forced into strange routines. She was eating unfamiliar food and ingesting medications which she was unaccustomed to taking and had equated to making her feel ill. I allowed myself to experience the situation subjectively through her world view. Hospitalization was an identifiable source of stress for Elise. I experienced the apprehension that arises from being separated from familiar people, personal possessions, and the safety and security of home.

PHASE III: NURSE KNOWING OTHER SCIENTIFICALLY

I reflected on what I knew of Elise intuitively and examined the experience objectively. During our dialogue, I had observed her dilated pupils, her look of bewilderment, her trembling hands, and her guarded, withdrawn manner. I recalled the elevated vital signs and nausea. I analyzed the available data.

PHASE IV: NURSE COMPLEMENTARILY SYNTHESIZING KNOWN OTHERS

I compared Elise's experience with that of other patients with similar symptoms and with what I had read in the literature. I recalled what Gibson described as a "need/fear dilemma" (Berger, 1977). Patients who are out of touch with reality need others desperately to strengthen their inadequate egos. Yet they feel threatened by others and find it hard to maintain a clear picture of reality. Thus, they may try to avoid other people to escape their feeling of being engulfed by them, which explains the withdrawal that they manifest (Berger, 1977).

PHASE V: SUCCESSION WITHIN THE NURSE FROM THE MANY TO THE PARADOXICAL ONE

In relating to Elise's experience, I concluded that she was experiencing the phenomenon of fear. Once isolated, the nursing diagnosis of fear can be approached via the nursing process. McKinnon (1991) contended that the humanistic nursing process does not include the development of a plan of care or mutual goal setting with patients of any age. Humanistic nursing practice, however, does call for intersubjective relating where the patient expects to be helped and the nurse expects to give help (Paterson & Zderad, 1976). The plan includes the establishment of a therapeutic relationship which forms the basis of all other treatment that follows. The plan of care utilizing the humanistic model may be supplemented by other theories and approaches. Although phenomenological nursology, an empathic approach, continued to be an important therapeutic approach with Elise, an interdisciplinary treatment approach was critical to her care as well, which included the collaborative efforts between nursing, psychiatry, occupational therapy, social worker, and dietician. The treatment approach focused on reassuring her of her safety.

PLANNING INVOLVES THE PATIENT IN MAKING RESPONSIBLE CHOICES

The effectiveness of the phenomenological approach with Elise was validated through her admission of fear and through direct observation of her behavior. She did not react with hostility. She stated her agreement to continue to take the medication. She acknowledged that she was hearing voices and that she wanted them to go away. Through continued intersubjective encounters with Elise, combined with the other treatment modalities, one could notice a gradual improvement in her mental status. She stayed on the unit for a total of two months. As she was able to relax and to see her own progress; the aggressive behavior disappeared. She began to show trust in staff and to actively involve herself in unit activities. Her affect improved markedly. Although the planning, implementation, and evaluation stages of the nursing process are not directly addressed by Paterson and Zderad, these stages may be inferred. The planning involved eliciting the active involvement of the patient in making responsible choices. The therapeutic relationship that was one of collaboration not only was an important intervention, but facilitated the implementation of other treatment modalities. Evaluation occurred through validation with the patient. The goal of well-being was met through Elise's steady improvement in mental status and her participation in health maintenance behaviors. She was discharged from the hospital and returned to live with her family. As long as Elise can be functional and maintained within the community, there can be continual movement toward the goal of more-being or the maximization of her human potential.

PHILOSOPHY OF SCIENCE AND NURSING THEORY ARE IN A "STATE OF TRANSITION"

Traditionally, logical empiricism with its quantitative methodologies has dominated theory development and testing (Silva & Rothbart, 1984). However, the philosophy of science and nursing theory are in a "state of transition" (Silva & Rothbart, p. 294). According to

Silva and Rothbart (1984), a new philosophy of science known as historicism has emerged. While logical empiricism provides a logical explanation of the nature of scientific knowledge, historicism is a philosophy of science that provides a historical explanation (Silva & Rothbart, 1984). According to Silva and Rothbart, historicists attempt to understand science in terms of research traditions. The authors defined a research tradition as "a broadly based foundation of many theories and [as] an accepted way of viewing fundamental phenomena within a discipline" (p. 295). Further, the authors noted that research traditions are global and changeable within the boundaries of an ontological commitment or nature of being. According to these authors, a methodological commitment which defines the legitimate method of inquiry suitable to a research tradition's ontology is essential. For example, Silva and Rothbart (1984) questioned whether the case study method of inquiry may be better suited to the ontological commitment of holism than a traditional experimental design method of inquiry with its built-in reductionism. Theories based on research traditions view the person as a holistic being as opposed to looking at parts. Thus, according to the authors, the logical empiricists with their deductive approach emphasize science as product, whereas, the historicists place emphasis on science as process.

In addition to the shift in the philosophy of science espoused in the nursing literature, Silva & Rothbart (1984) identified a shift in emphasis from quantitative to qualitative methodologies as another trend. Grounded theory research is an example of a current break from tradition. In grounded theory research, the researcher becomes immersed in the world of the research subject (Bowers, 1988). According to Bowers, the researcher attempts to discover how subjects experience their world. Through bracketing, researchers are able to temporarily relinquish their perspectives and assume the perspective of the research subject (Bowers, 1988). The similarity between grounded theory research and the phenomenological approach proposed by Paterson and Zderad is clearly evident. Moreover, there are other methodologies such as ethnomethodology and ethnography that employ a strategy which allows researchers to apprehend experiences as they are perceived by those who live them (Swanson-Kauffman & Schonwald, 1988).

Further, Silva and Rothbart (1984) suggested that historicism and alternative research methodologies hold promise in helping to bridge the gap to contend with phenomena dealing with humanism and holism. Thus, phenomenological nursology may serve as a valuable tool for qualitative research and for the identification of concepts and further theory development.

Interestingly, Paterson and Zderad published their conceptual framework in 1976, but their model received little attention in the nursing literature (Silva & Rothbart, 1984). Silva and Rothbart (1984) speculated that this may be due to its existential-phenomenological perspective and ontological commitment, which was out of the mainstream of current thinking about philosophy of science at that time. Thus, Paterson and Zderad's humanistic nursing model reflected progressive thinking in keeping with the historicist philosophy.

The humanistic nursing model must not be dismissed due to its unique perspective and nontraditional approach. The model serves as a valuable framework in the development of knowledge through esthetic and personal patterns of knowing. Empathy is an important mode in the esthetic pattern of knowing (Carper, 1978). Further, through the "therapeutic use of self," the nurse develops personal knowledge. Without question, phenomenological nursology is an empathic process which requires the "therapeutic use of self." More-

over, Carper (1978) stated that the more skilled the nurse becomes in empathizing, the more knowledge will be gained in alternative perceptions of reality.

According to Chinn and Kramer (1991), there should be an integration of all patterns of knowing. The authors suggested that there has been little attention given to developing forms of expression for personal and esthetic knowing. Further, they asserted that all patterns of knowing are legitimate sources of knowledge for a collective body of nursing knowledge and for nursing practice.

HUMANISTIC NURSING COMPLEMENTS OTHER APPROACHES IN PATIENT CARE

There is no one theory that serves as a panacea for all nursing problems. All paradigms have their particular strengths and weaknesses. A model is neither all good nor all bad. The phenomenological approach serves as a form of expression for the development of knowledge acquired through esthetic and personal patterns of knowing. The humanistic nursing approach complements other approaches in patient care. It offers a philosophical framework in the therapeutic nurse-patient relationship. Further, the model provides a methodology for qualitative research and for describing human phenomenon derived directly from the lived experiences of patients which is important to clinical nursing practice.

REFERENCES

Berger, M. (1977). *Working with people called patients.* New York, NY: Brunner/Mazel Publishers.

Bowers, B.J. (1988). Grounded theory. In B.S. Sarter (ed.), *Paths to knowledge* (pp. 33–59). New York, NY: National League for Nursing Press.

Brouse, S.H., & Laffrey, S.C. (1989). Paterson and Zderad's humanistic nursing framework. In J.J. Fitzpatrick & A.L. Whall, *Conceptual models of nursing: Analysis and application* (2nd ed.). Norwalk, CT: Appleton and Lange.

Carper, B.A. (1978). Fundamental patterns of knowing in nursing. *Adv Nurs Sci*, 1(1): 13–24.

Chinn, P.L., & Kramer, M.K. (1991). Nursing's patterns of knowing. *Theory and nursing: A systematic approach* (3rd ed.). St. Louis, MO: Mosby-Year Book.

McKinnon, N.C. (1991). Humanistic nursing: It can't stand up to scrutiny. *Nursing and Health Care*, 12(8): 414–416.

Oiler, C. (1982). The phenomenological approach in nursing research. *Nursing Research*, 31(3): 178–181.

Paterson, J., & Zderad, L. (1976). *Humanistic nursing*. New York, NY: John Wiley & Sons, Inc.

Silva, M.C., & Rothbart, D. (1984). An analysis of changing trends in philosophies of science on nursing theory development and testing. In L.H. Nicoll (ed.), *Perspectives on nursing theory* (pp. 293–302). Glenview, IL: Scott, Foresman and Company.

Swanson-Kauffman, K., & Schonwald, E. (1988). Phenomenology. In B.S. Sarter (ed.), *Paths to knowledge* (pp. 97–105). New York, NY: National League for Nursing.

22

A Multiparadigm Approach to Nursing

JOAN ENGEBRETSON, DrPH, RN

Nursing theory development has made good progress in differentiating the domain of nursing from medicine; many of these theories are categorized as holistic theories. Nursing classification systems are also being developed to organize extant nursing practice. The dissonance between the two has been one of the most difficult contemporary issues for the leadership of nursing. A framework is proposed that would account for these disparate approaches. This proposed framework for the domain of healing is in keeping with the metaparadigm of health and uses a multiple paradigm approach. Nursing interventions are discussed in relation to the framework. It invites a dialogue in keeping with the scholarship of holism. Practice and scholarship implications are discussed. [Keywords: Classification systems, Culture, Holism, Paradigm, Theory]

Nursing theory has, since the 1960s, sought to define the profession of nursing and to differentiate its scope of practice from that of biomedicine.[1] This search has led to some discrepancies between theory development that differentiates nursing action from biomedical nursing practice, the latter of which uses many nursing actions derived from biomedicine. Differentiating autonomous nursing practice was a necessary step, because historically many nursing functions were derived from biomedicine, since nurses have practiced in biomedically dominated settings.

One primary differentiating feature was holism, which was contrasted with biomedical reductionism. The movement to declare nursing holistic is now well accepted; however, a holistic framework must be inclusive of, not only differentiated from, biomedicine. In alignment with holism, the appropriate construct for the nursing profession is healing. Health is a derivative of healing, or making whole, and part of the metaparadigm of nursing.

Another element of professional evolution is the development of diagnostic, intervention, and outcomes classifications systems. These are often grounded in nursing practice and thus reflect both nursing activities as well as predominant sociocultural ideologies. There is often a disjuncture between the differentiating and defining theories and the more pragmatic classifications systems.[2] In an effort to reconcile grand conceptual models and practice, this article presents a conceptual framework for discussion as a step toward the consolidation of a holistic approach to nursing. The intent is to support both unique autonomous actions and to incorporate medically derived actions. Using the construct of healing, a multiparadigm model is presented to incorporate both

Source: Engebretson, J. (1997). A multiparadigm approach to nursing. *Adv Nurs Sci* 20(1):21–23. Reprinted with permission by from and copyright © 1997 Aspen Publishers, Inc.

the medical model and other cultural healing models on which nurses may ground their actions. This integration is at the level of paradigm, which allows the incorporation of and expansion beyond the biomedical model and avoids the pitfalls of the derivative–differentiation polarity.

Nursing has over the past 30 years made great strides in the development of nursing theories and conceptual models. These activities have been necessary to define the professional domain to its members and to society at large. Theory guides the practice and the activities that are unique to the profession, informs research efforts, and provides direction for future development.[3]

CONTEMPORARY CONTROVERSIES

Despite the progress made, the use of nursing theories in practice has been a matter of controversy. One area of controversy is the dichotomy between medicine and nursing, with many theories focusing on unique nursing functions and in some cases redefining actions associated with medical models. This position has often still held the medical model as the orthodox standard against which nursing defined itself by negation or differentiation, thereby maintaining dependence on the medical model.

Closely related to the nursing–medicine dichotomy is the rupture between academia and practice. Academia and much of theory development focused on the autonomous nature of nursing, differentiating it from medicine. Extant nursing practice often eschewed the nursing theories learned in school, and practicing nurses functioned in a more pragmatic manner reflective of the medical model.[4] Many times the praxis of nursing is covertly, if not overtly, aligned with the medical model. This

alliance with the medical model is understandable considering the hegemony of the medical bioscientific model in U.S. culture. Barnum[4] noted that normative theory evolves from practice rather than academic theory development and that inconsistencies develop when practice (theory) is not intellectually analyzed and scrutinized according to logical coherence.

A third, related problem area is the disjuncture between nursing theories and the diagnosis, intervention, and outcome classification systems. The two strongest competitors in the theory business are holistic theories and nursing process,[1,4] which often represent opposing philosophies regarding content, methodology, and interpretation. Holistic theories are global, espouse a transcendental view of humans, and are committed to not viewing subject matter as an accumulation of parts.[4]

Nursing process approaches are much more concrete and practice based and have focused on nursing action and classification systems.[5] The International Council of Nurses,[6] the Omaha Project,[7] the Iowa Project,[8] and separate projects by Grobe[9] and Saba[10] have recently developed nursing classification systems.

Recent debates in nursing have also reflected controversies over the usefulness of a unified theory vs multiple theories. Reed[11] proposed an approach that links science, philosophy, and practice in the development of nursing knowledge. She advocated a metanarrative that involves a dialogue of practice and philosophy. This metanarrative provides an excellent format for the development of nursing theory that is holistic in nature and can integrate multiple paradigms from the patient's perspective and from the nurse. It is in this spirit of inviting a dialogue and providing a format for a dialectic discussion between paradigms that the author presents the multiparadigm model.

HOLISM AND NURSING

Grand theory, or the concept level of theory development, has evolved into a metaparadigm with four propositional statements related to the concepts person–health, person–environment, health–nursing, and person–environment–health.[12] The global level defines the frameworks within which the more restricted structures develop.

Consistent with the concept heal–health, the related ideologies for nursing theory development would come from healing, rather than be restricted to medicine. Healing and health stem from the root word *hale*, or to make whole.[13] This etymology grounds the concept heal–health in holism. Barnum[4] identified holistic theories as the fastest growing trend in nursing. Holistic concepts in nursing have been evident since the time of Florence Nightingale and evolved in nursing theories through the influence of Teilhard de Chardin, Jan Smuts, and Ludwig von Bertalanffy.[14] Anthropology, another discipline based on holism, provides another source of information on healing that can inform nurses in the development of holistic theory. Traditionally, in many cultures, healers, shamans, and medicine people reflected the broader concept of healing rather than the science-based concept of cure.

Holistic health has recently become very popular among both lay and professional groups. Characteristics of holistic health have been described in many studies.[15-19] Two common mistakes occur in the analysis of holism from a modernist perspective based in a scientific or reductionistic paradigm. Alster's[15] analysis of holistic health is an example of such an attempt; it reaches the syllogistic conclusion that holistic health cannot be studied scientifically because it is not scientific.

The opposite pitfall is to romanticize traditional or primitive healing systems and unfavorably compare science and biomedicine.

This antiscience position is often seen in lay literature that attributes all social ills to scientific–rational thinking while extolling a holistic framework as the alternative. A consistent holistic framework incorporates science but does not hold that paradigm as sufficient for explaining the human experience or for bringing about health or healing. The model proposed in this article recognizes the holistic nature of nursing and expands the domain from disease treatment to the broader concept of health by incorporating several paradigms and their adjunctive ideological perspectives on humans, health, and therapeutic actions.

HISTORICAL CONTEXT OF WESTERN MEDICINE

Healing systems reflect and influence the cultural values of the parent culture. Contemporary biomedicine has been informed by and influential in the development of modernism. Modernity had its philosophical origins in the 17th century with the emphasis on rationality by the protagonists Galileo and Descartes.[20] Kuhn[21] described the shift of vision that enabled people to see and think about phenomena in a different manner and that he labeled a "paradigm shift." Modernity is characterized by the development of science and technology, the valorization of reason and humanity's dominion over nature. The scientific paradigm of modernity has dominated medicine and health care.

The establishment of the scientific model as the foundation for biomedicine paralleled the development of modernity. The scientific paradigm is characterized by philosophical dualism between the material and nonmaterial, and the corresponding designation of matter as the subject of science and the nonmaterial or metaphysical as the domain of religion. Descartes is often credited with conceptualiz-

Positivist ← ───→ Metaphysical

Material	Modalities	Mechanical	Purification	Balance	Supranormal
↑	Physical manipulation	Biomedical surgery	Colonics Cupping	Magnetic healing Polarity	Drumming Dancing
	Applied and ingested substances	Pharmacology	Chetation	Humoral medicine	Flower remedies Hallucinogenics plants
	Energy	Laser Radiation	Bioenergetics	Tai chi Chi gong Acupuncture Accupressure	Healing touch Laying on of hands
	Psychological	Mind-body	Self-help (confessional type)	Mindfulness	Imagery
↓ Nonmaterial	Spirtual	Attendance at organized religious functions	Forgiveness Panance	Meditation Chakra Balancing	Primal religious Expedence Prayer

Figure 22.1. A Multiparadigm approach to healing.

ing the mind–body dualism and the corresponding value of the mind–soul as the superior demarcation of the human.

Throughout the following centuries, especially in England, increasing cultural value was placed on the scientific, material, rational, and technical.[22,23] Metaphysical and nonmaterial issues associated with religion were progressively devalued, especially among intellectuals.[24] Medicine, which historically had been based in a metaphysical model and supported by religion, became the domain of science and was severed from its metaphysical and religious roots. This split allowed medicine to make unprecedented technological advances through the application of scientific reason. But a contemporary surge of public interest in alternative healing modalities suggests that the biomedical scientific approach by itself is insufficient for healing.

DEVELOPMENT OF THE MULTIPARADIGM MODEL

The multiparadigm model was developed from the author's ethnographic work with healers and nurses. Field work, including participant observation, long interviews, free list-

ing, and pile sorts, was used in a study exploring and comparing the conceptual frameworks of health and healing between nurses and healers.[25] A matrix of healing modalities that incorporated biomedicine and examples of alternative models emerging in the United States in the late 1980s and early 1990s was developed to focus the study on healers using healing touch[26] and used to orient nurse practitioners to alternative healing modalities that their clients might be using.[27]

This matrix was then developed into the Heterodox Explanatory Paradigms Model for health practice that incorporated multiple healing modalities.[28] The philosophical coherence of the model and the related positioning of modalities was presented as a framework for developing integrated health care models. Because nurses and healers have similar conceptual frameworks of healing,[25] this model could be adapted for nursing as a possible framework toward a more holistic model.

Philosophical Design

The multiparadigm model (Fig. 22.1) developed from the author's previous work[25-28] represents a multiparadigm approach to healing. Philosophical dualism between the material and nonmaterial is represented on both axes. Four paradigms of healing are incorporated and philosophically arranged from the most material to the most nonmaterial along the horizontal axis, which represents a philosophical continuum from logical positivism to metaphysics. Consistent with the positivist–metaphysical continuum, the mechanical paradigm is on the extreme left, reflecting the logical positivism of its philosophical scientific foundation. The paradigms are progressively more nonmaterial, ending in the most metaphysical paradigm, supranormal, at the extreme right. The vertical axis represents the Cartesian body–mind dualism in healing activities. Activities that are most material or physical are at the top. Moving down, activities become progressively less material and more psychological or spiritual.

Horizontal Axis

The four paradigms are mechanical, purification, balance, and supranormal. The mechanical paradigm is best represented by examples from biomedicine, which is primarily a mechanistic, materialistic paradigm exemplified by the focus on discovering explanatory mechanisms to understand a healing activity. The positivist philosophy bases knowing on objective, material data perceived by the senses.[29] It is characterized by determinism, mechanism, and reductionism. Disease is assumed to be reducible to disordered body functions and a disease-specific etiology.[30] Treatment and intervention are disease specific.

The purification paradigm has examples cross-culturally and throughout Western history. This paradigm is characterized by healing actions that cleanse or purify. The name of the prestigious English medical journal *Lancet* is a remnant of the bloodletting and purges that dominated Western medicine before technical advances in surgery and antibiotics in the 20th century. Health and

healing activities related to cleanliness or purification either physically or symbolically have been documented in many ritual practices.[31] The hygienic health reform movement of the late 19th century[32,33] incorporated many practices that were understood as cleansing and keeping the body pure.

The balance paradigm is best represented by Eastern or humeral systems. In Eastern systems health–healing is viewed as the proper balance of yin and yang and unimpeded flow of Chi (or Ki or Qi).[34] Humeral medicine, or the balance of vital forces or humors, is evident in Hippocratic, Galenic, and Ayurvedic medicine.[35] Nineteenth-century vitalism also incorporated this approach. Health is attained or maintained by creating a balance in daily living through types of foods, activities, temperature, and so forth. Personality types, environment, and circumstances are considered in determining the corrective balance. One example is the hot and cold classification in Mexican folk medicine. The balance paradigm is on the right half of the model and therefore cannot be fully understood through a materialist mechanistic paradigm.

The supranormal paradigm incorporates all magicoreligious and psychic phenomena used to promote health or create healing. Spiritual, symbolic, and other nonmaterial understandings of healing are in this column. The supranormal paradigm is philosophically the most metaphysical, going beyond physics, sense experience, or any discipline and involving ultimates.[36] This paradigm incorporates psychic, spiritual, and other types of healing such as prayer, distant healing, and other spontaneous healing that cannot be explained by mechanistic models or one of the other paradigms.

Vertical Axis

The vertical axis describes types of healing activities that progress along the continuum from body to mind–soul, from material to nonmaterial. The first row contains physical manipulations, and examples are given for each paradigm. Physical manipulation may be performed either by the patient or on the patient by a healer.

In row 2 applied and ingested substances are listed according to each paradigm. Such substances include all foods, herbs, and pharmaceuticals that are ingested, inhaled, or topically applied.

Using energy, the third activity, is a concept that is poorly understood in biomedicine but important in other paradigms. Many healing activities are understood and conducted as an active manipulation of energy. The concept of energy, or the transfer from matter to energy to matter, has been proposed by some scientists (eg, Bohm, Capra[37]) as the basis for quantum physics and as a possible link in understanding the material and nonmaterial worlds. This could be a promising area in linking the material, physical body with nonmaterial thought, spirit, and so on. The concept of energy has been proposed by some nurses as the basis for understanding the benefits of touch therapies.[38–40]

Psychological activities deal with functions of cognition and of the mind. Mind to body medicine has been a rapidly growing area of research. With the discovery of neurotransmitters and hormonal–neural pathways, mechanisms have been discovered by which thoughts and feelings can manifest in physiological changes.[41] Theory has been developed and researched regarding the association of personality characteristics with illness, in particular hostility and heart disease.[42] Psychoneuroimmunology is another promising field where theory is developing. Associations have been demonstrated between various personality characteristics and mortality and morbidity.[43,44]

Spiritual activities are at the polar opposite of the continuum from physical manipulation. Spiritual actions are distinct from cognitive activities. Spirituality, being the most distant from the physical or material, is the least understood from a modernist perspective. Some studies have found that attendance at religious activities is related to improved health or healing.[45] Attendance at religious activities represents a mechanistic conceptualization of spiritual activity, whereas a primal spiritual experience as described by Cox[46] would be a more metaphysical approach.

The model has, at present, four paradigms, but others could be added along the continuum. Restriction to a two-dimensional format is often interpreted as containing mutually exclusive cells. A more appropriate geographic conceptualization would be as general areas on a double-axis continuum, with no specific boundary between areas. Modalities in the model are examples only, and many other modalities could fit in each location. The modalities describe healing activities only. An individual practitioner–healer could, and often does, use many modalities.

The positioning of modalities according to philosophical continuums also reflects the degree of passivity or activity of the healer. Starting from the upper left corner, where the modalities are most material, the healer is most active and the recipient most passive. Moving diagonally down and across, the person who is healing is progressively more active and the role of the healer increasingly that of facilitator, consistent with healing philosophy, which posits that real healing is done by the "healee."

One area that is a vital part of the nursing metaparadigm and other healing systems is the environment, especially social relationships. Although not specifically addressed in the model, an additional line at the bottom could be added to address social activities.

	Positivist ←				→ Metaphysical
Material	**Modalities**	**Mechanical**	**Purification**	**Balance**	**Supranormal**
	Physical manipulation	Positioning Exercise therapy Joint mobility	Bathing	Exercise promotion	Intuitive body work†
	Applied and ingested substances	Medication administration	Wound and bladder irrigation Leech therapy	Nutritional counseling	Homeopathic remedies
	Energy	Laser precautions	Phototherapy	Acupressure Acupuncture†	Therapeutic touch
	Psychological	Cognitive restructuring	Active listening†	Counseling*	Simple guided imagery
Nonmaterial	Spiritual	Activity therapy*	Forgiveness and purification rituals	Meditation	Spiritual support*

*NIC listed intervention that could be developed with understanding of the paradigm
†No NIC listing and should be considered as a potential referral or potential development for nursing action

FIGURE 28.2. Nursing activities and interventions.

APPLICATION TO NURSING

The multiparadigm model is holistic and avoids the medicine–nursing and practice– academia dichotomies by placing the Western biomedical model in context with other paradigms of healing. It speaks to the domain of healing, which is the stated domain of nursing. This model can provide a framework for nursing diagnoses and interventions that easily integrates biomedical model functions with complementary functions that either are autonomous nursing activities or might constitute appropriate referrals. The model also incorporates paradigms that can be useful in understanding cross-cultural healing practices and systems.

IMPLICATIONS FOR PRACTICE

Operating from a multiparadigm model allows nurses to adapt whatever paradigm or modality fits the situation. This flexibility is helpful in working with patients who practice health- and healing-related activities from other para-

digms. A multiparadigm approach that incorporates models of health–healing can help providers better understand beliefs and practices of patients that may be poorly comprehended in the biomedical model.

Most health practices originate in the popular sector,[47] which includes family and social networks. This sector has beliefs about health maintenance and hierarchies of resort that direct types of health–healing activities, healer consultants, and adherence to treatments. The orientation of the popular sector often incorporates other paradigms than the scientific–mechanistic approach of biomedicine. By understanding the explanatory paradigm of health practices, the practitioner is better able to communicate and collaborate with the client and family in the management of health–healing.

Many interventions listed in the various nursing classification systems may be positioned in this model. Examples from one of these systems, the Nursing Interventions Classification (NIC),[8] have been identified in Fig 28.2, along with other modalities that could be referral sources for the client. Examples are easily placed in the mechanistic and purification paradigms but more difficult to place in the balance and supranormal paradigms. Thus, the model can display areas where nursing has developed actions and where referrals are more appropriate. It is important to note that a holistic paradigm is impossible to implement in its entirety by any one person or discipline; therefore, nurses should be able to understand how other providers fit into an overall plan of care.

By understanding these modalities through the appropriate paradigm, practitioners may select whatever modality is appropriate for the client, either by interventions or referral to other providers. For example, existing NIC actions in the mechanical paradigm for physical manipulation could incorporate positioning, exercise therapy including range of motion, and ambulation. Applied and ingested substances include medication administration of all types. Although energy is poorly understood in the mechanical model, it is present on the NIC as laser precautions. Energy, if better understood, could have potential for much broader use.

Psychological interventions in the mechanical (medical) model include cognitive restructuring and reality therapies. Spiritual interventions may include assisting a patient with religious practices such as attending chapel or praying. This is not specifically listed in NIC but is covered under activity therapy.

Examples of nursing actions in the purification paradigm using physical manipulation include bathing and other hygiene activities. Wound and bladder irrigations are good examples of applied and ingested substances. Many medications have cleaning or purification action, such as emetics, expectorants, and purgatives. Psychological and emotional catharsis are examples of psychological purification. These are not specifically listed, although could be covered under the NIC active listening.

Spiritual purification includes a number of rituals that serve to purify and cleanse the individual, such as confession, seeking of forgiveness, ritual bathing, and use of incense. These would need to be developed or referred because there is no NIC entry related to this.

Nursing interventions are being expanded into the balance and supranormal paradigms through the work of nurses who have expanded their individual practice and those who are using many of the more recent nursing theories, such as Rogers,[48] Watson,[49] Parse,[50] or Newman,[51] to direct their practice. Exercise promotion is listed in NIC and could be expanded and developed with a better understanding of the balance paradigm. Nutritional counseling is based on providing a balance of nutrients and could also be expanded to incorporate use of some herbs for the promotion of health. Approaching these from the perspective of balance rather than mechanical cure allows for an expansion into health and attention to individual life systems. Acupuncture or acupressure are not on the NIC but could be a source of referral. While currently not part of the balance paradigm, counseling, simple relaxation therapy, or self-modification assistance have the potential for development into that paradigm. Meditation also has potential for development.

Nursing interventions in the supranormal paradigm cluster in the nonmaterial areas. Intuitive body work, if not done by a nurse, could constitute a referral. Likewise, activities using homeopathic remedies or flower essences are included as they are understood to work through the spiritual level.

Therapeutic touch is well developed in nursing and is understood as a supranormal use of energy. Guided imagery is a supranormal psychological technique that is listed in the NIC. Spiritual support, including prayer, could be further developed to fully express this paradigm.

IMPLICATIONS FOR RESEARCH AND SCHOLARSHIP

By constructing a paradigm map with health–healing activities, nurses can determine appropriate paradigms to guide their understanding and research of particular modalities. Locating it on the model can serve as a guide for better understanding a particular modality; it also provides a direction for further scholarship and research. An exploration of both axes can enhance understanding. For example, nursing actions in the mechanical paradigm are often best understood by a better comprehension of the medical–scientific model, and research using the positivist philosophy is often appropriate. Many of the NIC classifications can be understood from this paradigm.

Working with a modality such as guided imagery could be enhanced by exploring both the supranormal paradigm and the psychological literature. Healing touch, a modality with a rich history in nursing, is located at the nexus of energy and the supranormal, the two axes least understood by biomedical science. Nurses who have conducted research using this modality or the existential psychological theories can attest to the frustration in conducting research without documented material and measurable mechanisms of action that are compatible with the mechanical paradigm. Research in these areas can be enhanced by learning more about the approaches of anthropology, theology, some psychology, and other humanity disciplines consistent with the supranormal paradigm. Investigation of energy through quantum physics (energy) and Eastern healing are also proximal areas that can illuminate the understanding of touch therapies.

The model can serve as an agenda for research and scholarship. In some modalities, links have been or can be developed that enable more mechanistic studies. In others, their position invites more qualitative or naturalistic methodologies of inquiry. Nursing theories may develop links that connect modalities for practice. For example, some of the developmental theories may have links across paradigms on the psychological axis. Although methods may be successfully combined, caution must be taken in attempting to link paradigms. Many paradigms are based on contradictory beliefs that are impossible to adhere to simultaneously.[52]

The multiparadigm model provides a holistic approach to bridging the gulf between holistic theories and biomedical nursing praxis. The dialectic method is appropriate scholarship for holistic frameworks.[4,53] In this approach, the whole is seen as governing relationships and providing coherence to the parts. The dialectic process would describe a nursing issue from one position—for example, the mechanical paradigm—and then counter that description with an oppositional position, the supranormal. After debate and dialogue, a third position emerges. This position can, in similar fashion, be refined by the same process. Placing the polar opposites in one model invites a dialectic methodology, appropriate for holistic nursing scholarship. The challenge remains for nurses to continue to develop theory that links modalities and explanatory paradigms. These links are being developed along nursing themes of health, environment, and individual potentials for healing. The model could help to provide a geographic map to locate these dialogues.

REFERENCES

1. Chinn PL, Kramer MK. *Theory and Nursing: A Systematic Approach*. St. Louis, Mo: Mosby; 1995.
2. Fitzpatrick JJ, Whall AL. *Conceptual Models of Nursing Analysis and Application*. 3rd ed. Stamford, Conn: Appleton & Lange; 1996.

3. Newman MN. *A Developing Discipline: Selected Works of Margaret Newman.* New York, NY: National League for Nursing Press; 1995.

4. Barnum BJS. *Nursing Theory: Analysis, Application, Evaluation.* Philadelphia, Pa: Lippincott; 1994.

5. Snyder M. Defining nursing interventions. *Image J Nurs Schol.* 1996;28(2):137–141.

6. International Council of Nurses. *Nurses' Next Advance: An International Classification for Nursing Practice.* Geneva, Switzerland: ICN; 1993.

7. Martin KS, Scheet NJ. *The Omaha System: Applications for Community Health Nursing.* Philadelphia, Pa: W.B. Saunders; 1992.

8. McCloskey JC, Bulechek GM. *Nursing Interventions Classification (NIC).* St. Louis, Mo: Mosby; 1996.

9. Grobe SJ. The nursing lexicon and taxonomy: Implications for representing nursing care data in automated patient records. *Holistic Nurs Pract.* 1996;11(1):48–63.

10. Saba VK. The classification of home health nursing. *Caring.* 1992;11(3):50–57.

11. Reed, PG. A treatise on nursing knowledge development for the 21st century: Beyond postmodernism. *ANS.* 1995;17(3):70–84.

12. Fawcett J. *Analysis and evaluation of nursing theories.* Philadelphia, Pa: F.A. Davis; 1993.

13. *Webster's Ninth New Collegiate Dictionary.* Springfield, Mass: Merriam-Webster; 1990.

14. Owen MJ, Holmes CA. Holism in the discourse of nursing. *J Adv Nurs.* 1993;18:1688–1695.

15. Alster, KB. *The Holistic Health Movement.* Tuscaloosa, Ala: University of Alabama Press; 1989.

16. English-Lueck JA. *Health in the New Age: A Study in California Holistic Practices.* Albuquerque, NM: University of New Mexico Press; 1990.

17. Gordon, JS. The paradigm of holistic medicine. In: Hastings AC, Fadiman J, Gordon JS, eds. *Health for the Whole Person.* Toronto, Ontario: Bantam Books; 1980.

18. Lowenberg JS. *Caring and Responsibility.* Philadelphia, Pa: University of Pennsylvania Press; 1989.

19. Mattson PH. *Holistic Health in Perspective.* Palo Alto, Calif: Mayfield; 1982.

20. Toulmin S. *Cosmopolis: The Hidden Agenda of Modernity.* Chicago, Ill: University of Chicago Press; 1990.

21. Kuhn T. *The Structure of Scientific Revolutions.* Chicago, Ill: The University of Chicago Press; 1972.

22. Tarnas R. *The Passion of the Western World: Understanding the Ideas That Have Shaped our World View.* New York, NY: Ballantine Books; 1991.

23. Lavine TZ. *From Socrates to Sartre: The Philosophic Quest.* New York, NY: Bantam; 1984.

24. Johnson P. *Intellectuals.* New York, NY: Harper Perennial; 1988.

25. Engebretson J. Comparison of nurses and alternative healers. *Image: J Nurs Schol.* 1996;28(2):95–100.

26. Engebretson J. *Cultural Models of Healing and Health: An Ethnography of Professional Nurses and Healers.* Houston, Tex: University of Texas-Houston, School of Public Health; 1992. Dissertation.

27. Engebretson J, Wardell D. A contemporary view of alternative healing modalities. *Nurse Practitioner.* 1993; 18(9):51–55.

28. Engebretson J. Models of heterodox healing. *Alternat Ther Health Med.* In press.

29. Andrews MM, Boyle JS. *Transcultural Concepts in Nursing Care.* 2nd ed. Philadelphia, Pa: Lippincott; 1995.

30. Freund PES, McGuire MB. *Health, Illness and the Social Body: A Critical Sociology.* Englewood Cliffs, NJ: Prentice-Hall; 1991.

31. Douglas M. *Purity and Danger: An Analysis of the Concepts of Pollution and Taboo.* London, England: Ark Paperbacks; 1989.

32. Brown PS. Nineteenth-century American health reformers and the early nature cure movement in Britain. *Med History.* 1988; 32:174–194.

33. Whorton JC. *Crusaders for Fitness: The History of American Health Reformers.* Princeton, NJ: Princeton University Press; 1982.

34. Kaptchuk TJ. *The Web that Has No Weaver: Understanding Chinese Medicine.* New York, NY: Congdon and Weed; 1993.

35. Helman CG. *Culture, Health and Illness: An Introduction for Health Professionals.* 3rd ed. Wolburn, Mass: Butterworth-Heinemann; 1994.

36. Reese WL. *Dictionary of Philosophy and Religion: Eastern and Western Thought.* Atlantic Highland, NJ: Humanities Press; 1991.

37. Horgan J. *The End of Science, Facing the Limits of Knowledge in the Twilight of the Scientific Age.* Reading, Mass. Addison Wesley; 1996.

38. Dossey BM, Keegan L, Guzzetta CE, Kolkmeier LG. *Holistic Nursing: A Handbook for Practice.* Gaithersburg, Md: Aspen Publishers; 1995.

39. Slater VE. Toward an understanding of energetic healing, part 1: Energetic structures. *J Holistic Nurs.* 1995;13:209–224.

40. Slater VE. Toward an understanding of energetic healing, part 2: Energetic process. *J Holistic Nurs.* 1995;13:225–238.

41. Rossi E. The *Psychobiology of Mind-Body Healing.* New York, NY: W.W. Norton; 1993.

42. Orth-Gomer K, Schneiderman N. *Behavioral Medicine Approaches to Cardiovascular Disease Prevention.* Hillsdale, NJ: Erlbaum; 1996.

43. Dreher H. *The Immune Power Personality.* New York: Dutton; 1995.

44. Schneiderman N, McCabe P, Baum A. *Perspectives in Behavioral Medicine: Stress and Disease Processes.* Hillsdale, NJ: Erlbaum; 1992.

45. Larson DB. Religion and spirituality—the forgotten factor in public health: What does the research share? Presented at the 12th annual meeting of the American Public Health Association, November 18, 1996; New York, NY.

46. Cox H. *Fire from Heaven.* Reading, Mass: Addison-Wesley; 1995.

47. Kleinman A. *Patients and Healers in the Context of Culture.* Berkeley, Calif: University of California Press; 1980.

48. Rogers ME. *An Introduction to the Theoretical Basis of Nursing.* Philadelphia, PA: F.A. Davis; 1970.

49. Watson J. *Nursing: Human Science and Human Care: A Theory of Nursing.* New York, NY: National League for Nursing.

50. Parse RR. *Man—Living—Health: A Theory of Nursing.* New York, NY: Wiley; 1981.

51. Newman MA. *Health as Expanding Consciousness.* 2nd ed. New York, NY: National League for Nursing; 1984.

52. Nagle LM, Mitchell GJ. *Theoretic Diversity: Evolving Paradigmatic Issues in Research and Practice.* Gaithersburg, Md: Aspen Publishers; 1991.

53. McKeon ZK. *On Knowing the Natural Sciences.* Chicago, Ill: University of Chicago Press; 1994.

Part VI

INTERRELATIONSHIPS AMONG NURSING THEORY, RESEARCH, AND PRACTICE

Ideally, nursing theory develops from practice, is tested and validated in practice, and then serves to change or modify nursing practice. However, this ideal cycle rarely exists in the real world of nursing. Although the interrelationships of theory, research and nursing practice have been discussed for years, the advancement of nursing science depends on generating nursing theory, testing theory in practice, and modifying practice based on theory. Hopefully as more graduate nurses learn about the value of nursing theory and research, and take leadership positions in practice, they will utilize nursing theories and research more consistently.

Knowledge of nursing theories, models, and principles, along with critical thinking skills, is essential for nurses to determine the congruence, or 'goodness of fit' between a client's health problems and selection of an appropriate theory or model. Advanced practice nurses need to understand the theorist's definitions of concepts, underlying assumptions and beliefs, and the interrelationships among the concepts of a variety of theories and models before deciding which one to use with an individual or family client.

In his article, "A Nursing Perspective on the Interrelationships Between Theory, Research and Practice," Steven Pryjmachuk discusses their meaning and relevance to nursing, and proposes a model illustrating a learning cycle for the acquisition of knowledge. He acknowledges the existence of a knowledge gap between theory and practice, and suggests using both formal and informal research to reduce the gap. Pryjmachuk also compares levels of knowledge acquisition to Benner's levels of nurse's expertise, and their role in research, along with the nursing process. He believes that for continued development of nursing's body of knowledge, nurses must be encouraged to use theories and models to guide their practice, and to test and refine them in practice.

A recent trend in nursing is to use 'evidence-based' practice to supposedly enhance nurses' accountability and show that their nursing care is supported by research. In her article, "Evidence-Based Practice," Dr. Gail Mitchell presents convincing arguments that such nursing practice is ill conceived. She claims that such evidence is non-existent in the first place, and would reduce nursing practice to using procedural or technical protocols. Dr. Mitchell critiques the effects of using evidence-based practice in relation to four specific issues. She concludes that theory-based knowledge requires effective nurse-client interactions, and guides making more appropriate decisions to enhance a client's health and quality of life.

In her article, "Critical Thinking and Theory-Based Practice," Ellen Birx emphasizes the importance of using both analytical and synthesis skills to identify client's patterns and select appropriate theories to guide nursing practice decisions. She discusses ways that nurses use both metacognition and metatheory in theory-based practice. Dr. Birx believes that critical thinking fosters nurses' empowerment through inquiry, reflection, exploration of creative alternatives, and articulation of nurses' insight, which lead to effective theory-based practice and high quality nursing care.

The last chapter of this book, "Theory-Based Advanced Practice Nursing," was written by the editor, Janet Kenney, based on many years of teaching graduate students to apply theories in their nursing practice, and from her textbook, *Nursing Process: Application of Conceptual Models*. Dr. Kenney explains why and how theories are essential to provide the rationale for holistic, systematic, individualized professional nursing care instead of rote, cookbook, medical-dependent technical nursing care. She describes the broad knowledge base of theories, types of theories from various disciplines, and the need for critical thinking skills nurses must continuously use for effective theory-based practice. Guidelines for choosing appropriate theories, congruent with client's health problems and lived experiences, are provided, along with related suggestions from other nurse scholars. Theory-based practice enhances nurses' autonomy, creativity, and effectiveness and is based on nursing knowledge and science.

23

A Nursing Perspective on the Interrelationships between Theory, Research and Practice

STEVEN PRYJMACHUK RMN, MSc

This paper is concerned with the interrelationships between the three concepts of theory, research and practice. In the course of discussing the interrelationships between these concepts, research is identified as the link between theory and practice on both a formal (explicit) and informal (tacit) level. The role of formal and informal research in the development of nursing expertise is also given some consideration.

THEORY, PRACTICE AND RESEARCH IN NURSING

Most nurses have some familiarity with the concepts of 'theory', 'research' and 'practice'. Many, however, find clarification of these concepts somewhat difficult, in that they lack a true understanding of the importance of theory, research and practice to the continuing development of nursing as a profession. Moreover, and more significantly, most nurses perhaps fail to acknowledge the importance of interrelationships between the three concepts.

What of these interrelationships? With regard to the theory–research diad, there appears to be some, albeit tentative, evidence for the existence of a relationship, in that academics view theory development and research as mutual, coexisting activities. With regard to the theory–practice diad, the fact that much

Source: Pryjmachuk, S. (1996). A nursing perspective on the interrelationships between theory, research and practice. *Journal of Advanced Nursing* 23, 679–684. Reprinted with permission by Blackwell Science Ltd.

has been written about the so-called 'theory–practice gap' implies that, at the very least, a relationship between these two concepts *should* exist. The evidence for a relationship between research and practice is, however, rather less clear.

Nonetheless, when the three concepts are examined in detail, explicit interrelationships between the three concepts are found to be manifest. It is possible, moreover, to illustrate the nature of these relationships by means of a model. Such a model is proposed by the author later in this paper.

To begin the discussion, there is a need to consider one of the concepts in detail. A logical choice is 'theory'.

What is 'Theory'?

'Theory', like most terms, has a number of different meanings. Whilst various taxonomies of its meanings are available (see McCaugherty 1992a, for a taxonomy of its meanings within nursing), a simple consideration of its formal

TABLE 23.1 Descriptions of the 'formal' and 'informal' arenas

Formal	Informal
Public	Private, personal
Academic	Practical
Explicit	Implicit, tacit
'Macro'	'Micro'
Exogenous	Endogenous
External	Internal

and informal meanings will suffice for the purposes of this discussion.

Used informally, theory describes an idea or hunch, a hypothesis, about the world. More formal interpretations of the term, on the other hand, tend to see a theory as a set of ideas, hunches or hypotheses that provides some degree of prediction and/or explanation of the world. (Formal definitions of theory within nursing can be found in Dickoff & James, 1968a; Stevens, 1984, and Chinn & Jacobs, 1987.)

The Formal and Informal Arenas

Reference was made above to formal and informal theories. These terms have significance throughout this paper (a significance which stems from the applicability of the proposed theory–research–practice model to both the formal and the informal arenas). To help the reader gain a better understanding of what is meant by the terms 'formal' and 'informal', some qualities of both arenas are listed in Table 23.1. All of the concepts discussed in this paper (including concepts introduced at a later point, such as 'learning', 'knowledge' and 'education') have both formal and informal connotations.

THEORY AND PRACTICE

Given that theory has undergone some degree of clarification, its relationship to practice and research can be considered.

Its relationship to practice appears to have some substance, in the formal arena at least. (Formal practice is the collective, public actions of a specific discipline; informal practice merely our day-to-day actions.) Disciplines with an established body of formal knowledge (broadly speaking, the sciences) frequently seek out practical applications for that knowledge: every pure science has its applied counterpart. Moreover, it is the theories of the pure scientists that dictate the actions of those in practice, the applied scientists. Though the relationship between theory and practice appears to exist, it seems somewhat unidirectional in nature.

Further evidence for a unidirectional relationship comes from the activities of the practice-based disciplines. Of the practice-based disciplines that have sought out theoretical justifications for their actions, most (and nursing has to be included here) have merely borrowed theories from other (usually more powerful, scientific) disciplines, using those theories to define their practices.

There are, however, some practitioners, notably social workers (Howe 1987), who argue the converse: that in a practice-based discipline foreign theories cannot dictate practice; if theory is to have any relevance, it has to be extracted from practice.

There is, as such, some justification in assuming that the relationship between theory and practice is, in the formal arena at least, bidirectional. If a bidirectional relationship between theory and practice exists in the formal arena, is such a relationship evident in the informal arena? Is there a relationship between informal theory (thought) and informal practice (action)? To answer this question, the discussion has to enter the realms of cognitive

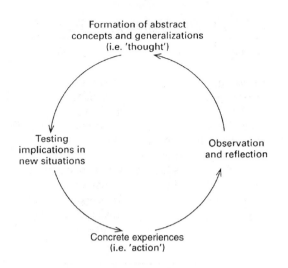

Formation of abstract
concepts and generalizations
(i.e. 'thought')

Testing
implications in
new situations

Observation
and reflection

Concrete experiences
(i.e. 'action')

Formal theory

Theory testing
via deductive
research

Theory generation
via inductive
research

Formal practice

FIGURE 23.2 A learning cycle for the acquisition of formal knowledge.

FIGURE 23.1 Kolb's learning cycle (adapted with permission from Kolb *et al.*, 1991 *Organizational Behavior: An Experiential Approach* 5th edn. Prentice Hall, New Jersey, p. 59).

psychology. Learning theorists, in particular, have something to say on the matter.

Kolb's Learning Cycle

One leading learning theorist, Kolb (see, for example, Kolb *et al.*, 1991), has not only speculated on the interrelationships between thought and action, he has also addressed the nature of these interrelationships. Consider Kolb's model of learning, adapted in Figure 23.1.

Learning is, according to Kolb, a cyclical process; a continual dialogue between thought and action that is effected via two processes: testing and reflection. Preconceived ideas, i.e., thoughts, about the world are tested against reality (ideas are put into practice; action is taken), after which the relative successes or failures of these actions are reflected upon. These reflections, in turn, lead to the refinement and development of our thoughts about the world.

Because Kolb's learning cycle considers the relationships between thought and action, rather than theory and practice, it is essen-

tially a model of informal learning; it is a model depicting the acquisition of informal (personal, implicit, 'micro') knowledge.

Though Kolb uses the terms 'testing' and 'reflection' to describe the processes linking thought and action, these processes can be described using a single word, 'research'. This comment becomes all the more meaningful if an analogous learning cycle for the formal arena is considered (see Figure 23.2).

A Universal Model of Knowledge Acquisition

Given that knowledge is acquired in the same manner in both the formal and the informal arenas, it is possible to delineate a universal model of knowledge acquisition. Such a model, as proposed by the author, is depicted in Figure 29.3.

Several points need to be made about this model. Firstly, the model stresses the importance of experience ('applying') in the acquisition of knowledge. Secondly, it acknowledges that knowledge has both cognitive and practical dimensions: it is both a model of theory (thought) development and of practice

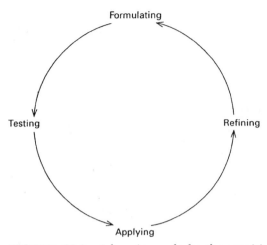

FIGURE 23.3 A learning cycle for the acquisition of knowledge.

TABLE 23.2   A Typology of 'research'

'Testing'	'Refining'
Analysing	Interpreting
Experimentation	Reflecting (I)
Deducing	Inducing
Deductive research (F)	Inductive research (F)
Quantitative research (F)	Qualitative
The scientific method (F)	research (F)
Theory/hypothesis testing	Phenomenological
'Assaying' (Dickoff &	research (F)
James 1968b)	Theory generation
	'Divining'; 'heuristic'
	research (Dickoff &
	James 1968b)

F, a term employed mainly in the formal arena.
I, a term employed mainly in the informal arena.

(action) development. It is, as such, a holistic model of knowledge acquisition. Thirdly, it sees the acquisition of knowledge as a dynamic process. Finally, learning is only complete when formulating and applying fuse, that is when there is no 'theory–practice gap'. (This point is discussed in more detail later.)

Research as the Link Between Theory and Practice

Research plays a key role in the acquisition of both formal and informal knowledge: testing and refining are the links between formulating and applying. In other words, learning cannot occur without research.

Though the author has labelled the two types of research 'testing' and 'refining', a variety of terms have been employed to describe these two processes. These are summarized in Table 23.2.

It is worth remarking that the universal model of knowledge acquisition proposed has striking similarities to Lewin's model of action research (see, for example, Lewin's 'change spiral' in Lewin, 1958). These similarities, however, are to be expected, as learning is an inherent part of 'change', a key concept in Lewin's work.

THE THEORY–PRACTICE GAP IN NURSING

The notion of the theory–practice gap has caused much debate within nursing (Vaughn, 1989, Lindsay 1990, Cook, 1991, McCaugherty 1991, McCaugherty, 1992b, Nolan & Grant, 1992). Two interrelated factors appear to be at the centre of this debate: (a) the necessity of a theory–practice gap if learning is to commence, and (b) its attenuation if learning is to progress.

The necessity of a theory–practice gap in nursing has been recognized by several authors (Lindsay, 1990; Cook 1991). As such, these authors argue that those (like Vaughn, 1989) who propose 'solutions' for the theory–practice gap are barking up the wrong tree.

Nevertheless, knowledge development, both formal and informal, can by definition only occur if the theory–practice gap narrows.

As such, much of the debate on the theory–practice gap (both within and outside nursing) has centred on the factors thought to hinder the narrowing of this gap. The major hindrance appears to be the cultural dominance of 'technical rationality' (Schön 1988).

The Dominance of Technical Rationality

Technical rationality is an objective approach to the discovery of 'truth'; an epistemology that unashamedly sees the relationship between theory and practice as unidirectional; theory precedes practice. Theory is, as such, afforded a greater status than practice or, to use the framework of the universal model of knowledge acquisition, formulating is afforded a greater status than applying. Technical rationality, furthermore, prides itself in its objectivity: testing (deductive experimentation) is seen as the superior research method, whereas refining (reflection and inductive research) is derided because of its subjective nature.

The dominance of technical rationality is evident in the organization of higher education and in a consideration of the professions. Those disciplines with a well-established body of theoretical knowledge (obtained largely from experimentation) are afforded the greatest status. Similarly, those disciplines distinguished enough to be called a profession are usually grounded in science. Consider, for example, the status of the pure sciences over the social sciences, and the status of medicine over nursing and social work.

Technical rationality, however, gives a very biased and artificial view of the world. Appleyard (1992) writes:

> . . . scientific knowledge is fundamentally paradoxical . . . all of science's 'truths' about the 'real' world are based upon the most flagrant distortion. In creating an understandable universe, we have committed ourselves to the most gross and obvious oversimplification. We have excluded the understanding mechanism, the self. (p. 208)

Schön (1988) suggests that this paradox can be resolved by acknowledging the importance of subjectivity in the acquisition of knowledge; for example, by reflecting on our actions, and by granting inductive research an equal status with deductive research. He calls for

> . . . an epistemology of practice which places technical problem solving ['science'] within a broader context of reflective enquiry . . . (p. 76)

Theory–practice gaps fail to narrow, therefore, because technical rationality denies subjectivity a place in the acquisition of knowledge. For knowledge to be acquired effectively, both forms of research—testing and refining—need to be in place. Adherence solely to technical rationality or, indeed, to its converse, reflective inquiry, serves only to deflect the acquisition of knowledge.

APPLICATION OF THE MODEL TO NURSING

Three messages become apparent when the universal model of knowledge acquisition is applied to nursing.

Firstly, a theoretical component is essential if a practice-based discipline, like nursing, is to develop. Nursing only really develops if improvements in patient care become manifest. As such, Nolan and Grant (1992) are justified in making the salient point that the ultimate benefit of theory in nursing is the improvement in patient care.

Secondly, research, being the link between theory and practice, is the key to the development of a discipline. Research should, furthermore, be carried out on both a formal and an informal level. Whilst informal research (putting ideas into practice and reflecting on them) is the key to individual development, the qualities of individual practitioners will also be reflected in the make-up of the discipline as a whole. And whilst formal (deductive and inductive) research is the key to the development of a discipline as a whole, the outcomes of such research (a change in formal theory and/or practice) will, in turn, influence the individual members of that discipline.

Thirdly, the research process has to be bidirectional. There is indeed a need for reflective skills and for formal, deductive research in nursing. Refining, however, has to coexist with testing; if nursing is to develop, it has to be both a science and an art.

From Novice to Expert: Nurse Education

In order to discuss the relevance of the universal model of knowledge acquisition to nurse education, a brief consideration of the work of Benner is required.

In her seminal book *From Novice to Expert*, Benner (1984) examines the acquisition of 'expertise' in nursing. She argues that there are five levels of nursing proficiency: novice, advanced beginner, competent, proficient and expert. Given that these levels are hierarchical, a continuum of nursing expertise is implied.

In her glossary, Benner defines expertise as a hybrid of theoretical and practical knowledge. Given that the universal model of knowledge acquisition is essentially a model of the acquisition of theoretical and practical knowledge (the two are, after all, intrinsically linked), the model can be incorporated into

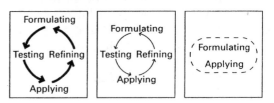

THE NURSING EXPERTISE CONTINUUM

Novice Advanced beginner Competent Proficient Expert

FIGURE 29.4 The universal model of knowledge acquisition and the transition from novice to expert in nursing.

Benner's theoretical framework with relative ease (see Figure 23.4).

In the novice, the gap between formulating and applying (theory and practice) is understandably and necessarily wide. The gap reduces as expertise develops, to the extent that the gap no longer exists when expertise is attained. At this point, the boundaries between theoretical and practical knowledge become blurred: action effectively becomes intuitive.

The thickness of the arrows in the novice learning cycle indicates that the cycle is highly active; novice nurses have a lot to learn. As the novice progresses towards expertise, the learning cycle becomes less active (hence the thinner arrows) until, when expertise is achieved, it grinds to a halt (hence the absence of arrows).

This is not to say that experts cannot learn. Expertise develops only in certain discrete areas of nursing; the cycle of learning must recommence whenever the expert is faced with new situations. It could, as such, be argued that expertise is never truly achieved.

The Role of Research

Though not making explicit reference to the role of research in the acquisition of expertise, Benner does nevertheless imply the necessity of research. She writes:

Expertise develops when the clinician *tests* and *refines* propositions, hypotheses, and principle-based expectations in actual practice situations. (p. 3; emphasis added)

Though informal research is the key to developing the personal expertise of a practitioner, note that formal research can play a similar role in developing the expertise of a discipline as a whole.

USES AND ABUSES OF NURSING MODELS

Novice nurses literally have no idea of how to practice. Whilst the novice nurse may well have informal theories (that is, ideas) of how to act in a particular situation, the nurse cannot feasibly test those theories (and indeed reflect on them) because of the risks to patients if the nurse blunders.

Novice nurses, therefore, require some guidelines for practice. This is where the value of formal models (such as hospital rules, standard procedures, the nursing process, nursing models and models borrowed from other disciplines) comes into play. Gordon (1984) writes:

For the individual lacking mastery, formal models can serve as *a substitute for personal knowledge and experience*. (p. 230)

She adds:

Let formal models . . . be regarded as training wheels, essential for the first safe rides, unnecessary and limiting once replaced by greater skill. (p. 243)

This latter quote from Gordon has a far-reaching implication for nursing, namely that expert nurses need only their own informal, internalized, personal theories to guide practice (subject, of course, to ethical and legal constraints). This remark may alarm those in the nursing profession who believe in the sanctity of one or other of the many nursing models, but it is concurrent with Benner's notion of an expert as an intuitive practitioner.

The Nursing Process

Whilst expert practitioners in other disciplines (in the medical profession, for example) enjoy the autonomy granted by informal theories, there is a need to ask why nurses continue to be passive and rule-bound. Take the nursing process, for example. As a simple set of rules for systemizing nursing care, it provides a particularly useful guide for the novice nurse. However, the nursing process soon becomes internalized in most nurses (most reasonably experienced nurses intuitively carry out the nursing process), so why does the nursing profession insist on documentation under discrete titles like 'assessment', 'plan' and 'evaluation' and why does every nursing action have to be rigidly recorded?

Why nurses are passive and rule-bound is a complex question, for which there are no immediate answers, though Meleis (1991) speculates that historical and cultural paternalism are largely to blame. Meleis suggests, furthermore, that the passivity of nurses has hindered theory development in nursing, because theory development (and, indeed, practice development) are, as we have seen, part of the same active process.

CONCLUSION

If the body of knowledge, both theoretical and practical, of a practice-based discipline is to develop, then research has to play a key role. Furthermore, if individual practitioners are to develop expertise, they too must undertake research, even if on an informal, personal level.

The successful education (and continuing education) of nurses is, as such, dependent on the opportunity both to test and refine, and to experiment and reflect. Nurse educators may well need to provide novice nurses with a range of formal models and theories to guide practice initially, but they equally need to encourage nurses to test and refine those models and theories so that they might develop their own personal models of practice.

As a final comment, the author urges nurses to heed the advice of Lindsay (1990), who notes that:

> Each nurse needs to recognize that the theorist, researcher . . . and practitioner exist to some extent in all of us. (p. 35)

REFERENCES

Appleyard B. (1992) *Understanding the Present: Science and the Soul of Modern Man.* Pan, London.

Benner P. (ed.) (1984) *From Novice To Expert: Excellence and Power in Clinical Nursing Practice.* Addison-Wesley, Menlo Park, California.

Chinn P.L. & Jacobs M.K. (1987) *Theory and Nursing: A Systematic Approach* 2nd edn. C.V. Mosby, St. Louis.

Cook S.H. (1991) Mind the theory/practice gap in nursing. *Journal of Advanced Nursing* 16, 1462–1469.

Dickoff J. & James P. (1968a) A theory of theories: A position paper. *Nursing Research* 17, 197–203.

Dickoff J. & James P. (1968b) Researching research's role in theory development. *Nursing Research* 17, 204–206.

Gordon D.R. (1984) Research application: Identifying the use and misuse of formal models in nursing practice. *In From Novice to Expert: Excellence and Power in Clinical Nursing Practice* (Benner P. ed.), Addison-Wesley, Menlo Park, California, pp. 225–243.

Howe D. (1987) *An Introduction to Social Work Theory: Making Sense in Practice.* Wildwood House, Aldershot.

Kolb D.A., Rubin I.M. & Osland J. (1991) *Organizational Behavior: An Experiential Approach,* 5th ed. Prentice-Hall International, London.

Lewin K. (1958) Group decision and social change. *In Readings in Social Psychology* 3rd ed. (Maccoby E., Newcomb T.M. & Sanford N. eds), Henry Holt, New York, pp. 197–211.

Lindsay B. (1990) The gap between theory and practice. *Nursing Standard* 5(4); 34–35.

McCaugherty D. (1991) The use of a teaching model to promote reflection and the experiential integration of theory and practice in first-year student nurses: an action research study. *Journal of Advanced Nursing* 16, 534–543.

McCaugherty D. (1992a) The concepts of theory and practice. *Senior Nurse* 12(2): 29–33.

McCaugherty D. (1992b) The gap between nursing theory and practice. *Senior Nurse* 12(6): 44–48.

Meleis A.I. (1991) *Theoretical Nursing: Development and Progress,* 2nd ed. Lippincott, Philadelphia.

Nolan M. & Grant G. (1992) Mid-range theory building and the nursing theory-practice gap: A respite care case study. *Journal of Advanced Nursing* 17, 217–223.

Sch{auo}n D.A. (1988) From technical rationality to reflection-in-action. *In Professional Judgement: A Reader in Clinical Decision Making* (Dowie J. & Elstein A. eds), Cambridge University Press, Cambridge, pp. 60–77.

Stevens B.J. (1984) *Nursing Theory: Analysis, Application and Evaluation* 2nd edn. Little Brown, Boston.

Vaughn B. (1989) Two roles—one job. *Nursing Times* 85(11), 52.

24

Evidence-Based Practice: Critique and Alternative View

GAIL J. MITCHELL, RN; PHD

Recent calls to promote evidence-based practice in nursing raise serious concerns. It has been suggested that evidence should be the primary source of knowledge for nurses. The general literature supporting evidence-based practice indicates that evidence will take nurses away from tradition, intuition, and anecdote to factual, scientific practice. The suggestion is that evidence can provide nurses with directives about how to think and act with patients, families, and groups. However, I contend that the notion of evidence-based practice is not only a barren possibility but also that evidence-based practice obstructs nursing process, human care, and professional accountability.

Prior to presenting arguments against evidence as the guide for nursing practice, let me state up front that evidence, defined here as conclusive statements based on findings from randomized controlled trials, has two areas of relevance. First, evidence may provide direction for development of procedures, techniques, and protocols that nurses and others

Author's Note: Please send comments regarding this column or ideas for future Practice Applications columns to Gail J. Mitchell, RN; PhD, Chief Nursing Officer, Sunnybrook Health Science Centre, 2075 Bayview Ave., Office-D404, Toronto, Ontario, M4N 3M5 Canada; phone: (416) 480-6100 extension 2778; fax: (416) 480-5207; e-mail:gail.mitchell@sunnybrook.on.ca.
Nursing Science Quarterly, Vol. 12 No. 1, January 1999. 30–35 Reprinted by permission of and copyright © (1999) Sage Publications, Inc.

are asked to perform. Healthcare professionals and nonprofessionals require such knowledge to guide their performance of tasks, and large systems require protocols to coordinate hospital-based care. Naturally, people who require knowledge and skill in these areas value the most effective techniques for preventing complications or performing tasks such as delivering medication, for instance. But evidence about procedure or service delivery is different from knowledge that informs the nurse-person process. Nurses may use techniques and technologies, but the knowledge base of nursing is not technical.

Second, evidence may provide one more resource for clients and nurses to consider the latest developments in the diagnosis and treatment of illness and disease. This information is available to any person who has access to libraries or to the Internet. Television broadcasts regularly offer the latest developments about links between heart disease and smoking or drug trials and side effects, for example. Health-care professionals no longer control access to health-related information, and the general public will have increasing opportunities to consider the latest developments and to weigh their relevance in light of personal life circumstances.

In a general way, evidence may well be useful to people for making decisions about how they wish to approach their care and what options are available. Pharmacological or medical information may be a launching pad for discussions with people as they figure things out—but evidence will not build a knowledge base for nursing practice. The usefulness of evidence has been wrongfully cast in the context of legitimizing nursing as a profession instead of describing evidence as one possible resource for supporting clients' processes of decision-making.

Rather than legitimizing nursing, evidence-based practice entraps nurses in the role of medical extender or medical technician. But even in these roles, evidence will not provide a foundation for practice. The idea that nurses in practice can access the relevant literature, make the required judgments about credibility of findings, interpret the significance of the findings in light of the guiding theory, and implement changes in practice is inconsistent with current realities. For one thing, nurses are expected to follow procedures written by multidisciplinary groups that are responsible for updating clinical practice in particular medical specialties. In the more technical practice contexts, nurses are rewarded for complying message is that nurses are the experts who intervene (try to manage and control) to create change toward provider-defined goals.

The term evidence-based practice, rather than being restricted to its technical and medical context where it may have some relevance, is being applied to the nurse-person process as the primary mode of knowing for relating with patients and families. Nursing practice happens in the nurse-person process, and to suggest that this process can be directed by evidence is not a supportable position; it is actually inconsistent with professional ethical codes, with current philosophical thought, and with what people say they want from nurses. Once again, it is obvious that nurses require current knowledge and skill for guiding activities involved in the delivery of

healthcare, especially in hospitals. However, the nurse-person process is not data based—it is human based and must be guided by values and theoretical principles.

SPECIFIC ISSUES OF CONCERN

Specific issues, then, about evidence and its use for guiding nursing practice are as follows. First, there is no body of evidence that can justify nursing as an applied science; current evidence is contradictory, tentative, unethical, and in some instances absurd. Second, proponents of evidence-based practice do not sufficiently acknowledge that all evidence is value laden and theoretically driven. Third, evidence-based practice is inconsistent with nursing's societal mandate to serve others rather than nurses themselves. Fourth, proponents of evidence-based practice oversimplify and misrepresent the complexities of human relating and the realities of multiple competing values, including those of the client, in the nurse-person process. Each of these points deserves thoughtful and scholarly attention by the nursing community. The following is an attempt to initiate discussion about these four issues.

WHERE IS THE EVIDENCE?

Proponents of evidence-based practice suggest that there is a body of knowledge that, if accessed by nurses, could provide clear direction about how to benefit others. In reality, the evidence does not exist. What does exist are multiple calls for more research and multiple reports that offer generalized statements that in many instances merely confirm the obvious. For instance, research findings about crisis intervention have led to recommendations that nurses should listen to people experiencing crisis. Or studies of quality of life have suggested that people with more resources have different health patterns than those who have no resources at all. This confirmation of the obvious is absurd. It should be a fundamental assumption that listening to all clients is essential in nursing practice—listening should be a core value of the nursing discipline. Directives for listening should be explicit in theories and standards that guide nursing practice. As a nurse leader, I prefer directing my time and energy to promoting practices that ensure that all persons experience being listened to by nurses so that the patient's reality provides the foundation for any care offered. If nurses began by listening, they would know how to be helpful and what actions and information might help people in light of their personal health experiences. The unsettling reality is that patients and families consistently report that many nurses, similar to other professionals, do not listen.

Most nursing philosophies specify nursing's commitment to treat all patients as unique human beings who define and live health differently; therefore, should not nurses already know and expect that all people have unique health patterns, not just those reported in research studies? Do we need evidence to know that some percentage of unemployed, single mothers with several children would benefit from more resources in the community? How will the evidence from these sorts of studies help nurses to practice with a particular mother and her children? Will nurses share with the mother that research evidence suggests that if she just had more money or more support she would be better off and her health patterns might improve? Nurses should be offended by the presentation of the obvious; it insults the knowing of both patients and nurses.

I am very concerned that nurses are being portrayed as empty (thoughtless) beings who must be directed when to speak, what to think, and when to listen—based on research evidence. The idea that nurses require evidence to know they should listen or be open to unique patterns of health, for instance, is a dangerous notion—if one can take it seriously at all. It is possible to imagine that evidence-based practice could propel nursing toward a purely technical vocation, which questions the need for professional nurses. Unregulated workers can certainly follow menu-driven directives based on evidence. I concur with White (1997), who suggests that evidence-based practice may represent one more example of how nurses embrace what they think will liberate them when, in reality, the initiative ensures their subservience to other interests and other disciplines.

Professional nursing practice requires the risk to embrace the inherent ambiguity of the moment and to be with others with explicit commitment, responsiveness, openness, compassion, and the intent to serve. Professional practice demands an engagement with the unknown in light of a broad knowledge base and understanding of lived experience and not the enforcement of predefined directives based on generalized and often meaningless statements of evidence. Beneficial outcomes for patients surface in genuine engagements with nurses—as persons (clients) themselves clarify meanings, ask questions, explore concerns, discover strengths, and make plans to change health and quality of life. Patients and families indicate that they want to be treated as human beings, and the essence of this kind of human relationship is unscripted engagement in which nurses live the commitment to be with clients and to listen, respect, provide, and be involved as directed by clients. Knowledge about how to be with others in ways that respect the client's power and direction can only be found in nursing theories, because theories direct the "how" of nursing in light of its human context. Unfortunately, evidence-based practice obscures the critical links among practice, theory, and the client's experience of nursing.

OBSCURING THE THEORY-PRACTICE LINK

Contemporary scholars endorse the belief that all thinking is theoretical and value laden. Yet, many supporters of evidence-based practice fail to acknowledge that nursing practice requires thought and is therefore also guided by theory. All the thinking and acting that happens in nursing moments are already guided by theory. Moments with nurses help or hinder persons as they struggle and plan to change patterns of health. In evolving as a discipline, nursing has relied on theory from other disciplines to guide practice, but it is becoming increasingly obvious that nurses require nursing theories to fulfill their societal mandate to provide a service that enhances health and quality of life. Introducing evidence as the guide for practice obscures the linkages that already exist between practice and theory. This is a critical omission in the literature promoting evidence-based practice because the reality is that, despite evidence, some theories are not appropriate for professional nursing because of what people experience when the theory is used and because the goals of some theories are not consistent with nursing's ethic.

For instance, there may be research evidence to support the use of behavior modification to make patients comply with medical directives, but this evidence does not justify the nurse's choice to reward and punish patients in a paternalistic model of care. In this example, there are clear directives from the theory that shape the nurse-person process and the patient's experience of nursing. Behavior modification, a theory borrowed from psychology, does not uphold nurses' commitment

to a dynamic (open and changing), nonjudgmental process that respects human freedom. I have heard nurses describe both the burden of policing patients and the harm to relationships that can accompany behavior modification. Any evidence that is unexamined in light of the guiding theory and uninformed about the client's experience is not consistent with nursing. One need only listen to patients describe what it is like to be on the receiving end of rewards and punishments to know that behavior modification is inconsistent with the mandate of nursing. In my opinion, it is essential to question who is being served when punitive interventions are used by professionals to bring about desired change.

SELF-SERVING OR OTHER SERVING

I have heard claims that disciplines are merely self-serving. Much of this antidisciplinary sentiment emerged a decade ago in North America when it was discovered that disciplines created large departments and complex care processes that had questionable benefit to the persons being served. Many health disciplines wanted to ensure a holistic approach to care and so their members developed extensive multisystem assessments for problem identification. Meanwhile, patients were being subjected to multiple, redundant questions and interventions that may or may not have been relevant to their immediate concerns and interests. The question of whether disciplines are self-serving is legitimate, and nurses especially must question whose interests they serve in day-to-day practice.

For instance, some nurses perform assessments and use tools that may harm patients or that diminish their quality of living. Nurses may lose sight of the client's experience and focus more on collecting evidence than on satisfying or comforting patients. There are multiple examples of this self-serving phenomenon, but two that are particularly meaningful are linked with nurses doing routine Mini Mental State Examinations (MMSE) and pain scale ratings. The MMSE is a tool for detecting problems with orientation and memory. In some institutions, nurses routinely complete the MMSE daily or weekly to collect evidence of change. Fluctuations in scores, however, are not usually explainable even from a medical perspective, and there is no clear direction about what nurses should do in the nurse-person process in light of any particular score. Furthermore, many patients find the MMSE unsettling at best, and for some, it leads to crying and upset as they try to find the right answer to please the healthcare professional. Nurses must begin to question this routine collection of data that does not inform their practice and that often leads to embarrassment for clients.

Similarly, frustrations have been reported by patients who are asked to rate their pain on a scale of 1 to 10. I recently heard a very compelling story from a patient who was being pressured to rate his pain on a scale of 1 to 10 before staff would respond to his requests for medication. He expressed frustration and anger about being treated as if he were wrong and having to say the right things to get pain medication. The message being given to patients who prefer not to rate their pain on a scale of 1 to 10 is that their language does not count as credible evidence. If a patient prefers to use the word terrible to describe pain, and if the person can only say that the pain is "somewhat" or "mostly better," it should be enough for nurses. From my view, we are already bordering on negligence by forcing patients to comply with our tools so that we can collect numerical evidence instead of attending to patients' concerns and issues with compassion and respect for their choice of words and descriptions. The above examples about patient

dissatisfaction lead one to the following question: Who are nurses serving in their day-to-day practice?

I support the belief that nursing practice should integrate particular values and principles to structure the nurse-person process. The only evidence that can help nurses understand the benefit of nursing will come from clients' personal descriptions of how health and quality of life change with nursing care. The notion of evidence-based practice should be clearly limited to the technical/procedural realm of clinical care so that nurses are not expected to relinquish their responsibility to live certain values and theoretical principles with all human beings. Nurses must begin to ask clients what difference nurses' attitudes, actions, and expressions make to their experiences of health and quality of life.

There are extensive reports from patients that indicate that they want to be accepted, listened to, involved, respected, and treated as unique human beings (see e.g., Gerteis, Edgman-Levitan, Daley, & Delbancho, 1993; Young-Mason, 1997). One man who spent a great deal of time with healthcare professionals developed his own principles that helped him deal with a medical belief system that consistently ensured staff had power and control (Macurdy, 1997). Macurdy's four principles, which are echoed in many stories from patients, are as follows:

1.   As the person with the greatest stake in my healthcare, I make the decisions, and no health professional can overrule my preferences.

2.   I am the only legitimate decision-maker, and no one else is permitted to speak for me.

3.   I must have complete information.

4.   Healthcare is a means to a full and meaningful life; it is not an end in itself. I will not allow the medical agenda to rule my life. I choose to lead my life and accept the risks and consequences of a meaningful existence.

The knowledge base for ensuring that all patients have experiences that support their being listened to, involved, respected, and treated like human beings flows from guiding nursing theories rather than evidence. Theories guide how nurses think and act with individual persons and families as clients provide direction by identifying concerns, what is helpful, what information might be useful, what things mean, what is possible, and what choices are most important. The nurse-person process is very complex, and proponents of evidence-based practice have, in my view, grossly oversimplified and misrepresented the process of nursing.

THE MISREPRESENTATION OF EVIDENCE

To say nursing is evidence based misrepresents what is in reality a complex, intimate, and multidimensional process of interhuman relating. Despite claims to the contrary (DiCenso et al., 1998), evidence-based practice does indeed promote a routinized process of care that is dehumanizing. Nurses want and need to know how to practice with people in open, nonjudgmental, participative relationships that enhance quality from the client's perspective. If nursing is to remain a human science concerned about quality of life and lived experience, then it is essential that nurses identify the specific values and theories that will guide the nurse-person process toward this goal. Proponents of evidence have not explicitly addressed the influence of values, assumptions, interpretations, intentions, and desired outcomes in practice.

It is also essential that nurse leaders acknowledge that there are higher values in the discipline of nursing (such as respect for self-determination, mutual process, and individual uniqueness). Any evidence or theory selected by nurses should be coherent with such values. The very term evidence flows from certain assumptions that are not consistent with nursing practices that honor situated freedom, human uniqueness, and client as leader. Nursing's responsibility should be first and foremost to develop and sustain knowledge that honors the client's meanings, realities, possibilities, wishes, and choices. The nurse-person process must be informed by values and theories that provide nurses with the knowledge to participate with human beings in changing health and quality of life as directed by people themselves.

Also underestimated by proponents of evidence-based practice is that hospitals, clinics, and other service-oriented centers already embrace some philosophy for practice that influences decisions made by frontline providers. Nurse leaders are responsible for creating settings that nurture specific values and beliefs about patient care. As a chief nursing officer, I want nurses to practice patient-focused standards that are consistent with the human becoming school of thought (Parse, 1998). The notion that individual nurses could or should practice in ways supported by any evidence is inconsistent with the expectation that nurses should represent specific values and principles when it comes to human care.

Research involving human beings is infinitely complex, open to interpretation, and value laden. If research expands and informs the guiding theory, then findings must be considered in light of the practice prescribed by the theory. The most challenging aspect of nursing is the reasoning and thinking required to be with others in open, participatory, nonjudgmental relationships in which multiple forces and struggles come into play. Therefore, nurses should be given opportunities to look at their practices in light of the values and beliefs of nursing philosophy and theory. Changes in practice happen through personal insights about the linkages among beliefs, values, and actions—not through presentation of data.

The responsibility of all nurses should be to continue to integrate and develop theories that assist practitioners to be helpful and to have meaningful relationships with clients. Evidence in the absence of values and theories about human care and participative relationships is meaningless unless nursing is to be reduced to a purely technical, menu-driven enterprise. It is unfortunate that some nurses have failed to be guided by the concerns and wishes of those served by nursing—patients and families—because there are opportunities for professionals to create practices that enhance quality of life and consumer satisfaction. Some people are coming to hospitals with extensive knowledge and with a greater understanding of their health situations than many professionals. People want dialogue that is relevant to their personal lives. Evidence-based practice does not support the shift to patient-focused care, and it is inconsistent with the values and interests of consumers. This gap between what evidence-based practice promotes and what consumers want raises this question: To what end? This question may indeed hold the essential seed of controversy that is fueled by the evidence-based initiative.

Proponents of evidence-based nursing practice contend that the initiative is consistent with practices that are patient focused and with qualitative research methods. I respectfully disagree. The ultimate goal of evidence-based practice is control. No matter what patient-friendly words are picked up along the way and no matter what research methods are employed, the values and assumptions embedded in evidence-based practice lead to a particular place—prescriptive interventions aimed at managing patients. Nurses and other professionals have been trying to manage people for many decades, and people have indicated that the management approach is not wanted. It is folly to think that people will embrace professionals who judge them and who do not recognize their knowledge and their investment in the healthcare process.

It is my hope that nurses will seriously consider the complex issues surrounding the evidence-based initiative. Debate will continue to shed light on how nursing is evolving as a human science. There are alternative views and different roads that lie in nursing's path. The call issued here is for nurses to choose a path that ensures a value-specific, theory-guided knowledge base that clearly places the client as the expert about health and change—a path that places nurses as accountable to clients for the quality of nursing care.

REFERENCES

DiCenso, A., Cullum, N., & Ciliska, D. (1998). Implementing evidence-based nursing: Some misconceptions. *Evidence-Based Nursing, 1*(2), 38–40.

Gerteis, M., Edgman-Levitan, S., Daley, J., & Delbancho, T. L. (Eds.). (1993). *Through the patient's eyes.* San Francisco: Jossey-Bass.

Macurdy, A. H. (1997). Mastery of life. In J. Young-Mason (Ed.), *The patient's Voice: Experiences of illness* (pp. 9–15). Philadelphia: F. A. Davis.

Parse, R. R. (1998). *The human becoming school of thought.* Thousand Oaks, CA: Sage.

White, S. J. (1997). Evidence-based practice and nursing: The new panacea? *British Journal of Nursing, 6*(3), 175–178.

25

Critical Thinking and Theory-based Practice

ELLEN CLARK BIRX, PhD, RN

Critical thinking is an essential and ongoing process in using theory to guide nursing practice. Theory involves seeing patterns that bring order to chaos. Chinn and Kramer define theory as "a systematic abstraction of reality that serves some purpose."[1(p20)] This definition emphasizes the idea that theory is an abstraction and not reality itself. From a different perspective or for a different purpose an alternate theory might be developed and found to be useful. The purpose of nursing theory is the description, explanation, and prediction of phenomena within the domain of nursing with the ultimate aim of guiding nursing practice.

A key question in using theory to guide nursing practice is, "What theories are useful in particular nursing situations?" Critical thinking on the part of each nurse is required to select or develop theories to guide practice in diverse clinical settings. While theories can be useful in organizing and guiding our practice, they can also be blinders that limit us from seeing things as they are. Critical thinking helps us gain awareness of how we are viewing and creating our world of practice.

There is a large body of literature in the fields of psychology, education, and nursing about critical thinking, what it is, how it is learned, and how it is applied in practice. The

National League for Nursing (NLN)[2] mandates that nursing programs emphasize the development of critical thinking and independent decision making. However, there is a lack of clarity about just what critical thinking entails. In a national survey of 470 deans or directors of NLN-accredited nursing programs, 51% of whom responded, Jones and Brown[3] found that most of the respondents conceptualized critical thinking as an objective, rational, linear problem-solving process similar to the nursing process. They concluded that most of the sample defined critical thinking in a rather narrow way, excluding aspects of critical thinking like imaginative speculation.

Experts have defined critical thinking in various ways. Ennis defines critical thinking as "reasonable reflective thinking that is focused on deciding what to believe or do."[4(p10)] While this definition includes reasoning and decision-making processes, it is not limited to these. It also incorporates reflective thought and creative thinking processes.

Smith[5] views critical thinking within the context of thinking in general. Smith describes thinking as "a single, continual, all-embracing operation of the mind, powered by an imagination that never rests, not a collection of disparate skills . . ."[5(p124)] Smith's holistic view of critical thinking as inseparable and overlapping with other natural thinking processes resonates with nursing's holistic world view. It is also consistent with the current trend in nurs-

Source: Birx, E. C. (1993). Critical thinking and theory-based practice. *Holistic Nurse Pract.* 7(3):21– 27. Reprinted with permission by from and copyright© 1993 Aspen Publishers, Inc.

ing toward integrating multiple types of thinking or patterns of knowledge—empirical, ethical, aesthetic, and personal—to guide clinical decision making.[6]

Smith's[5] emphasis on the role of imagination in our thinking processes is also especially pertinent. Critical thinking not only involves rational, linear thinking processes, but also intuitive, imaginative thinking processes. The ability to imagine an alternative leads us to question the current system and move toward more humanistic health care environments and relationships.

Viewing or defining critical thinking in a broad way, rather than limiting it to linear problem-solving processes encompasses the many aspects of critical thinking that are needed to select or develop theories to guide nursing practice. Increasing our awareness of various critical thinking processes facilitates our ability to use these processes in the complex world of practice.

ATTITUDE OF INQUIRY AND OPENNESS

Smith[5] suggests that critical thinking is facilitated by an attitude of doubt. An attitude of doubt involves questioning what is happening within and around us and a comfort with uncertainty or not knowing. According to Smith, "Thought flourishes as questions are asked, not as answers am found."[5(p129)] An open and inquiring mind is needed to question the way things are in our clinical practice and to be open to new possibilities.

Through research and theory development, the profession is engaged in developing knowledge on which to base our clinical practice. The knowledge on which we base our practice is not just an accumulation of facts and theories, but also a dynamic, ongoing process of awareness, inquiry, investigation,

integration, imagination, and openness to realities and possibilities. Our knowledge base is not static; it is constantly evolving.

KNOWLEDGE OF THE DISCIPLINE OF NURSING

Critical thinking involves both process and content. We must have something to think about. In a practice discipline like nursing, we have a body of knowledge gleaned from our literature and the direct experience of clinical realities from our everyday practice to think critically about. While the undergraduate student and beginning nurse are able to think critically at a beginning level with freshness of vision, the graduate student and experienced nurses are able to think critically at an advanced level due to an expanded familiarity with nursing literature and a rich background of clinical experience.

Most of the nurses in the graduate course in nursing theory that the author teaches are currently practicing nurses from diverse clinical settings. Two major objectives of the course are to familiarize the students with a broad range of nursing theories in as interesting a manner as possible and to encourage critical thinking about the relevance of these theories to their own clinical practice. Students often comment that they were not looking forward to taking a course in nursing theory and expected it to be dry and tedious. However, by the end of the semester, they express much enthusiasm for the course and find it to be a real eye-opener. They state that they have become more aware of the theories that, whether they realized it or not, have been guiding their clinical practice; they are able to critique and select useful theories to improve their practice; and they are inspired to imagine what new theories are needed to guide practice in their specialty area.

METACOGNITION AND METATHEORY

Another type of critical thinking process used in selecting or developing theories to guide clinical practice includes metacognition and metatheory. These terms refer to the processes of thinking about thinking and thinking about theory, respectively. Metacognition involves the awareness of the thought processes we are using and the ability to select appropriate thinking strategies to accomplish our task.[7] Metatheory focuses on philosophical and methodological issues related to nursing theory, such as questioning the type of theory needed in nursing, critiquing nursing theories, and analyzing nursing theories to identify recurring themes and trends.[8] Both of these critical thinking processes require that we step back from our clinical practice and reflect about the theories we need to guide our practice and the thought processes we need to use to select or develop these theories.

Metatheory involves asking questions such as

- "What are the values of the nursing profession?"
- "What are the assumptions we are making when we approach nursing situations in a particular way?"
- "What are characteristics of nursing's world view?"

The ability to identify underlying values, assumptions, and perspectives is an essential critical thinking skill.

INTEGRATING MULTIPLE LEVELS OF THEORY

Selection of theory to guide nursing practice involves multiple levels of theory, including metatheory, grand theory, and midrange theory. Grand theory "deals with broad goals and concepts representing the total range of phenomena of concern within a discipline."[1(p199)] Midrange theory is more specific and limited in scope, dealing with a single phenomenon or a limited number of phenomena within the domain of nursing.

The use of theory to guide clinical practice involves selecting, adapting, or developing a grand-level nursing theory or conceptual framework. This conceptual framework then guides the selection, adaptation, or development of midrange theories that are specific enough to guide nursing actions. The conceptual framework is like the two-by-fours that frame in a house, outlining where walls, windows, and doors will go. The midrange theories complete the house with various wall finishings and varieties of windows and doors. We first select the overall house plan, and then we select fixtures, colors, flooring, and so forth. Even when the house is finished, we are open to the possibility of remodeling to update or improve the house in various ways.

An example of this process is the use of Levine's[9] grand nursing theory to guide clinical practice in a neonatal intensive care unit. Levine's Conservation Principles provide a useful conceptual framework for organizing nursing care in this complex setting. The four conservation principles, (1) conservation of energy, (2) conservation of structural integrity, (3) conservation of personal integrity, and (4) conservation of social integrity, guide the nurse in providing holistic and comprehensive care for the neonate and family.

In addition to selecting this broad nursing conceptual framework, additional midrange theories must be selected to provide the specific knowledge to guide nursing action. Levine's conservation of energy principle guides the nurse in selecting or developing physiological theories and nursing theories related to temperature regulation, oxygenation, nutrition, fluids and electrolytes, and rest and activity aimed at conserving the energy of the neonate for growth and healing. The principle of conservation of structural integrity guides the nurse in selecting or developing theories related to immune response, positioning, range of motion, wound healing, and skin care. The principle of conservation of personal integrity guides the nurse in the selection of nursing theories and the adaptation of theories from related disciplines dealing with early psychological development. The principle of conservation of social integrity guides the nurse in the selection or development of nursing theories and the adaptation of theories from related disciplines, such as sociology and anthropology, to guide nursing care for neonates within the context of their family, community, and culture. Examples of midrange theories that are useful in neonatal intensive care that can be integrated within Levine's broad nursing conceptual framework are the synactive theory of infant development,[10] crisis intervention theory,[11] attachment theory,[12] and maternal role attainment theory.[13] A wide range of theories from nursing and related disciplines are organized within Levine's conceptual framework to provide theory-based care that is congruent with nursing's holistic, caring world view.

Cromwell proposes a definition of critical thinking as "the ability to apply disciplinary frameworks in personal, academic, and professional settings and to monitor and evaluate that activity."[14(p40)] As the nurse engages in metatheoretical inquiry, and in the evaluation of nursing conceptual frameworks and midrange theories for use in clinical practice, he or she is engaged in critical thinking. Critical thinking is an ongoing process in clinical practice as the nurse monitors and evaluates the usefulness of the theories he or she has applied. Critical thinking is a creative process as nurses identify areas within their clinical practice where new theories need to be developed.

In that critical thinking is both a rational and a creative process; the selection and application of theory to guide clinical practice is not performed in a mechanical way. It is a reflective, creative process. Johnston and Baumann[15] discuss a process for selecting and tailoring nursing models to meet the needs of particular clinical settings. Among the steps in the process they outline are reflection on the nurse's own values and ideas about person, environment, health, and nursing; categorizing the attributes of the client population served; and identifying effective intervention used on the unit. This is followed by the selection or development of a nursing conceptual framework that fits well with these considerations and that allows for collaboration with other disciplines practicing on the unit. Johnston and Baumann suggest selecting conceptual frameworks to guide practice at the unit level rather than at the level of an agency or institution as a whole. This allows the selection and development of theory that is most useful in guiding nursing practice in particular clinical settings.

PERSPECTIVE TAKING

A critical thinking process that is especially pertinent to the development of theory-based practice is the ability to view a situation from multiple perspectives. The discipline of nursing has a rich tradition of valuing not only the nurse's perception of a situation, but also the client's perception of the situation; of valuing subjective realities; and of valuing multicultural perspectives.[16-18] In addition, nursing practice requires consideration of multiple historical, philosophical, economic, and political viewpoints. Engaging in dialogue with nursing colleagues, colleagues from other disciplines, health care consumers, and families enhances perspective-taking ability.[19] Through critical dialogue, nurses can move toward a synthesis of multiple perspectives.[20]

Gebser[21] describes and predicts the evolution of human consciousness beyond the synthesis of multiple perspectives to an integral or aperspectival consciousness. According to Gebser, humankind has evolved through archaic, magical, mythical, and mental stages and is now on the verge of evolving to a stage of integral or aperspectival consciousness. He describes the awareness of a person in aperspectival consciousness in the following way: "For him them is no longer heaven or hell, this world or the other, ego or world, immanence or transcendence; rather beyond the magic unity, the mythical complementarity, the mental division and synthesis is the perceptible whole."[21(p543)] Aperspectival consciousness is characterized by integration rather than synthesis.

Lassalle emphasizes that in integral or aperspectival consciousness, "thinking is not determined solely by reason; in it intelligence, feeling, will, spirit, and the body play equally important roles."[22(p63)] In this new thinking, previous stages are not eliminated, rather they are integrated and brought into balance in an awareness of the whole. Ultimately, this level of holistic thinking is desirable to guide nursing practice.

EMPOWERMENT

A further consideration regarding critical thinking and theory-based nursing practice is empowerment. Smith[5] encourages examination of the extent to which individuals are allowed to be critical thinking in hierarchical, bureaucratic systems. He contends that a necessary ingredient in critical thinking is that people be given the authority to be independent thinkers. This he refers to as empowerment.

Empowerment that fosters critical thinking in nursing practice involves communicating to nurses that they have the authority, ability, and responsibility to think critically about their practice. The authority to think critically is conveyed by eliciting, listening to, and valuing the views and experiences of nurses engaged in clinical practice. Authority, is conveyed through an atmosphere of collaboration and equality with other disciplines. The ability to think critically is cultivated through role-modeling. Nurses grow in their ability to think critically when they work with and observe other nurses engaged in inquiry, critical reflection, exploration of creative alternatives, and articulation of what they are seeing.

Theory-based practice is not just a matter of latching onto the latest theory. It goes far deeper than this. We must critically reflect on the theories, whether implicit or explicit, we are using to guide our practice. As nurses, we have not only the authority and ability, but also the responsibility to question and work toward better health care systems.

While the present emphasis on critical thinking as the use of problem-solving skills in nursing practice is necessary, it is not sufficient or representative of the broad range of critical thinking processes required for theory-based clinical practice. An attitude of openness and inquiry, knowledge and clinical experience in nursing, metacognition and metatheoretical reflection, the integration of multiple levels of theory, perspective taking, and empowerment are all important critical thinking processes.

In addition to taking a holistic approach to critical thinking, it is important to view critical thinking as an ongoing process in using theory to guide clinical practice. As the nurse engages in clinical practice, there is the need to continually question, "What is going on here?" "Are the theories I am using to guide my practice really helpful or are they limiting my authenticity, creativity, and compassion in helping this person?" "What new theories need to be developed in this practice setting?" Through critical thinking, we continually become more open, more inquiring, more knowledgeable, more experienced, more reflective, more integrated, more sensitive to multiple perspectives, and more empowered to refine and develop theory to improve clinical practice. Critical thinking creates theory-based practice that is nursing at its best.

REFERENCES

1. Chinn PL, Kramer MK. *Theory and Nursing: A Systematic Approach*, 3rd ed. St. Louis, Mo: Mosby; 1991.
2. National League for Nursing. *NLN Self-Study Manual*. New York, NY: NLN; 1989.
3. Jones SA, Brown LN. Critical thinking: Impact on nursing education. *Journal of Advanced Nursing.* 1991;16:529–533.
4. Ennis RH. A taxonomy of critical thinking dispositions and abilities. In: Baron JB, Sternberg RJ, eds. *Teaching Thinking Skills: Theory and Practice. New York, NY*: W.H. Freemonk; 1987.
5. Smith F. *To Think.* New York, NY: Teachers College Press; 1990.
6. Carper BA. Fundamental patterns of knowing in nursing. *Advances in Nursing Science.* 1978;1(1):13–23.
7. Beyer BK. *Practical Strategies for the Teaching of Thinking.* Boston, Mass: Allyn & Bacon; 1987.
8. Walker LO, Avant KC. *Strategies for Theory Construction in Nursing.* Norwalk, Conn: Appleton-Century-Crofts; 1983.
9. Levine ME. The conversation principles: Twenty-years later. In: Riehl-Sisca J, ed. *Conceptual Models for Nursing Practice.* 3rd ed. Norwalk, Conn: Appleton & Lange; 1989.
10. Als H. Neurobehavioral development of the premature infant. In: Avery ME, First LR, eds. *Pediatric Medicine.* Baltimore, Md: Williams & Wilkins; 1989.
11. Aguilera DC, Messick JM. *Crisis Intervention: Theory and Methodology.* 5th ed. St. Louis, Mo: Mosby; 1986.
12. Klaus MH, Kennel JH. *Parent-Infant Bonding.* 2nd ed. St. Louis, Mo: Mosby; 1982.
13. Mercer RT. *First-Time Motherhood: Experiences from Teens to Forties.* New York, NY: Springer; 1986.
14. Cromwell LS. Assessing critical thinking. In: Barnes CA, ed. *Critical Thinking: Educational Imperative.* San Francisco, Calif: Jossey-Bass; 1992.
15. Johnston N, Baumann A. Selecting a nursing model for psychiatric nursing. *Journal of Psychosocial Nursing.* 1992;30(4):7–12.
16. Orlando I. *The Dynamic Nurse-Patient Relationship.* New York, NY: Putnam; 1961.
17. Watson J. Nursing: *Human Science and Human Care: A Theory of Nursing.* New York, NY: National League for Nursing; 1988.
18. Leininger M. *Transcultural Nursing: Concepts, Theories, and Practices.* New York, NY: Wiley; 1978.
19. Chaffee J. Teaching critical thinking across the curriculum. In: Barnes CA, ed. *Critical Thinking: Educational Imperative.* San Francisco, Calif: Jossey-Bass; 1992.
20. Lorensen M. Response to "Critical theory: A foundation for the development of nursing theories." *Scholarly Inquiry for Nursing Practice,* 1988;2(3):233–236.
21. Gebser J. *The Ever-Present Origin.* Athens, Oh: Ohio University Press; 1985.
22. Lassalle HE. *Living in the New Consciousness.* Boston, Mass: Shambhala; 1988.

26

Theory-based Advanced Nursing Practice

JANET W. KENNEY, RN, PhD

All professional disciplines are based on their unique knowledge, which is expressed in models and theories that are applied in practice. The focus of nursing knowledge is on humans' health experiences within the context of their environment and the nurse-client relationship. Theory-based nursing practice is the application of various models, theories, and principles from nursing science and the biological, behavioral, medical, and socio-cultural disciplines to clinical nursing practice. Conceptual models and theories provide a broad knowledge base to assist nurses in understanding and interpreting the client's complex health situation and in planning nursing actions to achieved desired client outcomes. "Explicit use of conceptual models of nursing and nursing theories to guide nursing practice is the hallmark of professional nursing"; it distinguishes nursing as an autonomous health profession (Fawcett, 1997:212).

This chapter describes the value and relevance of theory-based nursing for advanced practice nurses and discusses some underlying concerns about applying theories in nursing practice. The structure of nursing knowledge and the transformative process for theory-based practice are explained, along with the importance of critical thinking. An overview of various models and theories of nursing, family, and other disciplines is provided. Lastly, the process for selecting and applying

appropriate models and theories in nursing practice is thoroughly described.

RELEVANCE OF THEORY-BASED PRACTICE IN NURSING

The value of theory-based nursing practice is well documented in numerous books and journal articles. Although many articles illustrate the application of a nursing model or theory to clients with a specific health problem, Alligood (1997b) recently reviewed the nursing literature and found that about 68% of the articles reflect a medical approach to nursing. She also noted that most nurses described their practice in terms of a specialty area, types of care or health problems, and nursing interventions.

All nurses use knowledge they acquired during their formal education and clinical experience to guide their practice. Some nurse practitioners consistently use models and theories to guide their practice, but most nurses are unaware of existing theories and models or do not know how to apply them. Many nurses are not aware of what knowledge they use or where they learned it, thus, their implicit knowledge tends to be fragmented, diffused, incomplete, and greatly influenced by the medical model (Fawcett, 1997). Although graduate nurse practitioner students learn about nursing models and theories, their education often emphasizes application of medical knowledge as the base for their nursing practice. Thus use of medical knowledge and policies of health care delivery systems have replaced nursing knowledge and influenced some nurses to become "junior doctors," instead of "senior nurses" (Meleis, 1993).

Theories and models from nursing and behavioral disciplines are used by advanced practice nurses to provide effective, high quality nursing care. Many nurses believe that use of nursing theories would improve the quality of nursing care, but that they do not have sufficient information about them or the opportunity to use them (McKenna, 1997b). According to Meleis (1997), theories improve quality of care by clearly defining the boundaries and goals of nursing assessment, diagnosis, and interventions, and by providing continuity and congruency of care. Theory also contributes to more efficient and effective nursing practice, and enhances nurses' professional autonomy and accountability. Aggleton and Chalmers (1986) claim that providing nursing care without a theory base is like "practicing in the dark." Kenney (1996) reported that professional nurses can effectively use theories and models from nursing and behavioral disciplines to:

- collect, organize, and classify client data
- understand, analyze, and interpret client's health situations
- guide formulation of nursing diagnoses
- plan, implement, and evaluate nursing care
- explain nursing actions and interactions with clients
- describe, explain, and sometimes predict clients' responses
- demonstrate responsibility and accountability for nursing actions

- achieve desired outcomes for clients (p. 9)

As we enter the next millennium, the health care revolution requires that nurses demonstrate efficient, cost-effective, high quality care within organized delivery systems. "Nursing theory-based practice offers an alternative to the dehumanizing, fragmented, and paternalistic approaches that plague current delivery systems" (Smith, 1994:7). With changes in the current third-party reimbursement systems, nurses will be paid for effective theory-based practice that enhances clients' health and their quality of life. To accomplish this, nurse practitioners must use critical thinking skills combined with theory-based knowledge and clinical expertise to achieve desired client outcomes.

Issues related to theory-based nursing practice

In recent years, the enthusiasm for using nursing models and theories in practice has waned due to criticisms about the "theory-practice gap" and the lack of relevance to clinical practice. Also there are philosophical concerns about whether only nursing models should guide practice and whether models and theories of nursing and other disciplines may be integrated in practice. This section discusses some of these issues.

The "theory-practice gap" refers to the lack of use or inability of nurses to utilize nursing and other theories in clinical practice. McKenna (1997b) claims that theories are not being used in a systematic way to guide nursing practice, although using theories may improve the quality of care. He believes nurses do not use nursing theories because they do not know about them, understand them, believe in them, know how to apply them, or are not allowed to use them. Professional nursing practice more often reflects the medical or organizational model of care than application of relevant nursing models or theories.

According to Rogers (1989:114), "Nursing knowledge . . . is often seen as being unscientific, intuitive, and highly subjective." Some nurses believe that conceptual models and theories are too abstract to apply in nursing practice: they do not provide sufficient information to guide nursing judgments, are subject to different interpretations, are incomplete, and lack adequate testing and refinement (Field, 1987; Firlet, 1985). Others argue that some nursing theories were never meant to be directly applied in nursing practice but were intentionally abstract to stimulate thinking, provide new insights, and develop creative ways of viewing nursing (McKenna, 1997b).

As a practice discipline, nursing models and theories should be useful in practice, or their value is questionable. When models and theories are logical and consistent with other validated theories, they may provide the rationale and consequences of nursing actions, and lead to predictable client outcomes. There are numerous articles and chapters describing application of various models to clinical nursing practice. However, rigorous research studies on how nursing models and theories contribute to desirable nursing actions and client outcomes are lacking.

Another issue is whether only nursing models and theories are appropriate for the discipline, since nursing is an applied science. Most professional nurses are familiar with theories from other disciplines, such as systems theory, family theories, developmental theories, and others; in clinical practice, nurses often combine their nursing and medical knowledge with theories from other disciplines. Some nurse scholars argue that nursing practice must be based on nursing models and theories, since they are consis-

tent with nursing's view of human science and provide the structure for explaining nursings' unique contribution to health care (Cody, 1996; Mitchell, 1992). Since nursing models or theories represent the theorist's unique beliefs about persons, health, and nursing and guide how nurses interact with clients, McKenna (1997b) believes that an eclectic approach, combining theories from nursing and other disciplines, may compromise nursing theories if the concepts are removed from their original context and interwoven with other theories.

In contrast, Meleis (1997) argues that because nurses study other disciplines, nursing theory tends to reflect a broad range of perspectives and premises. Many nursing theorists have incorporated or "borrowed" theories from other disciplines, then transmuted them to fit within the context of nursing, so that their nursing theories comprise shared knowledge used in a distinctive way (Timpson, 1996).

A related issue is whether professional nurses should consistently use only one nursing model, or use various models and theories from nursing and other disciplines in their practice. Most professions, like nursing, have multiple theories that represent divergent and unique perspectives about the phenomena of concern to their practice. Within nursing, conceptual models and theories range from broad conceptual models, or grand theories, to specific practice theories. There are advantages and disadvantages to using one or more theories in clinical practice. Depending on the nurse's knowledge and clinical practice area, some nursing models and theories may be more appropriate than others. However, some would argue that use of only one nursing theory limits the nurse's assessment to only those things addressed by the theory, and the nurse may be forced to "fit" the client situation to the theory.

Others believe that nurses should consider a variety of nursing theories and select the model or theory that best "fits" the client's health problems. The majority of early nursing theories were based on traditional scientific methods and reflect a reductionistic perspective of humans as passive beings, consisting of elementary parts that respond to external stimuli in a linear, causal, and predictive way (Benner & Wrubel, 1989). Nursing models based on this perspective ultimately dehumanize individuals into disparate parts and systems and lead to fragmented, non-holistic nursing care (Aggleton & Chalmers, 1986). More contemporary nursing models view humans as continuously changing during reciprocal interactions with their environment, thus individual's reactions to nursing care are not predictable, nor can they be controlled. However, these newer nursing models are more abstract than earlier models and are less likely to offer specific guidelines for nursing actions. Professional nurses are expected to develop unique, creative nursing actions suitable for each client's health problem and lifestyle. And, theories from other disciplines may be integrated to complement and strengthen some limitations in both early and contemporary nursing models.

Cody (1996) contends that eclecticism, or selecting the best theory from other sources, is not necessarily wrong, but constantly borrowing theories from other disciplines does not contribute to the science of nursing or differentiate nursing from other professions. He believes that nursing practice ought to reflect a coherent, nursing theoretical base to guide practice in specific ways and contribute to the quality of care.

Since professional nurses provide health care for a variety of clients, each of whom is unique yet may have similar health concerns, nurses must use a broad knowledge base from nursing and other disciplines to select and apply relevent models and/or theories that are congruent with the client's situation. Health care, based on appropriate nursing models and theories, that integrates appropriate family, behavioral, and developmental theories, is most likely to achieve desired client health outcomes.

STRUCTURE OF NURSING KNOWLEDGE AND PERSPECTIVE TRANSFORMATION

Advanced practice nurses must first understand the structure of nursing knowledge and the process of transforming nursing models and theories into useful perspectives prior to implementing theory-based practice. In her recent book, Fawcett (1995) described the structural hierarchy of nursing knowledge, or nursing science. Nursing's metaparadigm, which includes the major concepts of person, health, environment, and nursing, provides the foundation from which nursing philosophies, conceptual models, and theories are derived. Each nurse theorist developed unique definitions of her major concepts, based on her education, practice, and personal philosophy (values, beliefs, and assumptions) about humans, health, nursing, and environment. The theorist's philosophy also influenced her conceptual model, which describes how the concepts are linked: the model explains the relationships among client-health-nursing situations (Sorrentino, 1991). Conceptual nursing models are usually called "grand theories," because they are broad and abstract and may not provide specific directions for nursing actions. Some nurse theorists have developed mid-range or practice theories from their models that describe specific relationships among the concepts and suggest hypotheses to be tested.

According to Rogers (1989), an individual's personal "meaning" perspective or conceptual model provides a frame of reference or lens that influences how one perceives, thinks, and behaves in the world. Yet, most people are not aware of how their perspective influences and affects their view of themselves, others, and their world because underlying beliefs are held in the unconscious mind. In practice, nurses' perceptions, thoughts, feelings, and actions are guided by their personal framework or perspective of nursing, which provides a cognitive structure based on their assumptions, beliefs, and values about nursing (Fawcett, 1995). Many nurses unconsciously use a medical or institutional model as their perspective for organizing care. The prevalent values of such models or perspectives are efficiency, standardized care, rules, and regulations, such as "critical care pathways" (Rogers, 1989). As nurses become aware of the differences between the present and potential possibilities of nursing practice, they experience a cognitive dissonance or discomfort from an awareness of "what is" versus "what could be" (Rogers, 1989). Thus, only when nurses experience cognitive dissonance in practice will they change their frame of reference and use nursing models and theories.

For professional nurses to apply conceptual nursing models and theories, a dramatic change, or "perspective transformation," must occur (Rogers, 1989; Fawcett, 1995). Perspective transformation is the process of moving from one frame of reference or perspective to another, when unresolved dilemmas arise and creat dissonance in one's current perspective (Mezirow, 1979). It is a process of critical reflection and analysis of other explanations or perspectives that might resolve the dilemma and explain or guide one's understanding and actions. The process involves gradually acquiring a new perspective that leads to fundamental changes in the way nurses experience, interpret, and understand their world and their relationships with others (Fawcett, 1995).

Fawcett (1995) describes nine phases leading to "perspective transformation." Initially, the prevailing *stability* of the current nursing practice is disrupted when use of a nursing conceptual model or theory-based practice is introduced. *Dissonance* occurs as nurses consider their own perspective for practice and the challenge of changing to a new conceptual model or theory. Some nurses identify discrepancies between their current practice and how the new model or theory could affect their practice. *Confusion* may follow as nurses struggle to learn about the model or theory and how to apply it in practice. Nurses often feel anxious, angry, and unable to think during these phases and may grieve the loss of familiar perspectives of nursing. Their former perspective no longer seems useful, yet they have not internalized the new model or theory well enough to use it effectively. While *dwelling with uncertainty*, nurses acknowledge that their confusion is not due to personal inadequacy, and as their anxiety diminishes, they begin to critically examine former practice methods and explore the possibilities of implementing a new model or theory (Rogers, 1989; Fawcett, 1995).

With the discovery that a new model or theory is coherent and meaningful, *synthesis* occurs. As ways to apply the new model become clearer, new insights assist nurses to understand the usefulness of the conceptual model or theory in nursing practice (Fawcett, 1995). *Resolution* occurs as nurses become comfortable using the new model; they may feel a sense of empowerment and view their practice differently. Gradually nurses consciously change their practice during *reconceptualization*; they shift from their former patterns to new ways of thinking and acting within the new model or theory. The final phase, *return to stability*, occurs when nursing practice is clearly based on the new nursing model or theory. Acceptance of a new perspective or paradigm, along with the corresponding assumptions, values, and beliefs concludes the transformation process.

Models and theories from nursing and other disciplines provide the cognitive structures that guide professional nursing practice. This body of knowledge helps nurses explain 'what they know' and the rationale for their nursing actions that facilitate the client's health (Fawcett, 1997). Theory-based nursing practice depends on the depth of nurses' knowledge of models and theories and their understanding about how to apply them in practice (Alligood, 1997a). Nursing models and theories represent ideal, logical, unique perspectives or 'maps' of the person and health. They provide a structure and systematic approach to: examine clients' situations, identify relevant information, interpret data for nursing diagnoses, and plan effective nursing care through critical thinking, reasoning, and decision-making ((Mayberry, 1991; Timpson, 1996; Alligood, 1997a).

Nurses must use *critical thinking skills* to apply models and theories to their clients' health concerns. Paul and Nosich's (1991) definition of critical thinking is a commonly accepted one:

> Critical thinking is the intellectually disciplined process of actively and skillfully conceptualizing, applying, analyzing, synthesizing, or evaluating information gathered from, or generated by, observation, experience, reflection, reasoning, or communication, as a guide to belief and action (p. 4).

According to Cradock (1996), it is *not what they know* that makes nurses advanced practitioners, but *how they use what they know*. They must make expert clinical decisions based on reflection, complex reasoning, and critical thinking to apply theoretically based knowledge to diverse client situations (Sparacino, 1991). Critical thinking incorporates ideas from both models or theories with clinical experience, and provides the structure for unique, creative nursing practice with each client (Alligood, 1997a; Field, 1987; Mayberry, 1991; Sorrentino, 1991). Several nurse authors believe that nursing theories will become the stimuli for reflection and critical thinking, leading to realms for creative expressions in nursing practice (Chinn, 1997; Marks-Moran & Rose, 1997). Theory-based nursing and critical thinking are the foundations of advanced nursing practice (Mitchell, 1992). Specific critical thinking skills for each component of the nursing process are identified in Table 26.1.

MODELS AND THEORIES APPLICABLE IN ADVANCED NURSING PRACTICE

Theory-based nursing practice is the creative application of various models, theories, and principles from nursing, medical, behavioral, and humanistic sciences. Models and theories from relevant disciplines provide the knowledge base to understand various aspects of the client's health concerns and guide appropriate nursing management. In advanced nursing practice, the client may be an individual, familys or an aggregate, such as a community or special population. Knowledge of relevant models and theories from nursing and other disciplines enables the nurse to select those that 'best fit' each client. This section provides a brief overview of some nursing, family, community, and other models and theories that may be relevant and useful to nurse practitioners.

Table 26.1. Application of Critical Thinking Skills to the Nursing Process

Components & definitions	Critical thinking skills & activities
Assessment	
An ongoing process of data collection to determine the client's strengths and health concerns	Collect relevant client data by observation, examination, interview and history, and reviewing the records
	Distinguish relevant data from irrelevant
	Distinguish important data from unimportant
	Validate data with others
Diagnosis	
The analysis/synthesis of data to identify patterns and compare with norms and models	Organize and categorize data into patterns
	Identify data gaps
	Recognize patterns and relationships in data
	Compare patterns with norms and theories
A clear, concise statement of the client's health status and concerns appropriate for nursing intervention	Examine own assumptions regarding client's situation
	Make inferences and judgments of client's health concerns
	Define the health concern and validate with the client and health team members
	Describe actual and potential concerns and the etiology of each diagnosis
	Propose alternative explanations of concerns
Planning	
Determination of how to assist the client in resolving concerns related to restoration, maintenance, or promotion of health	Identify priority of client's concerns
	Determine client's desired health outcomes
	Select appropriate nursing interventions by generalizing principles and theories
	Transfer knowledge from other sciences
	Design plan of care with scientific rationale
Implementation	
Carrying out the plan of care by the client and nurse	Apply knowledge to perform interventions
	Compare baseline data with changing status
	Test hypotheses of nursing interventions
	Update and revise the care plan
	Collaborate with health team members
Evaluation	
A systematic, continuous process of comparing the client's response with the desired health outcomes	Compare client's responses with desired health outcomes
	Use criterion-based tools to evaluate
	Determine the client's level of progress
	Revise the plan of care

From: Christensen, P.J. Kenney, J.W., eds: *Nursing process: Application of conceptual models,* ed 4, St. Louis, 1995, Mosby, p. 8.

Nursing Models and Theories

Numerous nursing models and theories have been reported in the literature since the 1950s. Some well-known nurse theorists' works are cited: readers are encouraged to seek other sources for more information about their models and theories. The early nurse theorists's conceptual models focused on individual clients and described nursing goals and activities. Peplau's "Interpersonal Model" described a goal-directed, nurse-client interpersonal process to promote the client's personality and living. Orlando's model explained a deliberative nursing approach to understand nurse-patient relationships and the communication process. Hall's "Core-care-cure Model" expanded and clarified nursing actions to promote clients' health. Levine's model identified four principles of human conservation to guide nursing activities.

More contemporary nursing theories have been published since 1970, when Rogers introduced her "Science of unitary man." She described mutually evolving relationships between humans and their environment that are expressed as changing energy fields, patterns, and organization. Orem's "Self-care Model" identified requisites for an individual's self-care, and specific nursing systems to deliver care according to the client's self-care needs. King designed a systems model that included the individual, family, and society, then developed her "Theory of Goal Attainment," which described nurse-patient transactions to achieve the client's goals. Roy's "Adaptation Model" identified three types of stimuli that affect a patient's four modes of functioning. She described how the nurse identifies maladaptive behaviors and alters stimuli to enhance the client's adaptation. Paterson and Zderad developed a model of "Humanistic Nursing." Leininger's "Transcultural Nursing Model" explained differences between universal and cultural specific views of

health and healing, and how nurses can provide culturally congruent health care. According to Watson, nursing is the art and science of human care: nurses engage in transpersonal caring transactions to assist persons achieve mind-body-soul harmony. Johnson's "Behavioral Systems Model" focused on nurturing, protecting, and stimulating the individual's seven subsystems to maintain balance and stability. Neuman designed a complex "Health Care Systems" model that identified different types of stressors and levels of defense: nursing actions were based on three levels of prevention. Parse developed a "Man-living-health Theory" in which nurses assist individuals to explore their past-present-future life experiences and illuminate possible lifestyle choices to enhance their health and lives. Newman's theory of "Health as expanding consciousness" considers disease as part of health, and explores time and rhythm pattern recognition with changes in life and health.

Family Models

Although most nursing models were originally designed to focus on individual clients, a few are applicable to families. King views the family as a social system or group of interacting individuals, and family health as dynamic life experiences. Roy views the family as part of the client's immediate social environment, whereas Neuman's concept of family is harmonious relationships among family members. These nurse theorists focused on the individual client with the family seen as context. If the family is viewed as the client, the nurse must decide what the model should focus on—family development, interactions and stress, family systems, structure and function, or a combination of these models, such as the Calgary Family Model.

Family development models are based on the premise that the life cycle of families follows a common sequence of events from marriage through childrearing, retirement, and bereavement. Most are based on the typical nuclear two-parent family and emphasize the stages and adult's responsibilities to accomplish desired goals. Duvall's (1977) model is well-known, and Stevenson (1977), a nurse theorist, also designed a family model.

Family interactional models view family members as a unit of interacting personalities within a dynamic life process. These models focus on how members' perceptions and interpretations of themselves and other family members determine their behaviors and actions. Also, these models consider how members' roles affect their interaction with others. Satir's "Family Interaction Model" is an example. Family stress and coping models, based on the work of Lazarus and Folkman, were developed by Moos and Billings (1984) to identify how the family appraised the situation, dealt with their problems, and handled the resulting emotions. McCubbin and McCubbin (1993) designed the "Double ABCX Model," which examines family life stressors and resources, along with changes that affect their adaptation to health problems, and ability to manage family crises. Curran's (1985) "Healthy Family Model" identified characteristics of healthy families and common stressors affecting families.

Family systems models view the whole family as greater than and different from the sum of its parts or members. These models focus on the family with a hierarchy of subsystems (mother-father, parent-child) and supersystems in the community (social, occupational, recreational, and religious networks) that interact with the family system. Olson, Russell, and Sprenkle's (1983) model identifies 16 types of family systems based on the premise that a balance must be maintained in family *cohesion*, so that members do not become too enmeshed or too distant, and *adaptability*, wherein too much change creates chaos and too little change leads to rigidity.

Communication between family members is the third dimension. The "Beaver's System Model" (Beavers & Voeller, 1983) examines the *structure*, *flexibility*, and *competence* of a family and its members. Centripetal families enjoy close family relationships, while centrifugal families seek satisfaction outside the family.

Family structural-functional models view the family as a social system composed of nuclear and extended family members, and their social-communicative interactions to achieve family functions. According to Friedman (1992), the structural components include family composition, values, communication patterns, members' roles, and the power structure. Functional components of this model include physical necessities and care, economic, affective, and reproductive behaviors, socialization and placement of family members, and family coping abilities. The structural and functional components are interrelated, and each part is affected by changes in other parts.

A model that combines many of the above models is the Calgary Family Model, developed by Wright and Leahey (1994). The major components include the internal and external family structure, similar to Friedman's (1992) model, along with family context, such as race, ethnicity, social class, religion, and environment. Family functions are viewed as "instrumental" or daily living activities, and "expressive" activities, including communication (emotional, verbal, and behavioral), problem-solving, roles, influences, beliefs, and alliances or coalitions. Family developmental stages and tasks, similar to Duvall's (1977), are also part of this comprehensive model.

Any family model may be combined with and complement a nursing model since nursing practice may involve individual clients or families. Nurses with knowledge of various family models are more likely to select the most appropriate and relevant one to meet the family's health concerns.

Community Models

There are many community models that are useful to nurses, but they differ according to whether "community" is considered a target population or aggregate or a geographical area. McKay and Segall (1983) described an aggregate model, in which the focus is on a group of individuals who share common characteristics, but may not interact with each other. Shamansky and Pesznecker (1981) identified three interdependent factors that constitute a geographical community: 1) *persons* who reside in an area; 2) *space and time*, which includes the community's history and environmental features; and 3) *purpose* factors that explain functional processes such as government policies, educational services, and forms of communication. The "Community-as-Client Model," designed by Anderson, McFarlane, and Helton (1986) combines both the aggregate and geographical community. It addresses the following eight subsystems of the aggregate in the community: physical environment, education, safety and transportation, politics and government, health and social services, communication, economics, and recreation. A community nursing process model was developed by Goeppinger, Lassiter, and Wilcox (1982) that examines the following eight processes in a community: commitment of members, awareness of others' views, articulation of community needs, effective communication within and among members, conflict containment and accommodation, participation in organizations, management of relations with the larger society, and mechanisms to facilitate participant interactions and decision-making. Knowledge of several community models facilitates selection of the most appropriate one.

Other Useful Models and Theories

Nurses, and theorists in other disciplines, have developed many relevant models and theories that are useful in advanced nursing practice. Some of these models include Maslow's Hierarchy of Needs, Erikson's "Stages of Development," Piaget's "Cognitive Development of Children," Pender's (1987) "Health Promotion/Disease Prevention" model, and Loveland-Cherry's (1989) "Family health promotion" model. In addition, there are numerous theories of stress, crises, coping, grief, berevement, death, and dying developed in psychology and behavioral disciplines. Nurses have transformed some of these theories to encompass a health-illness context. Nurses who are cognizant of a variety of nursing, family, community, and behavioral models and theories are more likely to select the "best fitting" model for their clients.

SELECTION OF RELEVANT MODELS AND THEORIES

This section provides an overview of several nurse scholar's criteria and guidelines for selecting models and theories. Meleis (1997) identified six criteria to guide selection of suitable models and theories for practice. McKenna (1997a) described seven selection criteria based on a review of the literature. Kim (1994) constructed a framework for practice theories with four dimensions to consider in selecting nursing models and theories. Fawcett and associates (1992) suggested that nurses consider three questions to determine the best "fit" between the client's health concerns and various models and theories. Relevant criteria from the above scholars' work were integrated with the author's prior work to delineate five guidelines for selecting appropriate models and theories (Christensen & Kenney, 1996).

Meleis (1997) wrote that selecting models and theories for nursing practice is both a subjective and objective process. She identified six criteria for nurses to consider in the selection process.

- *Personal* the nurse's comfort with the theory and congruency with the nurse's own philosophical views of life

- *Mentor* the model or theory learned from a nurse mentor or educator

- *Theorist* their reputation in the discipline and degree of recognition

- *Literature support* the amount of literature available about the theory and the theory's significance for one's specialty

- *Socio-political congruency* the model or theory's acceptability within the nurse's workplace and whether major structural or practice changes are required

- *Utility* the ease in which nurses can understand and apply the model or theory in practice settings.

McKenna (1997a) reviewed the literature and identified the following seven criteria for selecting models and theories.

- *Type of client* the client's needs should direct the choice since the theory provides guidelines to achieve the client's goals

- *Health care setting* the type of clinical setting and nursing practice are contextual factors that affect selection of theories

- *Parsimony/simplicity* simple and realistic theories are more likely to be understood and applied in practice

- *Understandability* nurses must understand a theory if they expected to use it

- *Origins of the theory* the credibility, prior use, and testing of the theory should also be considered

- *Paradigms as a basis for choice* nurses must decide between the totality or simultaneity paradigm, as each provides a different view of clients and nursing actions

- *Personal values and beliefs* the theory must be congruent with the nurse's own views about humans, health, and nursing.

In her article on practice theories, Kim (1994) defined two dimensions of theories, which include four "sets of practice theories" relevant to selecting models and theories. One dimension is the "target," which addresses both the philosophy of care for the person and the philosophy of therapy for the client's problems. The other dimension is the "nurse-agent," which includes two phases, deliberation, and enactment. The four "sets of practice theories" serve to guide nurses in choosing theories that will: 1) explain the patient's problems and ideas about therapy for the problems; 2) provide ideas about how the nurse should approach the patient, such as through communication, caring, or empowerment; 3) explain how to make decisions about appropriate nursing actions for the patient; and, 4) explain what happens during enactment of nursing actions. Kim proposed that a science of nursing practice could be developed from this framework.

Fawcett and associates (1992) identified questions to guide nurses' selection of appropriate theories and models. The nurse must understand the differences among various models and theories in nursing and other disciplines to answer these questions. The following three questions will help the nurse identify the most appropriate model:

1. Does the theory or model address the client's problems and health concerns?

2. Are the nursing interventions suggested by the model consistent with the client's expectations for nursing care?
3. Are the goals of nursing actions, based on the model or theory, congruent with the client's desired health outcomes?

These questions help nurses decide which models and theories will assist them to organize the data into patterns, identify other health concerns, and determine congruency of the client's and nurse's view of nursing and health.

The first step toward theory-based nursing practice is the *conscious decision to use theories in practice* (Fawcett, 1997). The second step is recognizing that use of conceptual nursing models and theories requires a major change in how the nurse thinks about and interacts with clients to alleviate their health concerns. This change, referred to earlier as a "perspective transformation," occurs gradually as the nurse discards one framework of practice and learns another perspective. Adopting and applying new models and theories in practice depends on nurses having knowledge of various models and theories and understanding how these models and theories relate to each other (Alligood, 1997a).

GUIDELINESF FOR SELECTING MODELS AND THEORIES FOR NURSING PRACTICE

After deciding to implement theory-based nursing practice, the author believes that each nurse must engage in the five steps described below.

1. *Consider your personal values and beliefs about nursing, clients, health, and environment.*

Each nurse has a personal frame of reference or perspective of nursing practice, based on his/her conscious or unconscious assumptions, beliefs, and values about nursing. One's perspective of nursing provides a cognitive structure that guides one's perceptions, thoughts, feelings, and nursing actions (Fawcett, 1995). Clarifying one's own values and beliefs about clients, health, and nursing practice is necessary before a "perspective transformation" can occur.

2. *Examine the underlying assumptions, values, and beliefs of various nursing models, and how the major concepts are defined.* After clarifying one's own values and beliefs, the nurse examines the definitions of major concepts in various models and theories to determine whether they are congruent with one's own beliefs (Alligood, 1997a). Nursing models and theories are based on different values and beliefs about the nature of the client's behaviors and abilities, what is health and environment, and what nursing actions facilitate clients' health.

Each nursing model and theory provides a unique view for specific nursing practice. Some nursing models reflect a "totality" paradigm, and view humans as having separate biological, social, psychological, and spiritual parts that respond to environmental stimuli or change, and the nurse's role is to facilitate adaptation or equilibrium to maintain health. Other nursing models reflect a "simultaneity" paradigm, and believe humans are intelligent beings, capable of making informed decisions about their lives, and that they continuously engage in a dynamic, mutual interaction with their environment. In this paradigm, the nurse's role is to guide clients in choosing lifestyles and/or therapies that are acceptable to them and facilitate their growth and life-health process.

3. *Identify several models that are congruent with your own values and beliefs about nursing,*

clients, and health. Each nurse must consider whether the theorist's underlying values are congruent with one's own personal values and beliefs about clients, health, and nursing because the theorist's values guide the nurse's critical thinking and reasoning processes (Alligood, 1997a). Models and theories reflect the theorist's views about people and nursing. They directly effect how nurses approach their clients, what information they gather, how that information is processed, what nursing activities are appropriate, and, what client outcomes are expected based on the model. For example, some traditional nursing models define the person as a bio-psycho-social being who responds to environmental stimuli, and health results from nursing actions that lead to predictable changes. These models would be incongruent for contemporary nurses who believe that people are free agents, dynamically interacting with their environment as a whole, and capable of making rational decisions, and that the nurse's role is to assist clients to explore various options and choose ones that are acceptable with their values and lifestyle.

4. *Identify the similarities and differences in client focus, nursing actions, and client outcomes of these models.* Nursing models and theories consist of concepts with specific definitions, and statements that describe how the concepts are interrelated. Some propose specific nursing actions and expected client outcomes. The major concepts guide what data is collected during the assessment and how the data is organized to identify and interpret bio-behavioral patterns and determine nursing diagnoses. Nursing models also guide development of the nursing care plans and designate desired outcomes to evaluate. By comparing various models, nurses recognize which ones are congruent with their values and beliefs about nursing and offer the best "fit" with the client's health concerns.

5. *Practice applying the models and theories to clients with different health concerns to determine which ones best "fit" specific situations and guide nursing actions that will achieve desired client outcomes.* The nurse explores specific models in depth, and may analyze their usefulness before implementing them. By comparing several models and examining the attributes of the client, the focus of nursing actions, and the proposed outcomes, the nurse will acquire a more in-depth understanding of different models. Each nursing model describes different areas for assessment, unique nursing diagnoses, and specific nursing interventions to assist the client toward health. The nurse must decide which models and theories are most appropriate for each client. Which one offers the best 'fit' for the client's health concerns? Selecting appropriate models and theories for each unique client health situation requires nurses to use their broad knowledge base from various disciplines, critical thinking skills, clinical expertise, and intuition to identify the best 'fit' between the client's health concerns and nursing models (Fawcett, et al., 1992).

APPLICATION OF THEORY-BASED NURSING PRACTICE

The choice of theories and models suitable to the client's health concerns occurs during the initial data assessment process. The initial data focuses on the client's primary expressed concerns and how they are related to or affect the client's lifestyle and patterns of living. These data assist the nurse to identify and understand the client's common and unique patterns. The client's view of health, along with past and present "lived experiences," and future lifestyle and health concerns, are also considered. Using this information, the nurse considers various models and theories from nursing and other disciplines that are relevant to the client's unique health concerns, and congruent with the nurse's own beliefs. Then,

TABLE 26.2.   Theory-Based Nursing Practice

	Nursing process	Nursing model
Component	*Use*	*Use*
Assessment	Describes *how* to collect data	Guides *what* data to collect
Diagnosis	Describes *how* to process data	Guides organizing, categorizing, and interpreting data
	Provides format for nursing diagnosis	Provides concepts for nursing diagnosis
	Describes *how* to plan	Guides *what* to plan
	Facilitates development of care plan unique to client	Designates appropriate types of nursing interventions
Implementation	Describes phases of implementation	Directs model-specific nursing actions
Evaluation	Identifies *how* to evaluate	Guides *what* to evaluate
General	Requires accountability through use of systematic approach to nursing practice	Enhances accountability of theory-based practice
	Process enhances continuity of care	Provides a comprehensive, coherent approach to care of client

From: Christensen, P.J., Kenney, J.W., eds: *Nursing process: Application of conceptual models*, 4th ed., St. Louis, 1995, Mosby, p. 21. Adapted with permission from Wealtha Y. Helland.

the nurse selects those models and other theories that best "fit" the client's situation and health concerns and will systematically direct nursing practice.

The major concepts of the chosen models and theories guide each component of the nursing process, as shown in Table 26-2. The concepts serve as categories to guide additional data collection. They suggest, either directly or indirectly, *what* information is relevant and should be collected. The models and theories assist the nurse to organize, categorize, and interpret pertinent data that illustrate the client's bio-behavioral patterns and identify appropriate nursing diagnoses that are linked to relevant etiological factors.

Nursing and other models and theories guide development of a care plan by suggesting appropriate types of nursing interventions and specific nursing actions. Desired client outcomes are derived from the models and theories and define what changes in the client

should be evaluated. For example, if Roy's model is chosen, data about the client's physiological needs, self-concept, role mastery, and interdependence, along with related stimuli would be collected, and used to identify adaptive and maladaptive behavioral patterns. The nurse who uses Orem's Self-Care Model would assess and judge clients' ability to meet their universal and developmental self-care requisites and whether they had any health deviations. From analysis of this data, the nurse would diagnose self-care deficits and determine appropriate nursing plans for partial, compensatory, or health education nursing care. Nursing care plans are based on the model and describe the client's desired outcomes, along with nursing actions to achieve the client's outcomes. Nurses who use Johnson's Behavioral Systems Model would consider ways to nurture, protect, or stimulate the client to facilitate health, whereas the Neuman's Health Care System's model assists the nurse to explore ways to reduce stressors within the three levels of disease prevention.

Some nurses believe that family models complement nursing models and provide a more holistic and comprehensive perspective of clients and their health concerns. Selection of a family model occurs after the nurse gathers preliminary data about the family and identifies its unique and common patterns. Then the nurse decides whether the "family as context" or "family as client" would be more appropriate and best "fit" the client's situation. Also the nurse's perception and definition of family and health guide the selection of a family model. For example, a pediatric nurse who works in an outpatient clinic may choose Orem's Self-Care Model to guide care of a nine-year-old child with an ear infection and the mother's treatment of the child. Friedman's Family System model may complement Orem's model and enhance understanding the family's structure and functions. The nurse may also use Erikson's Developmental Framework to help the mother recognize and encourage her child's normal developmental behaviors. Pain management theories may also be applied to reduce the child's earache.

This example illustrates how nurses examine and judge the value of various models and theories and select those which are most congruent and useful and best 'fit' the client's health concerns and the nurse's perspective of practice. Gradually nurse practitioners develop an expertise in selecting theories and models that are appropriate and relevant to their client's health concerns and congruent with their own views of advanced practice.

SUMMARY

This chapter described the importance and value of applying models and theories from nursing and other disciplines in advanced nursing practice. Issues related to the nursing theory-practice gap were discussed, along with concerns about using only one nursing model in practice and about integrating models and theories from other disciplines with nursing models and theories. The structure of nursing knowledge was explained and the need for a "perspective transformation" to occur prior to implementing theory-based nursing practice. Critical thinking, logical reasoning, and creatively applying nursing models and theories was emphasized. Different types of nursing, family, community, and other models and theories were discussed. Lastly, the process of selecting and applying models and theories was thoroughly described.

In the last few decades, the emergence of nursing models and theories has illuminated several nursing paradigms and explicated their underlying assumptions, beliefs, and values that guide nursing practice. The science of nursing and empirical patterns of knowing are represented by these nursing models and their theories. Application of models and theories from nursing and other disciplines depends on nurses having a broad knowledge base and understanding how models and theories are interrelated. Empowerment of nurses through 'perspective transformation' and the use of nursing models and theories is essential. They provide the framework for critical thinking within the context of nursing and guide the reasoning that professional nurses need to survive in an era of cost containment and evidence-based practice. Use of models and theories from nursing and related health disciplines enables nurses to demonstrate accountability for their decisions and actions through scientific explanation and provides a coherent approach to theory-based nursing practice.

REFERENCES

Aggleton, PJ, & Chalmers, H. (1986). *Nursing models and the nursing process.* Basingstoke: Macmillan.

Alligood, MR. (1997a). Models and theories: Critical thinking structures. In MR Alligood and A Marriner-Tomey, *Nursing Theory: Utilization & Application*, St. Louis: MO: C. V. Mosby. pp. 31–45.

Alligood, MR. (1997b). Models and theories in nursing practice. In MR Alligood and A Marriner-Tomey, *Nursing Theory: Utilization & Application*, St. Louis: MO: C. V. Mosby. pp. 15–30.

Anderson, ET, McFarlane, JM, & Helton, A. (1986). Community as client: A model for practice. *Nursing Outlook*, 3(5):220

Beavers, WR, & Voeller, MN. (1983). Family models: Comparing and contrasting the Olson circumplex models with the Beaver's systems model. *Family Process*, 22:85–98.

Benner, P, & Wrubel, J. (1989). *The primacy of caring*. Menlo Park, CA: Addison-Wesley.

Chinn, PL. (1997). Why middle-range theory? *ANS*, 19(3):viii.

Christensen, PJ & Kenney, JW. (1996). *Nursing process: Application of conceptual models*, 4th ed., St. Louis, MO., C. V. Mosby.

Cradock, S. (1996). The expert nurse: Clinical specialist or advanced practitioner? In Gary Rolfe, (Ed.) *Closing the theory-practice gap: A new paradigm for nursing*. Butterworth-Heinemann Ltd., Oxford, UK.

Cody, WK. (1996). Drowning in eclecticism. *Nursing Science Quarterly*, 9(3):86–88.

Curran, D. (1985). *Stress and the healthy family*, Minneapolis, MN., Winston Press.

Duvall, EM. (1997). *Marriage and family development*, 5th ed., Philadelphia, PA., Lippincott.

Fawcett J, Archer CL, Becker D, et al., (1992). Guidelines for selecting a conceptual model of nursing: Focus on the individual client, *Dimen Critical Care Nursing*, 11(5):268–277.

Fawcett, J. (1995). Implementing conceptual models in nursing practice. In J. Fawcett, *Analysis and evaluation of conceptual models of nursing*, 3rd ed. Philadelphia, PA., F. A. Davis.

Fawcett, J. (1997). Conceptual models of nursing, nursing theories, and nursing practice: Focus on the future. In MR Alligood and A Marriner-Tomey, *Nursing Theory: Utilization & Application*, St. Louis: MO., C. V. Mosby. pp 211–221.

Field, PA. (1987). The impact of nursing theory on the clinical decision making process, *Journal of Advanced Nursing*, 12:563–571.

Firlet, SI. (1985). Nursing theory and nursing practice: Separate or linked? In J. McCloskey & HK Grace (Eds.) *Current issues in nursing*. Boston: Blackwell Scientific Publications. pp 6–19.

Friedman, MM. (1992). *Family nursing: Theory and practice*, 3rd ed. New York, Appleton & Lange.

Goeppinger, J, Lassiter, PG, & Wilcox, B. (1982). Community health is community competence. *Nursing Outlook*, 30(8):464.

Kenney, JW. (1996). Relevance of theory-based nursing practice. In P. J. Christensen & J. W. Kenney, *Nursing Process: Application of Conceptual Models*, 4th ed. St. Louis, MO: C. V. Mosby. pp 1–23.

Kim, HS. (1994). Practice theories in nursing and a science of nursing practice. *Scholarly Inquiry for Nursing Practice: An International Journal*, 8(2):145–158.

Loveland-Cherry, CJ. (1989). Family health promotion and health protection. In P. Bomar (Ed.) *Nurses and family health promotion: Concepts, assessment, and interventions*. Baltimore, MD., Williams & Wilkins.

Mayberry A. (1991). Merging nursing theories, models, and nursing practice: More than an administrative challenge, *ANS*, 15:44.

Marks-Moran, D, & Rose, P. (Eds.) (1997). *Reconstructing nursing: Beyond art and science*. Philadelphia, PA., Bailliere Tindall.

McCubbin, MA, & McCubbin, HI. (1993). Families coping with illness: The resiliency model of family stress, adjustment and adaptation. In C. B. Danielson, B. Hamel-Bissell, & P. Winstead-Fry (Eds.), *Families, health and illness: Perspectives on coping and intervention* St. Louis, MO., Mosby (pp. 21–65).

McKay, R, & Segall, M. (1983). Methods and models for the aggregate. *Nursing Outlook*, 31(6):328

McKenna, H. (1997a). Choosing a theory for practice. In Hugh McKenna, *Nursing theories and models*. New York, Rutledge, pp. 127–157.

McKenna, H. (1997b). Applying theories in practice. In Hugh McKenna, *Nursing theories and models*. New York: Rutledge, pp. 158–189.

Meleis, AI. (1993). *Nursing research and the Neuman model: Directions for the future*. Panel discussion conducted at the Fourth Biennial International Neuman Systems Model Symposium, Rochester, NY.

Meleis, AI. (1997). *Theoretical nursing: Development and progress*, 3rd ed. Philadelphia, PA. Lippincott.

Mezirow, J. (1979). Perspective transformation. *Adult education*. 28(3):100–110.

Moos, RH, & Billings, AG. (1982). Conceptualizing and measuring coping resources and processes. In L. Goldberger & S. Breznitz (Eds.) *Handbook of stress*. New York, Free Press.

Mitchell, G. (1992). Specifying the knowledge base of theory in practice. *Nursing Science Quarterly,* 5(1):6–7.

Olson, DH, Russell, CS, & Sprenkle, DH. (1983). Circumplex models of marital and family systems: VI. Theoretical update. *Family Processes,* 22:69–83.

Paul, RW, & Nosich, GM. (1991). Proposal for the national assessment of higher–order thinking (revised version). The United States Department of Education Office of Educational Research and Improvement, National Center for Education Statistics.

Pender, NJ. (1987). *Health promotion in nursing practice.* New York, Doubleday.

Rogers, ME. (1989). Creating a climate for the implementation of a nursing conceptual framework. *Journal of Continuing Education in Nursing,* 20(3):112–116.

Shamansky, SL & Pesznecker, B. (1981). A community is . . . . *Nursing Outlook,* 29(3):182–185.

Smith, MC. (1994). Beyond the threshold: Nursing practice in the next millennium. *Nursing Science Quarterly,* 7(1):6–7.

Sorrentino, EA. (1991). Making theories work for you. *Nursing Administration Quarterly,* 15(3):54–59.

Spiracino, P. (1991). The reciprocal relationship between practice and theory. *Clinical Nurse Specialist,* 5(3):138.

Stevenson, J. (1977). *Issues and crises during middlescence,* New York, Appleton-Century-Crofts.

Timpson, J. (1996). Nursing theory: Everything the artist spits is art? *Journal of Advanced Nursing,* 23:1030–1036.

Wright, LM, & Leahey, M. (1994). *Nurses and families: A guide to family assessment and intervention,* 2nd ed. Philadelphia, PA., F. A. Davis.

Frederickson, et al. (1997). Nursing theory-guided practice. *Nursing Science Quarterly,* 10(1):53–58.

Gioiella, EC. (1996). The importance of theory-guided research and practice in the changing health care scene. *Nursing Science Quarterly,* 9(2):47.

Huch, MH. (1988). Theory-based practice: Structuring nursing care. *Nurs Science Quarterly* 1:6.

Huch, MH. (1995). Nursing science as a basis for advanced practice. *Nursing Science Quarterly,* 8(1):6–7.

Huckabey, LH. (1991). The role of conceptual frameworks in nursing practice, administration, education, and research. *Nurs Admin Quarterly* 15(3):17–28.

Jacobs, MK, & Huether, SE. (1978). Nursing science: The theory-practice linkage. *Advances in Nursing Science,* 1(1):63–78.

Kappeli, S. (1994). Why not practice-based theory? *Clinical Nursing Research,* 3(1): 3–6.

Koziol-McLain, J, & Maeve, MK. (1993). Nursing theory in perspective. *Nursing Outlook,* 41 (2):79–81.

Kristjanson LJ, Tamblyn R, & Kuypers JA. (1987). A model to guide development and application of multiple nursing theories. *J Adv Nurs,* 12:523.

Oberst, MT. (1995). To what end theory? *Research in Nursing & Health,* 18:83–84.

Rolfe, G. (1996). Nursing praxis: Integrating theory and practice. In Gary Rolfe, *Closing the theory-practice gap: A new paradigm for nursing.* Butterworth & Heinemann Ltd.: Oxford, UK.

Wardle, MG, & Mandle, CL. (1989). Conceptual models used in clinical practice. *Western Journal of Nursing Research,* 11(1):108–114.

Wilkinson JM. (1992). *Nursing process in action: A critical thinking approach.* Menlo Park, CA.: Addison-Wesley.

ADDITIONAL REFERENCES

Birx, EC. (1993). Critical thinking and theory-based practice. *Holistic Nursing Practice,* 7(3):21–27.

Chinn, PL, & Kramer, MK. (1995). *Theory and nursing: A systematic approach,* 4th ed., St. Louis, MO., Mosby Year Book Co.

Cody, WK. (1994). Nursing theory-guided practice: What it is and what it is not.*Nursing Science Quarterly,* 7(4):144–145.

Derdiarian, AK. (1991). Effects of using a nursing model-based assessment instrument on quality of nursing care. *Jr of Nurs Admin,* 15(3):1–16.

Index